Essentials
of
Pharmacology

Essentials
of
Pharmacology

P. MICHAEL CONN, Ph.D.
Professor and Head
Department of Pharmacology
The University of Iowa
College of Medicine
Iowa City, Iowa

G. F. GEBHART, Ph.D.
Professor and Director of Graduate Studies
Department of Pharmacology
The University of Iowa
College of Medicine
Iowa City, Iowa

ESSENTIALS OF MEDICAL EDUCATION SERIES

DAVID T. LOWENTHAL, M.D., Ph.D./Editor-in-Chief
Professor of Medicine and Pharmacology
University of Florida College of Medicine
Gainesville, Florida

 F. A. DAVIS COMPANY • Philadelphia

Printed in the United States of America

Last digit indicates print number: 10 9 8 7 6 5 4 3 2 1

NOTE: As new scientific information becomes available through basic and clinical research, recommended treatments and drug therapies undergo changes. The author(s) and publisher have done everything possible to make this book accurate, up-to-date, and in accord with accepted standards at the time of publication. However, the reader is advised always to check product information (package inserts) for changes and new information regarding dose and contraindications before administering any drug. Caution is especially urged when using new or infrequently ordered drugs.

Library of Congress Cataloging-in-Publication Data

Essentials of pharmacology/[edited by] P. Michael Conn, G.F. Gebhart.
     p.   cm.—(Essentials of medical education series)
    Bibliography: p.
    Includes index.
    ISBN 0-8036-1973-1
    1. Pharmacology.   I. Conn, P. Michael.   II. Gebhart, Gerald F.
III. Series.
    [DNLM: 1. Pharmacology   QV 38 E78]
RM300.E83   1989
615'.1—dc19
DNLM/DLC
for Library of Congress   89-1068
                                              CIP

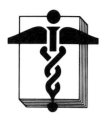

Preface

Essentials of Pharmacology was developed to fulfill the needs of medical, dental, and graduate students for a concise, easy-to-read reference to complement larger pharmacology textbooks. It will also be helpful to students and practitioners in nursing, pharmacy, and other allied health professions. In addition, medical residents and clinicians will find it useful as a quick bookshelf reference.

Our primary goal is to aid the student in developing an overview of principles and key concepts for understanding lectures during most pharmacology courses, but the text also serves as a useful review in preparation for course and national examinations. To that end, self-assessment questions (and answers) have been consolidated at the back of the book. Selected references and bibliographic recommendations are also listed at the end of the text for individuals interested in more detailed treatment of particular subjects.

The content in this volume has been constructed around current educational recommendations for pharmacology curricula nationally. In order to support our goal of conciseness, figures and tables have been carefully selected to consolidate information. Emphasis is placed on drugs having the widest clinical applications and those that illustrate scientific principles. Meanwhile, discussions of underlying anatomy, physiology, and pathophysiology have been limited to those areas where this foundation is most complex and critical to understanding basic mechanisms of drug action and interaction, such as the peripheral nervous system.

In order to meet the direct need for more clinical information related to frequently encountered drugs, an accompanying pocket handbook of the 100 most commonly prescribed drugs for hospitalized patients is included with *Essentials of Pharmacology*. This supplement is intended to be a quick, convenient reference to specific drugs, their primary action, recommended dosages, therapeutic effects, and precautions in administration.

We want to thank our colleagues for their participation in this effort; in many cases, chapters reflect a distillation of over twenty-five years of individual research and teaching experience. Also, thanks to our office staff, notably Marilyn Kirkpatrick and Elizabeth McDonald, for their efforts in the multiple revisions that this volume has undergone.

P. MICHAEL CONN, PH.D.
G. F. GEBHART, PH.D.

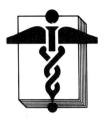

Contributors

From:
The University of Iowa
College of Medicine
Iowa City, Iowa

R. K. BHATNAGAR, Ph.D.
Professor of Pharmacology

MICHAEL J. BRODY, Ph.D.
Professor of Pharmacology

P. MICHAEL CONN, Ph.D.
Professor and Head of Pharmacology

G. R. DUTTON, Ph.D.
Professor of Pharmacology

ROSS D. FELDMAN, M.D.
Associate Professor of Internal Medicine and Pharmacology
Currently: R. W. Gunton Professor of Therapeutics
University of Western Ontario
London, Ontario, Canada

G. F. GEBHART, Ph.D.
Professor and Director of Graduate Studies of Pharmacology

R. KENT HERSMEYER, Ph.D.
Professor of Pharmacology
Currently: Director of Cardiovascular Research
Chiles Research Institute
Providence Medical Center
Portland, Oregon

WILLIAM R. HUCKLE, Ph.D.
Student, Department of Pharmacology
Currently: Fellow
Lineberger Cancer Center
University of North Carolina
Chapel Hill, North Carolina

J. P. LONG, Ph.D.
Carver Professor of Pharmacology

SEAN MURPHY, Ph.D.
Assistant Professor of Pharmacology

TIMOTHY J. NESS, M.D., Ph.D.
Student, Department of Pharmacology
Currently: Resident
Department of Anesthesia

ROBERT J. ROBERTS, M.D., Ph.D.
Professor of Pharmacology and Pediatrics
Currently: Professor and Chairman
Department of Pediatrics
Children's Medical Center
University of Virginia
Charlottesville, Virginia

THOMAS K. SHIRES, Ph.D.
Professor of Pharmacology

M. D. SOKOLL, M.D.
Professor of Anesthesia

REYNOLD SPECTOR, M.D.
Professor of Pharmacology and Internal Medicine
Currently: Executive Director
Clinical Sciences
Merck Sharp and Dohme Research Laboratories
Rahway, New Jersey

JAMES L. SPRATT, M.D., Ph.D.
Professor of Pharmacology

WILLIAM STEELE, Ph.D.
Professor of Pharmacology

THOMAS R. TEPHLY, M.D., Ph.D.
Professor of Pharmacology

H. E. WILLIAMSON, Ph.D.
Professor of Pharmacology

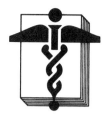

Contents

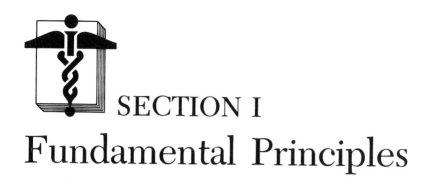

SECTION I
Fundamental Principles

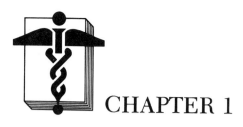

CHAPTER 1

General Principles of Drug Action and Pharmacokinetics

H. E. WILLIAMSON, Ph.D.

Pharmacology is concerned with the study of substances (**drugs**) that affect living systems. This discipline is sometimes subdivided into **pharmacodynamics,** the study of the effect and mechanisms of action of substances on living systems, and **pharmacokinetics,** the study of how such substances are handled by the body. Pharmacology involves both desirable and undesirable actions of drugs (**toxicology**). Substances producing adverse effects are often referred to as poisons or toxins. The use of drugs clinically to treat, prevent, or diagnose diseases and develop dosage regimens is called **therapeutics**.

RECEPTORS

The intensity of action of a drug depends upon the concentration of the drug at its site of action. The site of action for most drugs is a receptor, which is a specific site on a macromolecule located on a cell membrane or within a cell. The interaction of drug and receptor results in altered cellular function (response or effect). (However, not all drugs act *via* a receptor mechanism. Some are substrate analogs that are incorporated into macromolecules or cellular components [6-mercaptopurine, 5-fluorouracil], while others are chelators [penicillamine], or osmotic agents [mannitol]).

Different types of chemical bonds are involved in drug-receptor interactions. A covalent bond is the strongest drug-receptor interaction, as electrons are shared between the drug and receptor. This bond is seldom reversible, and accordingly, interactions of this type are more apt to lead to toxicity. Ionic bonds and hydrogen bonds are reversible. Bonds involving van der Waals forces are the weakest of bonds and are readily reversible. The last three types of bonding are best for drugs because regulation is easier when bonding is reversible.

The chemical nature of receptors is currently a topic of major research interest. Several receptors have been characterized and found to be proteins, glycoproteins, or lipoproteins. Receptors recognize drugs with a high degree of selectivity, a single atom sometimes determining if a particular agent is recognized.

DOSE-RESPONSE INTERACTIONS

When the effect of a drug is plotted against log dose (dose-response curve), a sigmoid curve is frequently obtained (Fig. 1–1). A useful dose is that quantity of drug that produces half of the maximal response (ED_{50}).

Dose-response curves associated with drug actions are actually **graded dose-response curves,** such as measured responses of heart rate or blood pressure. This type of curve is necessary to determine **maximal efficacy** (E_{max}). Plotting responses on ordinate against log dose on abscissa decreases skewing

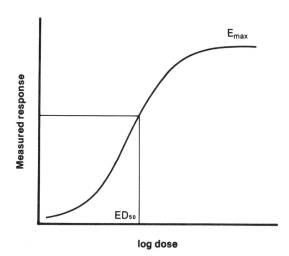

Figure 1–1. Semilog plot of a measured (or graded) response curve of a drug showing maximal response (E_{max}) and dose that produces half (ED_{50}) of the maximal response.

of curve. Another type of dose-response relationship is **quantal dose-response curve**. Here, log dose is plotted on the abscissa as just described, but fractional response is plotted on the ordinate (i.e., the fraction of a test group exhibiting a specified response such as hypnosis, toxicity, or death).

Therapeutic Index

If the ordinate of the dose-response curve is changed to multiples of the standard deviation (probits), the curve will be linear. With this type of plot, it is possible to calculate a **therapeutic index (TI)** for a drug. Dividing the **LD50** (dose that kills 50 percent of the animal population) or **TD50** (dose that produces toxicity in 50 percent of the tested population) by the **ED50** (dose that produces the desired effect in 50 percent of the tested population) will yield the TI, which can be viewed as an index of safety. The higher this ratio, the larger the margin of safety of the drug. Agents such as digoxin (a cardiac glycoside, **TD50/ED50** = <2) that have low therapeutic indices require great caution in their use.

Efficacy and Potency

Compounds that produce the same maximal effect are said to have equal **efficacy**. If one compound produces a smaller maximal effect than another compound, the first compound is less efficacious. Although different compounds may produce similar maximal effects, they may require different doses. Those requiring smaller dosages are said to be more **potent**. Of these two terms, **efficacy** is more significant than **potency** because the former is an expression of response, whereas the latter affects only the size of the dosage form (e.g., tablet size).

AGONISTS AND ANTAGONISTS

An agent that stimulates a receptor (e.g., morphine) is called an **agonist**. A **full agonist** is a drug with maximal efficacy relative to other agonists. In contrast, a **partial agonist** produces a less than maximal effect compared with other agonists. Such agents may also inhibit other agonists. Partial agonists usually have high affinity for a receptor and thus produce an effect when they initially bind to the receptor. However, they are not readily released from the receptor and thus are able to block the action of other agonists. Pentazocine, an analgesic, is an example of a partial agonist. It can interfere with the actions of the agonist, morphine. Dose-response curves of agonists of differing efficacy and potency are presented in Figure 1–2A.

While some drugs activate receptors and produce a response (i.e., agonists), others, known as **antagonists,** are capable of blocking responses. Some agents compete for the same site as agonists but do not produce a response. These substances are **competitive antagonists**. Although they alter the ED_{50}

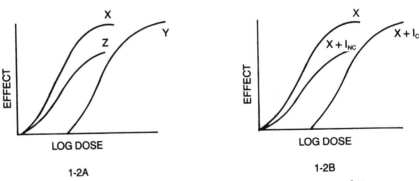

Figure 1–2. Representative log dose-response curves. *A*, Curves X and Y are two agonists with similar efficacy but differing potency (X more potent than Y). Curves X and Z are two agonists with similar potency but differing in efficacy (X: full agonist, and Z: partial agonist). *B*, An agonist (X) in the absence and presence of a competitive antagonist (I_C) and a noncompetitive antagonist (I_{NC}). (Adapted from Ross, EM and Gilman, AG: Pharmacodynamics. In: Goodman, LS and Gilman, AG (eds): Goodman and Gilman's The Pharmacological Basis of Therapeutics, ed 7. Macmillan, New York, 1985, p 42.)

of a drug, they do not alter its maximal effect (E_{max}). Thus, a given agonist will require a greater dosage to produce its effects in the presence of a competitive antagonist (i.e., its dose-response curve will be shifted to the right). Naloxone is an example; it antagonizes the actions of morphine.

Other antagonists are said to be **noncompetitive**. These agents generally act on the same molecule as the agonist. They may act at a site distinct from the agonist binding site or bind irreversibly to the receptors. Often these agents produce an irreversible antagonism. They do not markedly affect the ED_{50}, but they decrease the E_{max}, as no amount of agonist will restore activity. Naloxonazine (an experimental drug) is an example of a noncompetitive antagonist. It antagonizes the actions of morphine because it binds irreversibly to the opioid receptors. Dose-response curves of agonist, agonist plus competitive antagonist, and agonist plus noncompetitive antagonist are presented in Figure 1–2B.

The antagonists described here are **pharmacological antagonists** (i.e., they interact with the same receptor or molecule as do agonists). Other types of antagonists are classified as **physiological** or **chemical**. Physiological antagonists produce an opposite response but do so by acting on different receptors. Thus, while the increase in blood pressure produced by norepinephrine can be antagonized by pharmacological antagonists (e.g., phentolamine), an agent such as nitroglycerin, which dilates blood vessels directly, will also antagonize the increase. Chemical antagonism may occur if the antagonist acts directly upon an agonist to alter it and thus prevent a response.

SYNERGISM AND POTENTIATION

Two drugs may also interact to produce effects that are more than additive. If both drugs when given separately produce a similar response but when given together produce a greater than additive response, this is referred to as **synergism** (e.g., ethanol and phenothiazines together produce a greater than predicted depressant action). **Potentiation** often refers to an inactive substance increasing the response of an active drug (e.g., physostigmine inhibits the enzyme acetylcholinesterase, which results in an increase in the activity of acetylcholine). Drug interactions are discussed further in Chapter 3.

TOLERANCE

Tolerance refers to a diminishing response to a drug with repetitive administration of the same dose. Thus, dosage must be increased to maintain the desired response. **Tachyphylaxis** is tolerance of such rapid onset that it occurs after only one dose of a drug. This is frequently seen with drugs that act by releasing an endogenous substance (e.g., tyramine, which releases catecholamines). If a second dose of tyramine is given shortly after the first dose, a lesser response is seen, as the catecholamine stores have not been repleted.

PHYSIOLOGIC DISPOSITION OF DRUGS

To produce an effect, a drug must reach its site of action in an adequate concentration. After a drug is administered, the rate at which it is absorbed from its site of administration, how it is distributed in the body, the rate of its metabolism, and the rate of its excretion all influence the activity of the drug. The manner in which a drug is handled by the body is referred to as its physiological disposition, and the study of this is **pharmacokinetics**.

Absorption, distribution, metabolism, and excretion are influenced by the movement of a drug across cellular membranes, which are lipoprotein structures. These membranes may also contain pores, which vary in number and size with various tissues. Drugs may cross membranes by (1) filtration, (2) diffusion, (3) active transport, (4) facilitated diffusion, or (5) pinocytosis. The molecular size and shape of a drug, degree of dissociation, and lipid solubility affect its interaction with other substances, movement across membranes, and hence disposition.

Filtration

This occurs at pores in cellular membranes and is generally limited to non-ionized small molecular weight substances that are water soluble. Pores vary in size but in most membranes are approximately 4 Å in diameter. Thus, only small molecular substances (100 daltons or less) will move readily through pores. As movement occurs with water, water solubility is necessary. Because of potential differences across membranes, only noncharged (non-ionized) substances move readily through pores.

Diffusion

This, like filtration, is a passive process. Movement is from high to low drug concentration. Because movement is through lipoprotein membranes, substances that are lipid soluble (lipophilic) will move across readily, whereas water-soluble (hydrophilic) substances will not cross to any great extent. Thus, non-ionized substances are more likely to cross membranes, whereas ionized substances will not move across readily.

Many drugs are weak acids or bases, and hence their degree of ionization is affected by the pH of the solution in which they are dissolved. With weak acids, ionization increases as pH increases (i.e., becomes more basic), whereas with weak bases, ionization increases as pH decreases. Since pH differences may exist across biological membranes, it is possible that the concentration of a weak electrolyte may differ on each side of the membrane. This can occur because of the different solubilities of the ionized and non-ionized drug in the membrane. The lipid-soluble non-ionized form of the drug will equilibrate on each side of the membrane. The ionized form, which does not readily cross the membrane, can have different concentrations on each side of the membrane. This occurs because of the different degrees of ionization of a weak electrolyte in solutions of different pH. A weak acid will be more ionized on the more alkaline side of the membrane than on the more acidic side. Thus, the total concentration (ionized and non-ionized) on the more alkaline side will be greater than on the more acidic side. The reverse will be true for weak bases, that is, total concentration will be greater on the more acidic side than the more alkaline side. These differences in concentrations occur without the expenditure of energy.

Active Transport

These processes require energy and can move a substance against a concentration or electrical gradient. The processes are selective and can be saturated (i.e., exhibit a maximal rate of transport).

Facilitated Diffusion

While the process utilizes a carrier, energy is not required and hence transport cannot occur against a concentration gradient. The process is more rapid than simple diffusion in moving substances.

Pinocytosis

This term describes the process whereby droplets of fluid are moved across cellular membranes.

The last two processes are less significant means of movement of drugs across biological membranes than the first three processes.

PHARMACOKINETICS

Absorption

Absorption refers to the movement of a drug from its site of administration into the blood. The rate at which a drug is absorbed determines the onset of action of the drug, the dosage, as well as the appropriate route for administration of the drug. A number of factors affect the movement of a drug from a site of administration into the blood. This includes the membrane permeability of the drug, that is, the processes involved in its movement across membranes surrounding the site of administration. Drug solubility or particle size is important, as smaller compounds are absorbed faster. Drugs in solution are generally absorbed faster than undissolved suspensions. Dissolution time markedly affects the rate of absorption. The onset of action of drugs with poor solubility is delayed because these drugs go slowly into solution. This is a useful means of lengthening the duration of action of a drug. The concentration of a drug at its site of administration is an important factor. The higher the concentration, the faster the drug will be absorbed. Blood flow to an area is also very important. In areas of high flow, the onset of action will be fast, whereas in areas of low flow the onset of action will be delayed but duration of action will be longer. The area of the absorbing surface is also a factor; the larger this area, the faster absorption will occur.

Routes of Administration

The **oral** route is most frequently employed because it is easiest to use, most acceptable to the patient, and more economical than other routes. Disadvantages can include slower onset of action than other routes, variable rates of absorption, and inactivation in the gastrointestinal (GI) tract. Furthermore, after absorption, drugs must pass through the liver, which can also metabolize them (**first-pass effect**). Irritating substances are difficult to give orally, as they induce nausea and vomiting. Such drugs may be given with food to reduce irritation. Absorption of drugs from the GI tract is primarily by passive movement across lipoprotein membranes.

After swallowing an oral drug preparation, it passes rapidly through the esophagus into the stomach where the pH is 1 to 2. In this environment, weak acids such as salicylates may be absorbed, as they will be predominantly nonionized. Weak bases, which are mainly in their ionized form at this low pH, as well as strong electrolytes are not absorbed appreciably from the stomach. Small molecular weight, water-soluble nonelectrolytes, such as ethanol, are absorbed throughout the GI tract. These substances are absorbed with water *via* pores. In the intestines, pH is considerably higher and near the mucosa may be 5.5 to 6. At this pH, conditions are more favorable for the absorption of weak bases than in the stomach, but they are less favorable for the absorption of weak acids. Strong electrolytes and other substances with poor lipid solubility are not readily absorbed from the stomach or intestines. Lack of absorption of some substances can be a useful property when there is a need to limit drug activity to the GI tract. For example, streptomycin, which is not absorbed, can be used to sterilize the GI tract prior to surgery or to treat infections of the GI tract.

A number of other factors can also affect absorption from the GI tract. For example, if gastric emptying is delayed, absorption of drugs will be delayed. The reason for the latter phenomenon is because of the large surface area of the intestines. Thus, most drugs given orally are absorbed primarily in the intestines, even if they are weak acids. Food present in the stomach usually delays absorption because it delays stomach emptying. When food is in the stomach, the time to empty half of the stomach contents is 20 to 25 minutes. For most of a drug given with food to pass into the intestines, three to four times the $t_{1/2}$ for emptying may be necessary. On an empty stomach, if a preparation is taken with a full glass of water, it could pass directly into the intestines. Thus, there can be considerable variability in the rate of passage through this portion of the GI tract. In addition, food may also interact to form nonabsorbable complexes (e.g., tetracyclines and Ca^{2+}). Digestive enzymes as well as bacterial enzymes may interact with drugs to inactivate them. Drug breakdown may also occur as a result of contact with the various pHs of the GI tract. Water solubility is a factor, as a drug that is to be absorbed must be in solution in the fluid adjacent to the mucosa. Thus, some degree of water solubility is essential to facilitate absorption.

In order to prolong activity, a number of oral preparations are formulated so that the drug is released slowly. There is, however, considerable variation in rates of absorption with these preparations. Irritating substances may be given in enteric-coated preparations. Because such preparations require the higher pH of the intestines to remove the outer coating of the tablet, they pass through the stomach without coming in contact with this organ.

After drugs are absorbed from the GI tract, they pass through the liver before entering the general circulation. Here, metabolism can inactivate the drugs. Thus, with oral administration, the action of some drugs may be markedly limited.

Sublingual absorption of drugs also may occur when they are placed under the tongue or in the cheek pouch. Absorption occurs across a lipoprotein barrier, thus limiting this route to lipophilic substances. In addition, irritating and unpleasant-tasting agents are not well tolerated. The advantage of sublingual administration is that the onset of action is within minutes. Furthermore, the liver is bypassed, thus avoiding the first-pass effect. Nitroglycerin is an example of a drug given by this route.

Rectal absorption across the membranes of the rectal mucosal may occur, and this has led to the development of drug forms such as suppositories and enemas. This route may be advantageous for certain drugs when a patient is vomiting or unconscious. Also, with this route, drugs do not pass through the liver before entering the general circulation. Disadvantages of this route include erratic absorption, irritation of mucosa by drugs, and a lack of acceptability by patients.

There are a number of injection sites (called **parenteral sites**) into which drugs may be administered. Generally, drugs given by these routes exhibit more rapid absorption than by the oral route and have a more predictable action. The injection routes can minimize the influence of the metabolic enzymes of the liver as well as bypass the bacterial enzymes of the GI tract. When the oral route cannot be used, as when patients are unconscious or vomiting or uncooperative, an injectable site is preferred. There are many disadvantages to injection routes. The drug preparations must be sterile; thus, they are more expensive. There may be pain involved in administration, and self-administration by the patient is more difficult. Drugs may inadvertently enter a blood vessel directly and produce a more sudden or greater effect than desired. In general, there is a greater risk involved in the use of an injection site.

The processes involved in absorption of drugs from injection sites into the blood include diffusion and filtration. Lipid-soluble substances pass through capillary membranes, whereas hydrophilic substances pass through pores in capillaries. Large molecular weight substances, such as proteins, may be picked up by the lymphatics. The rate of absorption from injection sites is dependent upon blood flow. As discussed under individual sites, drug action may be prolonged by choice of site. In addition, measures may be taken to alter blood flow to a site to change rates of absorption.

Subcutaneous injections are administered just under the skin. Solutions should be isotonic to minimize pain. They should also be nonirritating, or damage to the site with subsequent sloughing of skin may occur. At subcutaneous sites, the area of absorption is limited and blood flow is low. Hence, absorption of drug is slow, and duration of action is longer compared with other injectable sites.

It is possible to slow absorption and thus create long-term reservoirs at subcutaneous sites. By including epinephrine in the injection, blood flow may be markedly decreased and duration of drug action prolonged. Substances given in oil will also have their duration of action prolonged. Also, substances placed under the skin in solid pellets may have durations of action of weeks or months.

Absorption rates can be increased if the site of injection is massaged or heat is applied. These measures increase blood flow to the area. It should also be noted that injections given subcutaneously when a patient is in shock will be poorly absorbed because of diminished blood flow to the skin. To obtain a response, larger doses of drugs must be given. If blood pressure is restored, blood flow to the injected sites will increase and it is then possible to see the drug produce a greater than desired response.

Intramuscular injections can be made into muscular tissue. Somewhat more irritating substances may be given by this route than the subcutaneous route. Absorption from intramuscular sites is generally faster than from subcutaneous sites. Since the organization of muscle is in planes, surface area is large. Also, blood flow is high. Absorption can be delayed if an oily vehicle is used or if an insoluble drug is given as a suspension. Massage or application of heat will increase absorption rate.

Intravenous injection occurs when a drug is placed directly into a vein. Absorption is dependent only on the rate of infusion of the drug. Dosage can be adjusted as the drug is given, if it is infused slowly; thus, a high degree of accuracy is possible with this route. As opposed to subcutaneous and intramuscular injections, very irritating drugs or hypertonic solutions may be given, if they are given slowly or with sufficient dilution. Large volumes can also be given by this route. Undesired reactions may occur because high concentrations may be reached in tissues too quickly. Once given, a reaction is difficult to reverse. With other routes, applying cold compresses or occluding blood flow can deter absorption. Also, with repeated injections, veins are damaged and new injection sites may be difficult to find.

Intra-arterial injections (directly into an artery) may be made if there is a need to limit the action of a drug to a smaller area. Contrast media for x-rays or antineoplastic agents are given by this route.

Intrathecal injections into spinal fluid may be made to produce spinal anesthesia or to treat central nervous system (CNS) infections.

In addition to the aforementioned routes, a number of other sites of drug administration are possible.

Pulmonary absorption is very rapid because there is a large surface area and large blood flow. Volatile or gaseous drugs may be administered by this route. Agents of this type are widely used for general anesthesia. In addition, aerosol forms of several drugs that are administered into the airways have been developed for use in the treatment of asthma. A disadvantage of this route is the need for special equipment to give drugs. Also, because most substances are irritating to the lungs, very few agents can be administered by this route.

A number of preparations are applied to **musocal membranes** for local actions. These internal surfaces include nasal passages, oropharynx, conjunctiva, urethra, and vagina. In addition to local action, such topical preparations may be absorbed and exert undesirable systemic effects. Lipid solubility in the membranes is the most important factor involved in drug absorption.

Topical application of drugs to **skin** usually results only in a local action, as the several layers or cells of this organ limit absorption. However, lipid-soluble substances may be absorbed, and systemic effects are, therefore, possible. Absorption may be enhanced if a substance is dissolved in oil and rubbed into the skin, a process known as **inunction**.

Distribution

Following absorption into the blood, the area(s) or tissue(s) to which a drug is distributed varies with physical-chemical properties. Because cell walls contain lipoproteins, lipid solubility is a factor determining entry into cells. As the pH within cells is more acidic than the pH of the plasma (7.4) and interstitial compartments, weak organic bases will tend to concentrate in cells, whereas weak organic acids will be found in slightly higher concentrations outside of cells. If a drug is bound within cells, then distribution becomes more complex.

Volume of Distribution

The **volume of distribution** (V_d) of a drug is determined by dividing the amount of drug given by the concentration of the drug in plasma. This concentration is that attained when the elimination curve is extended back to zero time. The V_d does not necessarily represent a defined compartment in the body such as plasma or body water. If a drug has a very small V_d, this implies very high binding to plasma proteins; if a drug has a very large V_d (e.g., larger than body volume), this implies that the drug is highly concentrated in tissues or organs.

Only unbound drug (or free drug) is active or subject to metabolism or excretion. Thus, when a drug is highly bound, the bound drug serves as a reservoir for the active or free drug. Since the bound drug is in equilibrium with free drug, as free drug is metabolized or excreted, bound drug will be released. The drug-binding sites on plasma proteins, as well as other sites that do not produce an effect, are referred to as inert binding sites.

In general, drugs that are bound require higher doses, inasmuch as it is necessary to saturate binding sites before free drug is present in amounts adequate to produce a response. Because many drugs can bind to similar sites (e.g., plasma albumin), a drug that has higher affinity may displace another drug and hence increase its activity or toxicity.

Drug-Binding Sites

In plasma, albumin is the predominant binding site. There is considerable variation among drugs in their degree of binding to plasma proteins. Some drugs exhibit no albumin binding (e.g., caffeine), whereas some may be nearly 100 percent bound (e.g., suramin). When drugs are bound intracellularly, they will have large volumes of distribution. Certain drugs exhibit specialized sites of localization. The concentration of some drugs in sites such as kidney and liver is facilitated by the active uptake mechanisms of these organs. Lipid-soluble drugs may concentrate in fat cells, whereas heavy metals and tetracycline tend to concentrate in bone. When binding occurs at a site, that site serves as a reservoir. Another site that may serve as a reservoir is the GI tract. Any drug that is poorly absorbed from the GI tract will be present in the body for several days (the time for contents to traverse the length of the alimentary canal varies from 4 to 7 days).

Penetration of drugs into the CNS is limited by the **blood-brain barrier**. The capillaries in the CNS are engulfed by glial cells, and this results in smaller pores. Thus, drugs in plasma do not enter freely into the extracellular fluid of the CNS. Although movement of hydrophilic drugs through pores is severely restricted, lipid-soluble drugs may still move into the CNS by diffusion across the capillaries. Exit of drugs from the cerebrospinal fluid (CSF) is also limited. While lipophilic drugs may diffuse out, hydrophilic agents must be removed by active transport processes. There is a mechanism that actively secretes organic anions and another that actively secretes organic cations. These systems (located in the choroid plexus) are capable of removing such substances from the CSF and secreting them into plasma. The active transport mechanisms found in the CNS appear to be similar to those found in the proximal tubules of the kidneys.

Movement of drugs across the placenta is limited to diffusion of lipid-soluble agents. Hence, fetal toxicity is possible with agents of this type.

The duration of action of drugs is usually terminated by metabolism, excretion, or both. **Redistribution,** however, is another possible means to end the action of a drug. For example, thiopental is a short-acting barbiturate administered intravenously to induce anesthesia. Thiopental is very lipophilic and readily leaves the circulation to enter the CNS where it acts. Its lipophilicity results in high affinity for fat cells. As blood circulates to fat stores (which have a low perfusion rate), the drug is removed from blood. This in turn causes it to diffuse out of the CNS. Hence, its action will diminish and terminate as it is redistributed. If thiopental is given repeatedly, it is possible for the drug to saturate fat storage sites. Thiopental would then exert an effect for a long period of time, as its action would have to be terminated by metabolism and excretion.

In the body, sites where drugs are found in the highest concentration are only occasionally related to sites of therapeutic action. More frequently, sites of highest drug concentration will be related to sites of metabolism, excretion, storage, or toxicity.

Metabolism

Metabolism (biotransformation) is a major means of terminating the action of drugs, although it may also activate drug from **prodrugs.** In general, metabolism usually results in the conversion to a more hydrophilic compound. This may occur in one or two phases: phase I—slightly more water-soluble compounds are formed (e.g., adding a —OH group); phase II—groups (e.g., glucuronic acid) are added that markedly increase the water solubility of the compound. Because many drugs are weak organic acids or bases that cross membranes readily in their non-ionized forms, metabolism to more hydrophilic forms limits their cellular access and hence activity. In addition, metabolism facilitates elimination from the body, since hydrophilic compounds can be more readily excreted by the kidneys and liver. While metabolism of drugs can occur in any cell, the liver is the organ principally involved in biotransformation.

There are four ways in which drugs are metabolized by the body: **oxidation, reduction, synthesis** (conjugation), and **hydrolysis**. Drug oxidation reactions occur in the endoplasmic reticulum of the liver. These cellular particles are isolated by centrifugation and are referred to as the microsomal fraction or microsomes. Drug oxidation reactions involving microsomes are also referred to as metabolism by the **mixed function oxidase system**. This system is involved in several types of reactions, including N-dealkylation, O-dealkylation, aromatic ring hydroxylation, aliphatic side-chain hydroxylation, desulfuration, sulfoxide formation, and dehalogenation. Requirements of these reactions are NADPH, O_2, and the endoplasmic reticulum. The smooth endoplasmic reticulum contains a family of enzymes (**cytochrome P-450 enzymes**) that are involved in the phase I biotransformations. These oxidative enzymes add or expose—OH or—NH groups on drugs, usually by adding oxygen. This generally results in a slight increase in water solubility, but probably more importantly, these reactions create sites for conjugation to occur (phase II reactions).

Oxidation reactions occurring without microsomes involve the soluble fraction (cell sap) and include enzymes for the metabolism of some alcohols (e.g., alcohol and aldehyde dehydrogenases), catecholamines (monoamine oxidase), and purines (xanthine oxidase).

Reduction is another phase I type of reaction. Azoreductase and nitroreductase reactions may occur. These two reactions involve an initial oxidation of the compound to an intermediate and then reduction by H^+ from $NADPH^+$.

The third type of reaction is synthesis or conjugation. In reactions of this type, an addition is made to a compound and this generally yields a highly ionized water-soluble substance that can readily be excreted by the kidneys or liver. These reactions require energy, usually ATP, and involve a step in which the drug or conjugation agent is activated. Types of synthesis reactions include acetylation; methylation; and glutathione, glucuronide, sulfate, or glycine conjugations. These reactions occur in various parts of the liver cells (cytosol, microsomes, or mitochondria).

Hydrolysis is the fourth type of reaction and can involve deamidation and de-esterification. Enzymes involved include pseudocholinesterase and peptidases in plasma and procainesterase in the liver and plasma.

A number of different factors can affect drug metabolism. The amount of enzyme can vary in different individuals. This can be due to age, sex, nutritional status, pathological state, or genetic background. In addition to these factors, there are a number of chemicals that can alter metabolism. More than 200 compounds have been identified that can increase drug-metabolizing activity following chronic administration. Most of these agents increase activity by increasing synthesis of drug metabolizing enzymes ("induction"). Various forms of cytochrome P-450 are induced by different substances and these forms exhibit different specificities for substrates. Such specificities may or may not include the inducer. Some agents can stimulate their own metabolism; this explains the tolerance that occurs with chronic use of such agents. Whereas many stimulators of activity have been described, a lesser number of inhibitors are known. Many agents, however, may decrease metabolism indirectly by decreasing blood flow to sites of metabolism. The blood supply of the liver is particularly dependent upon blood pressure, and small decreases in pressure can result in marked decreases in blood flow to this organ.

When a substance affects the metabolism of another agent, such drug-drug interactions will alter the dosage requirements of the affected agent. Failure to change dosage could result in an inadequate or enhanced drug effect. If the inducer or depressor substance is withdrawn, metabolism that was altered will be reversed, and consequently changes in activity of drugs previously affected will occur.

Excretion

Excretion, in addition to metabolism and redistribution, is a means of terminating the action of drugs. Drugs or foreign compounds may be excreted in the various secretion products of the body: urine, feces, expired air, sweat, tears, saliva, and milk. Penicillin is a drug that can be found in all of these. Although a drug such as penicillin may be excreted by more than one route, usually a drug will be excreted primarily by one route. In the case of penicillin, the kidneys are the principal organ of excretion. Because a drug is handled primarily by one organ, it is important to know the functional state of that organ. If it is deficient, then the duration of action of the drug will be prolonged and its activity will be enhanced if the frequency of administration is not reduced. Although a deficiency of an excretory organ can occur when the organ is diseased or damaged, a deficiency can also occur if blood flow to the excretory organ is reduced, as when the patient is in shock.

Since drugs tend to concentrate at their sites of excretion, this property can be exploited. Infections of excretory organs are best treated by antibacterial agents that are excreted by that organ. X-rays of excretory organs have been facilitated by using radiopaque compounds that are readily excreted by them.

Another generalization concerning routes of excretion is that the greater the volume of distribution of a substance, the longer it will take to excrete such an agent. Thus, drugs that are highly bound in tissues will have very long half-lives in the body. This occurs because only a small fraction of such agents will be present in plasma and, since an excretory organ can only excrete a drug that perfuses it, the drug will be eliminated very slowly.

Routes of Excretion

In the following sections, the various organs of excretion are discussed. The processes involved, types of compounds excreted, and overall importance of the route are reviewed.

Renal Excretion. The **kidneys** are the most important organ involved in the excretion of drugs since the greatest percentage of drugs employed are handled by this organ. The processes of filtration, diffusion, and active transport are involved in the renal handling of drugs.

Filtration is a very developed process in the kidneys in that all substances smaller than plasma proteins can be filtered at the glomerular membranes into the tubular lumens. Thus, practically all drugs will be filtered, as only a few have molecular weights greater than the plasma proteins. Since, in humans, 20 percent of the plasma volume that perfuses the kidneys is filtered at the glomeruli, a similar fraction of drug is filtered. Drugs that are bound to plasma proteins, however, will not be filtered. Agents freely filtered but not further handled by the tubules will have fairly fast rates of excretion, provided their volumes of distribution are low (Table 1–1). Generally, most substances filtered at the glomeruli will undergo some reabsorption and hence have rates of excretion longer than indicated in the table.

Movement across the tubules can occur in either direction and is based on the lipophilic properties of drugs. Because fluid filtered at the glomeruli is absorbed as it flows along the tubules (usually 99 percent), substances present in the filtrate will be concentrated. Hydrophilic substances will not be reabsorbed and their concentration will increase in the tubular fluid as water is reabsorbed. Lipophilic substances will diffuse across tubular cells back into

Table 1–1. EFFECT OF DRUG DISTRIBUTION ON RATE OF RENAL EXCRETION OF DRUGS

Drug Type and Renal Excretion Process	Area of Distribution		
	Extracellular Compartment	Body Water (Cellular and Extracellular Compartments)	99% Bound in Tissues
	Half-Life ($t_{1/2}$)		
Hydrophilic;* Active Secretion	15 min	50 min	50 days
Hydrophilic; Filtered	70 min	280 min	500 days
Lipophilic;† Passive Reabsorption	7 days	24 days	93 years

*Drug does not cross membranes, unless actively transported.

†Drug cannot achieve a concentration gradient across tubular membranes.

blood as their concentration increases; hence, their half-lives will be very long (see Table 1–1). Excretion of such substances can be increased by increasing urinary volume, as this decreases the concentration gradient. In the case of weak electrolytes, it is possible to see excretion rates change markedly as urinary pH is altered. Altering urinary pH changes the dissociation of weak organic acids and bases, thus altering the fraction of lipophilic (non-ionized) and hydrophilic (ionized) components of the drug. Such changes can change the direction of diffusion. For example, a weak organic acid in an acidic urine (i.e., with a pH less than that of plasma) will be less ionized in urine than in plasma, and its non-ionized concentration in urine will be greater than in plasma; this favors reabsorption of the lipophilic moiety. As non-ionized drug is reabsorbed, ionized drug in urine will become non-ionized and hence available for reabsorption. Thus, it is possible that nearly complete reabsorption of this drug can occur without the expenditure of energy.

On the other hand, if a weak organic acid is in a urine with a pH greater than that of plasma (alkaline urine), its ionized concentration will be greater than that in plasma and its non-ionized concentration less. Hence, diffusion of this drug into urine will occur. As secretion occurs, the non-ionized drug will be converted to its ionized form which, being hydrophilic, remains in the tubules and thus produces large concentration gradients. This is referred to as ion trapping. With large urine volumes it is possible to obtain marked losses of such agents without the expenditure of energy. With weak organic bases the opposite happens. In acidic urine, secretion of drug occurs, whereas in alkaline urine, drug is reabsorbed.

Half-lives of such agents in the body can be affected by altering their urinary excretion rates. Thus, if there is a need to increase excretion rates of such substances, as in the case of poisonings, urinary pH may be altered. Administration of sodium bicarbonate will alkalinize the urine and may increase the excretion of weak organic acids; administration of glutamine HCl or lysine HCl will acidify the urine and may increase the excretion of certain weak organic bases.

Active transport processes are also involved in the renal excretion of drugs. In the proximal tubules, there are active mechanisms for the secretion of organic acids and organic bases that are capable of completely clearing the plasma of drugs. Thus, agents handled by these systems may have very short half-lives in plasma. Protein binding may limit active secretion if binding affinity is great. While the system for organic acids handles many different organic acids (penicillin, Diodrast, glucuronides), not all organic acids are transported. For example, phenobarbital is not handled by this system. Similarly, many but not all organic bases are actively secreted by the organic base transport system. Within each system, there is competition for transport. Certain agents have higher affinity for the transport mechanism and can displace other substances. For example, **probenecid** has a high affinity for the organic acid transport system and displaces other substances. Thus, this agent increases the duration of action of substances it displaces. Probenecid was once used to prolong the action of penicillin.

Compounds excreted by the kidneys may be handled by more than one process. Thus, it is possible that filtration, active secretion, and passive reabsorption or secretion may be involved in the renal elimination of a single drug. It should be apparent from the foregoing that the more hydrophilic a drug, the more readily it will be excreted by the kidneys. Because the liver generally forms more hydrophilic substances when it metabolizes drugs, these two organs can be viewed as working in concert to hasten the elimination of drugs or foreign compounds from the body.

Hepatobiliary Excretion. The **liver** may also serve as an excretory organ for drugs that it transports into bile. It is also possible, however, that such substances may be reabsorbed from the intestines and thus returned to the liver *via* the portal vein, where they may be excreted again (**enterohepatic circulation**). This may serve as a reservoir for such substances. Thus, while glucuronides may be secreted by the liver into the bile, they may be acted upon by glucuronidases of bacteria in the intestines to yield compounds that can be absorbed from the intestines, which in turn can form glucuronides and be excreted again.

The processes involved in excretion by the liver are somewhat similar to those of the kidneys. Uncharged substances with molecular weights up to 500 can be filtered through hepatic cells. Thus, compounds such as sucrose and inulin may appear in bile.

Diffusion of lipophilic substances into bile may also occur. The primary processes for elimination, however, are active transport processes. There are transport mechanisms for organic anions and for organic cations. These systems are similar to those in the kidney, differing in that they are more specific for compounds with molecular weights greater than 600. This is not an absolute, since if either the kidneys or the liver should be deficient, then the fully functioning organ system can increase the transport of compounds usually handled by the deficient organ system. There is also a third active transport system in the liver. It is involved in the secretion of bile salts into the bile but is also capable of handling some other agents that also have steroid structures.

The loss of drugs by the liver is dependent on blood flow and, as hepatic blood flow (particularly portal flow) is variable, excretion of drugs by the liver can vary markedly. Also, in disease states such as congestive heart failure or cardiogenic shock, hepatic blood flow—and, hence, hepatic excretion as well—can be decreased.

Intestinal Excretion. Drugs excreted by the **GI tract** in the feces are from several different sources. They include drugs that are given orally but are incompletley absorbed, drugs excreted into the bile and not reabsorbed from the intestine, and drugs that diffuse across the GI epithelium into the GI tract. No active transport mechanisms are involved, but because final intestinal pH is more acidic than plasma pH, weak organic bases may be concentrated here as a result of ion trapping.

Pulmonary Excretion. The **lung** is an important excretory organ for gaseous and volatile substances. Agents with low solubility in plasma (lipophilic agents, e.g., ether) will be excreted rapidly in expired air, whereas agents with high solubility in plasma (hydrophilic agents, e.g., ethanol) will be excreted slowly. Anesthetic gases and volatile liquids that are administered *via* the lungs are excreted by this route as well. Although ethanol is only slowly excreted by the lungs, its concentration in expired air is related to its concentration in plasma, a fact that has led to the development of instruments to estimate blood alcohol levels for use by law enforcement agencies.

Other Routes of Excretion. Excretion of drugs by **mammary glands** in milk is not a major route of loss; however, it can serve as a source of toxic agents for a nursing infant. Compounds may move into milk by filtration or diffusion. Because pores in mammary ducts are small, only uncharged low molecular substances will appear in milk. Ethanol meets these criteria and is present in milk in the same concentration as in the plasma of the nursing mother. Since the pH of milk is acidic (about 6.5), weak organic substances may achieve concentrations in milk greater than in plasma because of ion trapping. Examples of such agents are erythromycin and morphine. Weak organic acids will be found in milk in concentrations less than in plasma and hence these are generally safer agents to employ in a nursing mother. However, allergic responses are possible. Some agents, such as antithyroid and antineoplastic agents, are simply too toxic at any level for a nursing infant. A few agents (e.g., tetracyclines) may be concentrated in milk owing to chelation with calcium. The chelate formed is a very strong one and passes through the GI tract of the nursing infant without any of the antibiotic being absorbed. It is evident that all drugs being taken by a nursing mother should be evaluated for possible effects on the breastfed infant.

Because saliva, the secretory product of the **salivary glands,** is swallowed, this is not a true route of elimination but may serve as a minor reservoir. Appearance of drugs in saliva is primarily by diffusion. Weak organic bases may be somewhat more concentrated than in plasma, as salivary pH is slightly more acidic than plasma pH. Blood levels of some compounds may be estimated by assaying concentrations in saliva. Another use of this route is the determination of circulation times. These may be estimated by administering a bitter substance (e.g., ascorbic acid) intravenously at different sites and noting the time it takes for the patient to report tasting it in the mouth.

In **sweat glands,** diffusion is the primary process involved and, because sweat is more acidic than plasma, weak organic bases may achieve higher concentrations in sweat than in plasma. Drugs that appear in sweat may cause contact dermatitis; thus, internally derived substances may be involved in this toxicity.

The presence of drugs in tears from the **tear glands** may result in eye irritation. Diffusion across the tear ducts is involved in their entry.

Rate of Excretion

The development of a dosage regimen for a drug requires a thorough study of the disposition and rate of excretion of the drug. The **clearance (Cl)** of the drug from the body and the time to eliminate **half of the drug** from the body (**half-life; $t_{1/2}$**) must be determined.

Clearance. Clearance represents the volume of blood or plasma from which a drug has been totally removed per unit time. It is determined by dividing **rate of elimination (K_{el})** by the concentration of the drug in blood or plasma (C) ($Cl = \dfrac{K_{el}}{C}$). Clearance is usually constant; thus, if the concentration of the drug increases, the rate of elimination will increase.

Total body clearance is a summation of various clearances. These include excretion by the kidneys, metabolism by the liver, and elimination or metabolism by other organs. If clearance is low, the drug has a high volume of distribution; if clearance is high, the drug has a very low volume of distribution.

Half-Life. The $t_{1/2}$ of a drug (i.e., the time for 50 percent of the drug to be eliminated) is determined by multiplying the volume of distribution (V_d) of the drug by 0.693 and dividing by the clearance of the drug ($t_{1/2} = \dfrac{0.693 \times V_d}{Cl}$). The resulting value is the time for the blood or plasma concentration (log scale) to fall to half of its initial level.

Single- and Two-Compartment Pharmacokinetics. If the concentration of drug is parallel in all tissues, then the drug is said to exhibit characteristics of single-compartment distribution. In this case, it is possible to administer the drug at intervals of its half-life and to attain a steady-state level after approximately four doses. At this time, the amount of drug entering the body and the amount being eliminated are equal. If administration of the drug is stopped, then it will take approximately five half-lives to reduce plasma concentration to negligible levels. Doubling of the dose should double the plasma concentration. If this does not occur, it means that some parameter has changed (e.g., saturation of binding sites, or exceeding metabolism or a different volume of distribution has occurred). If, during administration of multiple doses of a drug, a parameter such as metabolism is saturated, then a new steady-state curve will result. With single-compartment distribution, the concentration of drug in all tissues increases in a parallel manner. However, with nonparallel changes in different tissues, as drug in the body is increased, plasma concentration of drug may be very unpredictable. Various tissues will behave differently. If a process is saturated, then zero-order kinetics apply (i.e., relationship of uptake and time is arithmetic), whereas if a process is unsaturated, first-order kinetics apply (i.e., relationship of uptake and time is loga-

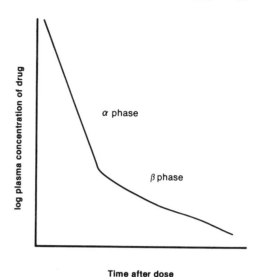

Figure 1–3. Drug disappearance from plasma in a two-compartment model showing distribution (α phase) and elimination (β phase) processes.

rithmic). If some aspect of saturation is involved in the half-life of a drug, then as a rule of thumb a small amount of drug (30 percent of prior dose) should be given when attempting to increase plasma levels. Plasma concentration should be determined and then the dose adjusted again if necessary.

Many substances exhibit **two-compartment pharmacokinetics** (Fig. 1–3). In plots of concentration versus time there is an initial steep fall in plasma drug concentration (α **phase),** which is referred to as the **distribution phase** of the drug. The slower second phase is referred to as the **elimination phase** (or β **phase**). With such drugs a loading dose may be necessary to fill the peripheral compartment, following which smaller doses will be sufficient to equal the rate of elimination.

DOSAGE REGIMENS

The use of pharmacokinetics to idealize drug regimens involves the manipulation of route of administration, dose, interval between doses, and the duration of therapy.

The ideal route of administration can be determined by administering a drug by different routes and plotting plasma concentration of drug against time. The dose for a drug for a given route will be determined by the peak concentration of the drug. This will be a concentration that produces the desired action. With some routes, this may not occur (e.g., first-pass effect by the liver, preventing action of drug after oral administration). The frequency of administration is determined by the minimal concentration of drug that produces the desired response. The lowest concentration of drug between doses of a drug is referred to as the trough. The peak and trough concentrations for a given drug will vary with different routes of administration. This is due to different rates of absorption as well as different degrees of absorption. Differences in total amount of drug absorbed (**bioavailability**) are reflected as differences in area under the concentration curve (AUC). If, however, absorption is similar by different routes, AUC will be the same even though curves will vary in times of peak or trough or both (i.e., flatter curves with routes that have slower rates of absorption).

The dosing rate of a drug may be derived by multiplying clearance of the drug by its desired blood or plasma concentration ($Cl \times C$). This indicates the quantity of drug lost per minute and hence the rate a drug should be administered to maintain a desired plasma concentration. If given by continuous intravenous infusion, a constant plasma level can be readily maintained. When given by other routes, maximal concentrations (peaks) and minimal concentrations (troughs) must be taken into account to determine frequency of administration. When long intervals between doses are used, peaks may be too high and lead to toxicity. Also, troughs may fall too low, resulting in long periods of no drug effect. Hence, a frequency of administration must be selected that maintains the level of the drug between maximal safe levels and minimal effective levels.

The **loading dose** of a drug is determined by multiplying the desired blood or plasma concentration by the volume of distribution of the drug ($C \times V_d$). Thus, a high dose may be given initially to achieve the desired blood levels.

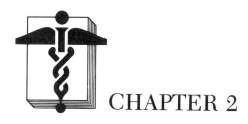

CHAPTER 2

Basic Concepts of Clinical Pharmacology

ROBERT J. ROBERTS, M.D., Ph.D.

Clinical pharmacology deals with the problems and the process of evaluation of drugs and drug therapy in the human.[1] In comparison with other disciplines of medicine, clinical pharmacology is relatively young. Although the roots began with the founding of the American Therapeutic Society in 1900, what we now call clinical pharmacology appears to have had its true beginning in the late 1930s and early 1940s. Dr. Walter Modell founded the first journal devoted to the discipline of clinical pharmacology, *Clinical Pharmacology and Therapeutics*, in 1960. The passage, in 1962, of the **Kefauver-Harris Amendment** to the United States Food and Drug law had a major impact on clinical pharmacology responsibilities. This amendment required, through the performance of properly controlled clinical trials, the demonstration of drug efficacy.

25

At about this same time an evolution began in clinical pharmacology research. Specific areas of drug effects in humans, including adverse effects and individual responses to drugs, began to receive attention. Tremendous inroads have now been made in understanding how and why individuals differ in their responses to drugs. This understanding has been an outgrowth of controlled clinical trials and the use of sophisticated technology for analysis of drugs in biological systems.

DEVELOPMENT AND CLINICAL TESTING OF PHARMACOLOGIC AGENTS

The average physician is obligated to have an understanding of the various processes involved in drug development in order to assess adequately the benefit-to-risk ratio of a drug used for therapeutic purposes. Prior to reaching the stage of clinical trials in humans, drugs must undergo extensive evaluation in several species of experimental animals and *in vitro*. These studies lay the groundwork in pharmacokinetic, pharmacodynamic, and toxic properties of the drug, which aid in the design and conduct of the human studies.

Clinical testing of drugs in man in the United States is divided into several phases, the first three of which must be completed under an **investigational new drug (IND)** application approved by the Food and Drug Administration (FDA). These initial three phases of clinical testing must be completed before a new drug application (NDA), involving a final, fourth phase of testing, can be submitted to the FDA. The IND should contain the following information:

1. A description of the chemistry and biological activity of the drug
2. The specific dosage forms to be given to humans
3. Specifications of the quality control measures employed in the manufacture of the drug, and identification of all ingredients
4. A description of equipment, procedures, and facilities used in manufacture of the drug
5. The names and qualifications of the individuals to conduct the initial studies
6. A signed statement of each investigator acknowledging his/her understanding of the drug, his/her responsibilities to personally supervise the studies, and his/her agreement to observe the requirements regarding use of volunteers in informed written consent
7. A description of the facilities available for the studies
8. Protocols concerning dose, route, and duration of drug administration, and the clinical laboratory examinations to be made, data sheets to be provided to each investigator for the studies detailing all that is known about the drug (indications and possible side effects)

9. Specified observations that should be reported to the FDA and manufacturer

An NDA based on the results of the clinical investigations must be approved before the drug can be made available for prescription use.

The four phases of clinical drug evaluation are outlined in Table 2–1. **Phase I** studies involve a limited number of volunteers and are primarily concerned with establishing a dosage range, including doses causing adverse effects. **Phase II** involves studies in a small number of patients afflicted with an illness that the drug is believed to be useful against. These study subjects have a known disease, in contrast to subjects in the phase I studies, who are generally healthy volunteers. The major emphasis of the phase II studies is to reaffirm safe dosage ranges, as well as to gain preliminary information on possible efficacy. In **phase III** clinical trials, hundreds to thousands of carefully selected patients receive the test drug under controlled conditions. Because the phase I, II, and III studies are conducted in a relatively small number of patients over a limited time period, only the most profound or overt toxicities are usually identified. Delayed or infrequent adverse effects (e.g., 1 in 1000 or more) are not apt to be identified. If safety and efficacy of a test drug can be established, an NDA can be approved by the FDA and the drug can be marketed (**phase IV**).

Although pharmacological efficacy and serious toxicity may be statistically established prior to NDA approval, true clinical effectiveness and incidence and nature of adverse reactions may not be appreciated until the drug is used

Table 2–1. PHASES OF DRUG DEVELOPMENT IN THE UNITED STATES

Phase I	Initial human trials conducted in a small number of healthy volunteers or occasionally in patients with certain diseases. Purpose of phase I studies is to ascertain safe or reasonable dosage tolerances for phase II and III studies.
Phase II	Limited human clinical trials in patients selected on the basis of disease potentially treatable by the drug. Purpose of phase II studies is to begin to establish the efficacy of the drug and further examine therapeutic dosage range (toxicity vs. efficacy).
Phase III	More extensive controlled clinical trials to establish the drug's efficacy and toxicity. Double-blind, placebo-controlled clinical studies are used as often as possible.
Phase IV	FDA approval granted for release of the drug for use in specific indications. Surveillance of efficacy and toxicity continues.

in the real market place (e.g., thalidomide). One of the major problems with the general marketing of drugs is the difficulty in monitoring and controlling its use. New uses of a drug and actual patterns of usage within different localities and medical specialities cannot be anticipated or regulated. For example, the IND studies may not adequately prepare for the use of drugs in pediatric or geriatric age groups. Additional challenges may come from a variety of sources such as special interests groups. Although well meaning, these organizations may demand removal of a drug with little appreciation of benefit-to-risk ratios. Drug recall as a result of an isolated incident or inappropriate use may result in the loss of a therapeutic agent with efficacy in appropriately selected patients.

Before marketing the drug, a package insert must be prepared by the pharmaceutical company in cooperation with the FDA. The package insert contains basic pharmacological information as well as essential clinical information regarding approved indications, contraindications, special warnings, precautions, adverse reactions, dosage and administration, drug interactions, and available dosage preparations. Largely because of legal implications, a package insert imposes restraints on the practicing physician, particularly with respect to adverse reactions and use in pediatrics and in pregnancy. Therefore, the physician should not ignore other sources of information, especially controlled clinical drug trials that provide evidence for new indications for an improved drug or, for that matter, newly reported adverse reactions.

CLINICAL EFFICACY

A constellation of pressures from numerous sources, including clinical pharmacologists and other scientists, practicing physicians and pharmacists, along with professional, consumer, legislative, and health care provider groups, has resulted in the introduction of a number of terms that are important for the student to understand. **Bioequivalence** can pertain to a pharmaceutical formulation of a drug being equal in chemical composition to another manufacturer's formulation (**chemical equivalence**). If the different pharmaceutical preparations yield similar concentrations of drug in the body, they are considered biologically equivalent and having equal bioavailability. **Therapeutic equivalency** implies equal therapeutic benefit of different pharmaceutical preparations in clinical trials. If there is equivalent chemical composition of two pharmaceutical preparations (**pharmaceutical equivalence**) but they differ in biological or therapeutic equivalency (**chemotherapeutic equivalence**), then the preparations must differ in bioavailability. Appreciation of this terminology is particularly important in understanding the issues involved in generic prescribing, generic substitution, and therapeutic substitution. **Generic prescribing** occurs when a physician prescribes a specific drug, leaving the choice of brand to the dispensing pharmacist. **Generic substitution** is a pharmacist-initiated act in which a different drug is dispensed from the drug product that was prescribed by the physician. This means that the same chemical entity and dosage form will be dispensed but it may be a product marketed or manufactured by a different company. **Therapeutic substitution** is a pharmacist-initiated act in which a pharmaceutical or therapeutic alternative for the physician-prescribed drug is dispensed. This denotes replacement of a prescribed drug with a chemically different drug albeit in the same therapeutic category, for example, antibiotic, diuretic, antihypertensive, and so forth.

VARIATION IN DRUG RESPONSE

Throughout the education of the physician, major emphasis is given to diagnosis and treatment of disease. The details accompanying the discussions of diagnosis are generally far more extensive than those associated with treatment, particularly drug therapy. It is important not only to select the appropriate "drug of choice" but also to recognize the possibilities of individualization of this therapy. Individual differences in responses or effects of drugs should be an anticipated event rather than an exception. A thorough understanding and knowledge of both the clinical status of the patient and the therapeutic agent chosen are necessary to achieve both identification of the treatment of choice and ideal individualized therapy with this treatment. Often the intellectual effort ceases after the selection of the therapeutic agent rather than continued considerations of the details of its pharmacology and administration (dose, route, interval, and duration), despite the fact that these considerations have a major impact on the patient realizing full therapeutic benefit.

Pharmacologic Factors Affecting Drug Response

The relationship between a patient taking a given drug and response to this drug can generally be associated with the amount of drug present in the patient at a given period of time. The **dose and frequency of administration** determine the amount of drug present. Manipulations of dose or interval of dosing, or both, can thus determine whether the resulting effects of a drug are therapeutic or toxic. Moreover, the **route of administration** may have a sizable impact on the onset, duration, and nature of the pharmacologic effect. The decision regarding duration of therapy must take into account the anticipated needs (e.g., short course of symptomatic pain relief versus lifetime anticonvulsant therapy) along with both financial and toxicity-related costs of the therapeutic program selected.

Dose, dosing interval, and route of administration differ among various therapeutic agents as well as among patients, as a number of other factors besides these can affect the amount of drug that reaches the site of action. For example, since the site of action of a drug is generally far removed from the site of administration, the drug must first be absorbed from the site of administration to travel to the site of action.

Clinical Factors Altering Drug Response

There is also a wide variety of clinical factors that can affect therapeutic outcome besides those outlined under Pharmacologic Factors. Lack of awareness regarding such clinical factors affecting drug action can result in "unexpected" effects being recognized only by the so-called trial-and-error approach or may even go unrecognized. Some of the more important clinical factors that can lead to altered drug response are listed in Table 2–2.

Disease States

Drug disposition refers to the absorption, distribution, storage, metabolism, and excretion of the drug in the body (see Chapter 1). Various disease states can significantly alter drug disposition by a variety of mechanisms. Deterioration or pre-existing dysfunction of organ systems involved in drug absorption, distribution, metabolism, or excretion will influence the amount of

Table 2–2. CLINICAL
FACTORS THAT CAN ALTER
DRUG RESPONSE IN HUMANS

Disease States
  Hepatic failure
  Renal failure
  Cardiovascular failure
  Pulmonary failure (hypoxemia)
  CNS abnormalities
  Severe trauma (drug metabolism, receptor response)
Genetic
  Drug metabolism (acetylation, hydrolysis)
  Hereditary diseases (hemolytic diseases, malignant
    hyperexia, jaundice, porphyria, glaucoma, hyper-
    uricemia)
Diet
Environmental Chemicals
Drug Interactions
Age (Infants, Elderly)

drug reaching the desired site of action. Altered drug disposition has been observed primarily in congestive heart failure or liver or renal failure. The explanation for these organs being primarily involved resides in the fact that they are major organs in drug distribution (heart) and metabolism and excretion (liver, kidneys). Pathophysiological states such as hypoxemia and acidosis have also been associated with alterations in drug disposition.[2] Although it is reasonable to generalize that organ failure can be expected to alter the disposition of drugs, organ failure is not the major or only contributor to qualitative or quantitative variability in drug actions. Individual variation in response to drugs continues to be a major factor that is not explained by disease or organ failure. Nevertheless, it is important to anticipate influences of organ failure on drug effects when the drugs used are known to have altered disposition with altered state(s) of organ function.

Hepatic Disease. The liver is the major site for drug metabolism. Although the majority of therapeutic drugs undergo some form of biotransformation prior to elimination from the body, administration of such drugs to patients with hepatic disease is not associated with a high incidence of unusual drug effect. Actual studies of the influence of hepatic disease on drug disposition have produced conflicting results, prompting some investigators to conclude that it is often difficult to predict, in a given patient with hepatic impairment, whether the effect of the drug will be retarded, unchanged, or increased.[3] There are drugs known to be subject to high hepatic extraction (**first-pass effect**), particularly following oral administration. Changes in hepatic blood flow (e.g., in those with liver disease, congestive heart failure) may substantially change the clearance of such drugs, resulting in increased availability. In these situations, reduction of the initial and subsequent doses may be necessary. Determination of serum drug concentration would be particularly helpful in individualizing drug dosage in these patients. Table 2–3 summarizes drug kinetics reported to be influenced by liver disease.

Protein binding of drugs is an important ingredient in drug distribution from the site(s) of absorption to the site(s) of action. Thus, the effect of liver disease can extend beyond modification of drug metabolism or clearance. The liver is the major organ for synthesis of circulating proteins involved in drug binding (albumin, α_1-globulin). For drugs greater than 90 percent protein-bound, significant changes in pharmacokinetics, particularly in volume of distribution, can occur as a result of changes in protein-binding.[4] A reduction in the amount of drug-binding capability can result in greater quantities of the drug reaching extravascular sites. Greater concentrations of drug may therefore occur at sites of effect, which may not be reflected in measurements of drug concentrations in plasma. Thus, there can be a shift in the relationship between plasma drug concentration and therapeutic and/or toxic effect(s) of the drug. Changes in pharmacodynamics may also occur secondary to liver disease. An increased sensitivity to drugs active in the CNS has been observed in adults with chronic **liver disease**.[5]

Table 2–3. EFFECTS OF HEPATIC DYSFUNCTION ON PLASMA CLEARANCE OF COMMONLY USED DRUGS

Drug	Hepatic Dysfunction*		
	Cirrhosis	Acute Viral Hepatitis	Obstructive Jaundice
Amobarbital	↓		
Ampicillin	↓ or 0		
Antipyrine	↓	↓	↓
Chloramphenicol	↓ or 0		
Clindamycin	↓		
Diazepam	↓	↓	
Digoxin	0	↑	
Heparin	↓		
Hexobarbital		↓	
Isoniazid	↓		
Lidocaine	↓	0	
Meperidine	↓	↓	
Pentobarbital	↓		
Phenobarbital	↓	↓ or 0	
Phenytoin		0	
Prednisolone	0		
Propranolol	0		
Theophylline	↓		
Tolbutamide		↑	
Warfarin		0	

Plasma clearance: ↑ = increased; ↓ = decreased; 0 = no change.

*Hepatic dysfunction includes a diverse group of clinical conditions such as hepatitis (acute) and cirrhosis (chronic).

From Roberts, RJ: Drug Therapy in Infants: Pharmacologic Principles and Clinical Experience. WB Saunders, Philadelphia, 1984, with permission.

It has been difficult to formulate general guidelines for the employment of drugs in patients with hepatic disease because liver disease itself is complex in etiology and pathophysiology. Liver disease can affect not only drug metabolism, excretion, and drug protein-binding but also tissue distribution and receptor responsiveness. In general, even with severe hepatic dysfunction, alterations in drug disposition beyond twofold to threefold are unlikely.[6] It is reasonable, in patients with serious liver dysfunction, to use drugs whenever possible that are eliminated by extrahepatic mechanisms with therapeutic activity unaffected by liver disease and not known to produce a pattern of toxicity themselves. In the absence of information on the use of a specific drug in hepatic failure, cautious and individualized therapy based on the known pharmacologic features of the drug and careful clinical observations of parameters of therapeutic effect are reasonable guidelines.

Renal Failure. The **duration** and **intensity** of pharmacological effect of many drugs can be associated with the status of kidney function. This association is a consequence of the major role of the kidneys in elimination of a large number of drugs and their metabolites from the body. In contrast to the liver, a number of very sensitive clinical laboratory tests are available for identification, characterization, and quantification of renal dysfunction. For drugs such as **digoxin** and the **aminoglycosides,** elimination depends almost entirely upon the kidneys; therefore, an estimation of the glomerular filtration rate (GFR) can accurately reflect the dosing requirements for these drugs under a variety of clinical situations of renal dysfunction. For example, if kidney function is 50 percent of normal, then the dosage requirements—dose or dosage interval or both—will be reduced comparably. In situations of rapidly changing renal function, including acute tubular necrosis and glomerular filtration, the onset of changes in BUN or creatinine clearance (indicator of GFR) may be significantly delayed or disproportionate to the effects on drug elimination. Some drugs do not depend at all on renal function for elimination; still others depend on both renal and nonrenal routes.

Renal failure can have a variety of influences on drug kinetics and dynamics similar to hepatic dysfunction. Renal failure has been reported to secondarily alter nonrenal elimination, protein binding, and volume of distribution of drugs.[7] If a drug is metabolized to a metabolite that is active as a therapeutic or toxic agent, then renal failure can lead to an increase in therapeutic or toxic effects unless the dosage of the parent drug is reduced. Drugs with this potential (e.g., procainamide) are best avoided in renal failure because of the complexity surrounding dosing considerations. Reviews[8] are available on the known influences of renal dysfunction.

Decisions on the need for or extent of dosage adjustment necessary for any given drug depend not only on the degree of renal dysfunction but also on (1) the percentage of drug cleared *via* the kidney; (2) the therapeutic index of the particular drug, especially under conditions of renal dysfunction; and (3) the extent of metabolism of the administered drug, including the pharmacological activity of the metabolite(s). Most penicillins and cephalosporins have wide therapeutic indices, and no dosage adjustment is necessary in cases of mild or moderate renal dysfunction. Table 2–4 represents a selected list of drugs that may require dosage adjustment with severe renal dysfunction. Unfortunately, none of the various nomograms, tables, or computer programs produced to deal with the problem of drug dosage adjustment in renal failure are uniformly successful. Individualized dosage adjustment based on drug blood concentration is the ideal approach in patients with renal dysfunction. This is especially important for drugs with high renal clearance (>90 percent) and for patients who have profound and sudden changes in renal function.

Table 2-4. MAINTENANCE DOSE INTERVALS FOR SELECTED DRUGS USED IN PATIENTS WITH SEVERE RENAL DYSFUNCTION

Drug	Major Route of Elimination	Increase in Dose Interval (Renal Function 10% Normal)
Ampicillin	Renal/hepatic	Unchanged
Caffeine	Renal	×2–?
Corticosteroids	Renal	Unchanged
Diazoxide	Renal	Unchanged
Digoxin	Renal	×2–?
Furosemide	Renal	Unchanged
Gentamicin	Renal	×3–6
Indomethacin	Hepatic/renal	Unchanged
Methicillin	Renal/hepatic	×1–2
Penicillin	Renal/hepatic	Unchanged
Phenobarbital	Hepatic/renal	×1–2
Phenothiazines	Hepatic/renal	×2–3
Procainamide	Renal	×2–3
Thiazides	Renal	Avoid use
Tubocurarine	Renal	Unchanged
Vancomycin	Renal	×10–20

Adapted from Roberts, RJ: Drug Therapy in Infants: Pharmacologic Principles and Clinical Experience. WB Saunders, Philadelphia, 1984.

Caution in the use of these techniques is required because the following assumptions are made in cases of renal failure: no change in drug availability, no active or toxic metabolites formed, no change in ability to metabolize the drug, no concentration-dependent kinetics, and no change in other aspects of drug disposition or dynamics.

Cardiac, Pulmonary, and CNS Disease and Trauma. Various other disease states have been associated with alterations in drug effects. **Cardiac function,** primarily cardiac output, is the basic means for drug movement from one site to another in the body. Cardiac insufficiency will disrupt the transport of not only critical nutrients including oxygen but also drugs. Slower rates of drug delivery or differences in absolute amounts of drug getting to sites of effect can change the expected relationships between drug dose and response or effect. For example, the amount of digoxin required for optimal effect may be influenced by the existing cardiac dysfunction. This may require that greater doses be given early in the course of therapy and lesser doses later when cardiac output has improved. **Pulmonary disease,** particularly that leading to hypoxemia, can be associated with changes in renal perfusion and thus clearance of drugs. Hepatic drug metabolism has also been shown to be influenced by hypoxemic states. Severe trauma such as that associated with major burns or accidents or with severe CNS abnormalities can alter hepatic drug metabolism and receptor response to drugs.

Adjustments in Dosage in Disease States. Regardless of the drug or causative situation involved, there are three adjustments in dosage possible: (1) alteration of the **dosing interval**, (2) alteration of the **maintenance dose,** or (3) change in both dosing interval and maintenance dose. When both dosing interval and maintenance dose are altered, some proportion of the usual maintenance dose (typically one-half) is administered at a dosing interval equal to the drug half-life in the patient.[9] Determination of which of the three possible dosage adjustments is best requires an appreciation of the likely drug plasma disappearance versus time curve resulting from each manipulation and a knowledge of the ideal peak and trough levels (**therapeutic window**) for the drug being given. Because diffusion of drug from one site or compartment in the body to another depends not simply on the drug concentration gradient but also on time or duration of that concentration difference, changes in dosage can significantly alter the usual relationships between plasma drug concentration and drug effect. The following information is needed to establish an ideal dosage regimen for a patient with organ failure: (1) the usual dose and dosage interval, (2) estimate of the existing organ dysfunction (percent of normal), (3) estimate of the effect of the existing organ failure on distribution and metabolism of the drug, and (4) percent of the unchanged drug or active metabolite normally eliminated by the organ in question. Changes in drug plasma concentration obviously will depend on the magnitude of the changes made in dose or interval of administration. The majority of published methods for dosage adjustment have as the major objective an average plasma drug level equal to that observed with normal organ function. In general, the **initial or loading dose** of drug should not be altered with organ dysfunction. It is the compromise in elimination from the body of the initial dose and subsequent doses that demands adjustment of the maintenance dosage.

Genetic Disorders

Genetic differences among individuals have been shown to explain a variety of quantitative and qualitative differences in drug response (see Table 2–2).[10] These genetic differences include influences on drug metabolism and receptor response to drugs, particularly toxicity. Some drugs are metabolized by acetylation, including **isoniazid** and **hydralazine.** Liver damage due to isoniazid is more common in rapid acetylators, whereas hydralazine-induced lupus erythematosus occurs almost exclusively in the slow-acetylator phenotype. A number of drugs that produce hemolytic anemia do so in an exaggerated fashion in individuals with inherited red blood cell enzyme deficiencies (**G-6-PD, GSH deficiency**). Individuals with certain **hemoglobinopathies** are more susceptible to oxidation of hemoglobin to methemoglobin by sulfonamides. Individuals with hereditary disorders of porphyrin and heme production show unusual sensitivity for aggravation of the disease state by barbiturates, sulfonamides, and estrogen-containing oral contraceptives. Genetically linked hyperbilirubinemia can produce slower elimination of drugs that undergo glucuronidation prior to elimination (**Crigler-Najjar syndrome**), or aggravation of their jaundice condition with the administration of oral contraceptives (**Dubin-Johnson syndrome**). Malignant hyperpyrexia can be precipitated in individuals with a genetically constituted predisposition by general anesthetics and muscle relaxants. **Glaucoma** can be triggered by the application of corticosteroids in individuals with this genetic predisposition. Topically applied mydriatics can also precipitate glaucoma in these individuals.

Diet

Interactions between drugs and nutrients have received increasing attention because of the enormous potential for such an occurrence, considering the frequency of drug use and the number and variety of nutrients involved in routine food consumption. Most **food-drug interactions** that occur are manifest as an alteration in drug disposition. Because the metabolism of drugs involves the utilization of many cofactors, including trace metals and vitamins, there are a variety of possible interactions between unusual dietary programs and drug use. Other causes of food-drug interactions exist that are much more complex in etiology, such as precipitation of hypertensive crises by tyramine-rich foods in individuals treated with monoamine oxidase inhibitor antidepressants.

Environmental Chemicals

Cigarette smoking has been widely appreciated as an inducer of mixed-function hepatic oxidases. This enhancement of drug metabolism has been associated with an increase in dose requirement with **theophylline**. Other **environmental contaminants,** including pesticides, have been associated with an alteration in drug biotransformation leading to alterations in therapeutic efficacy (e.g., oral anticoagulants).

Drug Interactions

Drug interactions are well known to affect drug pharmacokinetics and dynamics. This topic is discussed in detail in Chapter 3.

Age

Disposition of certain drugs changes dramatically throughout life.[11] Age groups in which there are notable changes include the young infant and the elderly. For example, **phenytoin metabolism** changes dramatically in the first few weeks of life—slow then rapid—then slows again and becomes rather constant for many years before again slowing in the elderly. Similar observations have been made for **phenobarbital**. Changes in metabolism of phenytoin and phenobarbital have been proposed as a mechanism for changes in dose requirements for maintenance of therapeutic efficacy. Renal function under-

Table 2–5. AGE-RELATED CHANGES IN DRUG DISPOSITION

Disposition	Age-Related Change (Newborn to Adult)	Possible Effect on Drug Disposition
Absorption	Change in intestinal absorptive surface area ($\uparrow$), splanchnic blood flow ($\uparrow$), gastric pH ($\uparrow$ acidity), and intestinal motility ($\uparrow$)	Increase in drug absorption (rate and extent) anticipated with all ($\uparrow$) with possible exception of pH which may affect the ionization status of certain drugs ($\uparrow$ ionization generally $\downarrow$ drug absorption)
Distribution	Change in body mass ($\uparrow$), tissue composition (fat, protein, CHO—fluctuate in percentage of total body weight, particularly during the first 20 years of life), % body water (in aged) ($\downarrow$), serum and tissue protein drug-binding ($\downarrow$ or $\uparrow$)	The distribution of drugs with large V_d (>1 l/kg) or high plasma protein binding (>95%) will be influenced by age related $\uparrow$ or $\downarrow$ in these parameters. Reduced plasma protein binding can result in increased drug distribution ($\uparrow V_d$). Increase in mass of adipose tissue mainly $\uparrow$ the V_d of lipophilic drugs
Metabolism	Change in proportion of organ to body mass, specifically in liver mass ($\downarrow$) and organ blood flow ($\uparrow$ or $\downarrow$); change in drug metabolizing enzyme activity ($\uparrow$ or $\downarrow$) and inducibility	Increase in drug metabolism or organ blood flow will generally increase the rate or quantity of drug eliminated from the body assuming the drug is metabolized and/or excreted by the organ undergoing changes
Excretion	Change in renal function (blood flow, glomerular filtration rate, and secretory function all increase)	Increases in renal function will generally increase the rate or quantity of drug eliminated from the body assuming the drug is handled by the kidney
Drug Receptor Response	Increases and decreases in receptor number, affinity, and response, which are both organ and tissue specific and age dependent	Increases in receptor number and/or affinity will generally be associated with $\uparrow$ drug response or effect

goes significant maturation in the first 12 months of life. Drugs that are predominantly cleared by renal mechanisms are therefore susceptible to influences of renal maturation (e.g., aminoglycosides). Individuals beyond 60 years of age have a progressive reduction in tissue mass as well as renal, hepatic, and cardiovascular function. Volume of distribution, half-life, systemic clearance, and receptor sensitivity have been shown to change with increases in age.[11] Table 2–5 outlines the general aspects of drug dispositon that are known to have age-related changes that affect drug action. Safe and more effective drug therapy in pediatric and elderly patients will depend on future research efforts in these age groups.

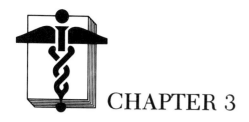

CHAPTER 3

Adverse Drug Reactions and Interactions

REYNOLD SPECTOR, M.D.

Three serious problems with **drug therapy** are apparent even when current drug therapy is optimally used. First, for many diseases there is no therapy. Second, many effective therapies, even when properly used, have significant adverse effects. Third, for many therapies there is very substantial interindividual and intraindividual variability in drug blood levels or response to a standard dose of a particular drug. The focus of this chapter is on the second problem. The various types of **adverse drug reactions** (ADR) and **adverse drug interactions** (ADI) will be defined and classified, and examples will be discussed. The chapter will also review how ADR and ADI are assessed in populations and in individuals.

ADR are frequent causes of hospitalization and also of serious iatrogenic morbidity in hospitalized patients. In outpatients, the magnitude of the problem of ADR is not clear. For example, a recent study[12] showed that 36 percent of patients on a general internal medicine service in a university hospital developed iatrogenic problems. ADR were a common form of these iatrogenic problems. In 9 percent of these patients, the adverse reaction threatened life or actually created disability. In 2 percent of these patients, the adverse reaction contributed to the patient's demise. What is clear from other studies is that the more drugs an individual receives, the more likely ADR or ADI are to occur. In the past, the evaluation and recognition of ADR and ADI have been difficult. This is due to many factors. For example, in some cases, a drug used to treat a clinical condition can actually cause the condition (e.g., antiarrhythmic drugs frequently cause arrhythmias). It is obvious that such occurrences greatly complicate the evaluation of ADR and cause clinical havoc.

ADVERSE DRUG REACTIONS

Definition

Throughout the literature, there are two general definitions of ADR. The first definition, the broad definition, states that an ADR is any type of unwanted consequence of drug use. Hence, such a definition would include drug overdose, drug abuse, medication errors (e.g., giving the wrong drug to the patient), or problems with medication bioavailability. Because of the extremely broad nature of this definition, however, it is not operationally useful. For example, if the wrong patient got a dose of insulin and became hypoglycemic, this episode would perhaps be best classified as a medication error. A better and less inclusive definition is that of the World Health Organization: An ADR is one that is "noxious and unintended and occurs at doses used in man for prophylaxis, diagnosis, therapy or modification of physiological functions."[13] This definition, which excludes many types of untoward reactions, including medication errors and purposeful overdoses, will be employed throughout this chapter unless otherwise stated.

Classification

The classification of ADR by general mechanisms is shown in Table 3–1.[14] **Pharmacological or toxic reactions** to drugs sometimes occur when stan-

**Table 3–1. TYPES OF ADVERSE
DRUG REACTIONS (ADR)**

Pharmacologic (or toxic)
Idiosyncratic
Allergic
Drug interactions
Miscellaneous including overdoses, drug abuse, medi-
cation errors, and bioavailability problems (see broad
definition of ADR in text)

dard doses of common drugs are employed. Frequently, such reactions may
be expected from the known pharmacologic or toxicologic properties of the
drug. For example, patients with renal or hepatic failure or at the extremes
of age may be unable to metabolize or excrete standard doses of common
drugs properly. Other patients may be slower metabolizers of such drugs.
Hence, these patients, although they may receive standard doses, may sustain
pharmacologic or toxic reactions. Frequently, such adverse reactions can be
anticipated (e.g., if renal function is known to be impaired) and the dose of
the drug decreased to avoid a toxic reaction (e.g., with gentamicin). Examples
of diseases that may promote pharmacological and toxic adverse drug reactions
are shown in Table 3–2.

So-called **idiosyncratic reactions** are a second type of ADR. These reactions occur infrequently and may be due either to quantitatively or qualitatively abnormal responses to drugs after average doses. In some cases, these
abnormal responses are due to genetic differences in the patients. Most reactions of this type are not understood. However, with time and increasing
knowledge, the number of idiosyncratic drug reactions is decreasing. Examples of idiosyncratic reactions due to both pharmacokinetic and pharmacodynamic causes are shown in Table 3–3. Prolonged paralysis due to
succinylcholine is caused by slow metabolism of the drug because of a deficiency of the hydrolyzing enzyme pseudocholinesterase.

By definition, **allergic reactions** are due to activation of some portion of
the immune system. A general (clinical) classification of allergic drug reactions
is shown in Table 3–4.

In general, ADR due to adverse **drug interactions** are less common clinical problems. ADI are clinical (pharmacologic) adverse responses that cannot
be explained by a single drug, but in fact are due to two or more drugs inter-
acting simultaneously in an adverse fashion. For example, drugs may interact
to alter plasma protein binding of each other and hence cause increased pharmacologic actions (e.g., many drugs interact with warfarin and cause bleed-

Table 3–2. DISEASES THAT MAY PROMOTE PHARMACOLOGICAL AND TOXIC ADVERSE DRUG REACTIONS—SELECTED EXAMPLES

Disease	Drug or Class of Drugs	Adverse Effects	Probable Mechanism
Renal Failure	Aminoglycoside antibiotics	Further renal damage and ototoxicity	Impaired drug and/or metabolite excretion
	Digoxin	Digitalis toxicity	
Liver Disease	Narcotics and sedative/hypnotics	Excess sedation and coma	Decreased drug metabolism and/or increased brain sensitivity
	Lidocaine	Seizures	
	Theophylline	Seizures	
Heart Disease	β-blockers	Precipitate or worsen heart failure	Decreased cardiac reserve
	Lidocaine	Seizures	Decreased metabolism
	Theophylline	Seizures	
Hypertension	Vasoconstrictors, e.g., phenylethanolamine	Raise blood pressure	Direct action on arterioles
Epilepsy	Phenothiazines	Increase seizures	Lower seizure threshold
Asthma	β-blockers	Asthmatic attack	Block adrenergic bronchorelaxing input

ing). Perhaps from 5 to 10 percent of all moderate or serious ADR are due to drug interactions, which are discussed later in this chapter.

The final type of ADR by the broad definition includes those due to **overdoses, drug abuse, medication errors,** and **bioavailability problems**. In many cases, these problems are caused by physicians, nurses, pharmacists, or the patient.

Assessment of Adverse Drug Reactions in Populations

It is frequently difficult to be certain that ADR are in fact real. Six approaches have been used to identify and quantify ADR in populations.[14] First, ADR are carefully monitored in initial drug trials. Second, the United States Food and Drug Administration (FDA) and pharmaceutical industry encourage voluntary reporting of ADR by physicians and other health care professionals.

Table 3–3. IDIOSYNCRATIC (GENETIC) ADVERSE DRUG REACTIONS

Pharmacokinetic Examples (Slow Metabolism)		
Drug	**Indications**	**Adverse Reaction**
Succinylcholine	Inducing muscle paralysis for surgery	Prolonged paralysis and apnea
Procainamide	Arrhythmias	Increased incidence of lupus–like syndrome
Isoniazid	Tuberculosis	Increased incidence of peripheral neuropathy

Pharmacodynamic Examples		
Drug	**Mechanism**	**Adverse Reaction**
"Oxidant" drugs, e.g., primaquine, nitrofurans, dapsone, quinine	Glucose-6-phosphate dehydrogenase deficiency	Hemolysis
Barbiturates, griseofulvin, sulfonylurea hypoglycemics	Induce aminolevulinic acid synthetase	Porphyria

Third, there has been intensive prospective monitoring of selected patients on inpatient wards. Fourth, epidemiological studies including inspection of national statistics have occasionally yielded important information about ADR. Fifth, case-control and cross-sectional studies have frequently been performed. Finally, animal toxicological studies have been helpful in assessing and predicting ADR in humans.

Table 3–4. CLASSIFICATION OF ALLERGIC DRUG REACTIONS

Anaphylaxis
Serum sickness
Tissue reactions
Skin reactions
Fever
Combination syndromes

Drug Trials

Before a new drug can be released for use by the general population, the FDA demands that the drug be carefully scrutinized for both suspected and unsuspected ADR.[14] These trials, often including thousands of patients, are frequently placebo-controlled. Hence, it is possible to make a prospective comparison with placebo-treated patients in many cases. The drug companies frequently seek both expected and previously unreported side effects. Therefore, especially if there is a hypothesis in advance about potential ADR, proper statistical analyses (taking into account multiple comparisons) can be made. Hence, in many cases, most if not all of the potential ADR and their frequencies are obtained before a drug can be released for general use. However, very rare ADR may not appear until the drug has been released for general use.

Voluntary Reporting of Adverse Drug Reactions

Physicians are strongly encouraged by both the drug companies and the FDA to report ADR. The FDA has a special form for this, and the information is held in confidence. Of course, one of the difficulties with this system is that ADR reporting is spotty. However, voluntary reporting has been a very useful method of assessing new ADR.

Drug Surveillance on Inpatient Units

Over the last 20 years, several valuable drug surveillance programs have been initiated. The most comprehensive of these programs is the Boston Collaborative Drug Surveillance Program, which monitors hospital wards in the United States and Europe.[15] In these programs, specially trained monitors are designated to follow prospectively all patients admitted to certain wards with regard to their history, drug exposure, side effects of drugs, efficacy of treatment, and many types of auxiliary data. These monitoring systems have yielded very important pieces of new data about ADR, much of which has been published. These publications are extremely useful in assessing ADR in hospitalized patients. However, such patients appear to have a much higher frequency of ADR than outpatients, and extrapolations to outpatients must be made with extreme caution.

National and International Statistics

In a few cases, data collected from national statistics have been very useful in suggesting the occurrence of new and serious ADR. For example, the sudden increase in a certain type of congenital limb disorder (phocomelia) caused an astute investigator to wonder if a new toxin had been added to the environment. Ultimately, this hypothesis led to the identification of the drug thalidomide as the toxin. When it was withdrawn, the incidence of phocomelia rapidly decreased.

Case-Control and Cross-Sectional Studies

Certain types of epidemiological studies including case-control and cross-sectional studies are frequently useful in assessing adverse drug reactions. In this approach, in general, the group of cases and controls (chosen scientifically) are investigated to see if antecedent drug usage can be implicated as the cause of the ADR. However, because these studies are retrospective, although frequently controlled, it is extremely important to avoid bias. Such studies have led to important suggestions of causal relationships (although case-control and cross-sectional studies can never establish causality). For example, the postulated causal relationship between the use of stilbestrol in women and vaginal carcinoma is an example of the successful use of these epidemiological methods.[14] Unfortunately, there have been many false-positive case-control studies that have wreaked substantial havoc. For example, reserpine, a very useful drug in the treatment of hypertension, was implicated in 1974 as being associated with cancer of the breast in women.[14, 16] However, subsequent careful study did not confirm these results.[16] The initial findings caused great anxiety in many patients and their physicians. Many women, whose blood pressure was successfully controlled on this rather safe, effective, and inexpensive medication, were withdrawn from reserpine because of, as it turned out, false concerns about induction of breast cancer. Hence, retrospective studies must be viewed with some caution. Controlled prospective studies when properly performed are almost always more useful.

Toxicological Studies

Toxicological studies in many cases have been useful predictors of certain types of ADR. For many drugs, particularly those that are nonmetabolized and excreted by the kidney, toxicological studies in animals are useful predictors of human toxicity. Of course, only studies in humans are definitive, however.

Assessment of Adverse Drug Reactions in an Individual Patient

In the last decade, methods have been developed to try to assess, in a standardized fashion, ADR. As noted previously, an ADR is one that is "noxious and unintended and occurs at doses used in man for prophylaxis, diagnosis, therapy or modification of physiological functions."[13] Hence, an ADR may be a symptom, a sign, an abnormal laboratory test, or even a fatal outcome.

There are a few so-called **pathognomonic ADR**. Some examples are shown in Table 3–5. When these occur, particularly with the corroborating evidence described in the table, arguments about cause of the ADR are generally straightforward. However, in the majority of cases, the assessment of causality is difficult.[13, 14] Therefore, a large number of investigators, both within and outside the pharmaceutical industry, have attempted to arrive at a consensus that a "standardized assessment of causality (SAC) of putative adverse drug reactions" is possible and desirable.[13, 17–19] Several SAC algorithms have been developed to attempt to assess adverse drug reactions.[13, 17–19] In general, the utility of these algorithms is based on an operational approach. When two assessors arrive at the same evaluation of causality using the same SAC algorithm and the same data, the causality is assumed to be correct. In many cases, it is not possible by rigorous inductive standards of causality to "prove" that the SAC assessment is correct. Rather, the operational definition of utility given above is employed.[13, 14]

An example of a SAC algorithm taken from *The Scientific Basis of Clinical Pharmacology: Principles and Examples* is shown in Table 3–6.[14] Proper use of this table depends on access to comprehensive textbooks of pharmacology

Table 3–5. EXAMPLES OF "PATHOGNOMONIC" ADVERSE DRUG REACTIONS

Drug	Adverse Reaction	Corroborating Evidence
Nonsteroidal anti-inflammatory drugs (NSAID), e.g., aspirin, naproxen, tolmetin, sulindac, ibuprofen	Asthma in a NSAID-sensitive patient	Rechallenge
Ergot	Ergotism (cyanosis, gangrene of extremities)	
Chloramphenicol	Gray syndrome	Elevated plasma drug levels
Warfarin	Bleeding	Prothrombin time
Chloroquine	Retinitis	Ophthalmological examination
Phenothiazines	Extrapyramidal syndromes	In some cases, rapid reversal with diphenhydramine
Hydralazine, procainamide	Lupus-like syndrome	
Diuretics (thiazides, furosemide)	Low serum K^+	
Tablets injected intravenously	Talc or silica lung	

Table 3–6. STANDARDIZED ADVERSE DRUG REACTION (ADR) ASSESSMENT (SAC) ALGORITHM*

	Yes	No
A) Documentation of ADR		
1) Is clinical history and/or laboratory tests convincing?	(Proceed)	(Stop)
2) Did the patient receive the suspected drug?	(Proceed)	(Stop)
B) History of Current ADR		
3) Was therapeutic dose exceeded?	(Stop)	(Proceed)
4) Was the drug given prior to ADR?	(Proceed)	(Stop)
5) If drug blood levels were measured, were they consistent with the ADR?	(+2)	(−4)
6) Was there other drug therapy prior to ADR?	(−1)	(+1)
7) Was the ADR a local reaction?	(+5)	(0)
8) Was the time interval after the ADR compatible with the ADR?	(+2)	(−3)
9) Was the onset of the ADR acute, i.e., immediately after the drug was given?	(+5)	(0)
10) Was a rechallenge positive?	(+7)	(−4)
11) Was dechallenge positive?	(+3)	(−2)
12) Were other drugs (if given) stopped at the same time?	(−1)	(0)
C) Patient's Past History of ADR		
13) Did the patient have the ADR before?	(+4)	(−1)
14) Did the patient have similar symptoms not related to drugs before?	(−1)	(+1)
15) Did the patient have the same ADR with other drugs?	(+1)	(0)
D) Literature About Suspected Drug		
16) Does the ADR-like event occur spontaneously?	(−1)	(+1)
17) Does the ADR-like event occur with the disease (or syndrome) being treated?	(−2)	(+1)
18) Are there contributory factors, e.g., other diseases, non-drug therapy, habits, environment?	(−1)	(+1)
19) Does the suspected drug cause this ADR?	(+3)	(−1)

Causality Assessment

Definite	>22
Probable	16–21
Possible	10–15
Unlikely	0–9
Unrelated	<0

*Questions that cannot be answered should be given a zero.

From Spector, R (ed): The Scientific Basis of Clinical Pharmacology: Principles and Examples. Little, Brown, & Co, Boston, 1986, with permission.

and clinical pharmacology that thoughtfully assess adverse drug reactions. There are several excellent source books.[15, 16, 20, 21]

The SAC algorithm shown in Table 3–6 is basically a series of questions with appropriate point scores associated with each question. Questions that cannot be answered are given a zero. At the end of the algorithm, a causality assessment is made by calculating the number of points. An ADR is then considered to be definite, probable, possible, unlikely, or unrelated, depending upon the point score.

Questions 1, 2, 3, and 4 of Table 3–6 deal with whether the history was convincing, whether the patient received the suspected drug in a standard dose, and whether the drug was given prior to the adverse drug reaction. Of course, if the patient received an overdose, the ADR is really an overdose and does not fit into the narrow definition of an ADR referred to earlier.

Question 5 deals with the issue of whether blood levels were measured. If they were, were they consistent with the adverse drug reaction? Suppose a patient was thought to have an ADR to lidocaine. However, if the blood concentration of lidocaine was subtherapeutic, this would argue against an ADR to lidocaine.

Question 6 suggests that if there was other drug therapy prior to the ADR, then that may confuse the issue. Of course, question 7 suggests that if the ADR was a local reaction (e.g., at an intramuscular injection site), the ADR is quite likely to be due to the injection. Question 8 depends upon knowledge of the time course of the ADR with the suspected drug.[15, 16, 20, 21] Question 9 deals with the issue of the acuteness of the ADR. For example, five to 10 minutes after an injection of penicillin, if an anaphylactic ADR occurred, this would be strong presumptive evidence for the ADR being caused by the penicillin.

Question 10 deals with the rechallenge. By definition, a rechallenge is giving the patient a drug after the patient has been off that drug for a period of time. This can be done only if rechallenging the patient is necessary for the patient's clinical care. It is not proper to risk a rechallenge in a patient for academic reasons. Frequently, in a patient with a putative ADR there are alternative drugs that may be used. For example, if a patient is allergic to ethacrynic acid, a structurally dissimilar but equally effective drug, furosemide, is available.

Question 11 deals with dechallenge, which means that when the drug was stopped, the ADR disappeared. Of course, if other drugs were stopped at the same time, this confuses the issue (question 12). Questions 13, 14, and 15 deal with the patient's past history of the ADR. If the patient had the ADR or similar symptoms before, this may clarify or confuse the assessment of the ADR substantially.

Finally, and very importantly, proper review of the literature about the suspected drug is crucial in order to answer properly questions 16, 17, 18, and 19. With the references described earlier, it is generally possible to discover the answers to questions 16 through 19.

An example of the application of the SAC algorithm follows:

> The patient, a 58-year-old man with a recent myocardial infarction, was treated prophylactically with lidocaine intravenously. The patient received two bolus doses of 50 mg each at 0 and 5 minutes, and then an infusion of 4 mg per minute. Thirty minutes after the lidocaine infusion was begun the patient suffered a grand mal seizure. The blood concentration at that point was 8 µg per ml (the therapeutic range is 1 to 5 µg per ml). The infusion was stopped and the patient had no more seizures. Application of the SAC system in Table 3–6 to this patient suggests that questions 5, 8, 9, 11, and 19 should be answered "yes." Question 10 cannot be answered, and all the remaining questions are answered "no." The total score equals + 19 (probable). The SAC system, as this case shows, yields a "probable" but not a "definite" assessment. Only a rechallenge would make the assessment "definite," but, of course, in this particular case a rechallenge is not indicated.

Clinically, if a SAC is "probable" or "definite," the drug should usually be stopped.[14] In other cases, a careful assessment of the risks and benefits must be made, depending upon the clinical circumstances, to determine whether to continue the drug.

Examples of Adverse Effects of Drugs

In this section, examples of adverse effects of drugs by organ systems are presented. The data are fairly convincing in terms of causal relationships, and specific details can be found in standard references.[14–16, 20, 21] Important ADR will be emphasized—that is, those that occur frequently or, if infrequently, are especially severe.

ADR due to excipients (pharmaceutical additives) in drug products are fairly infrequent but may be extremely difficult to detect, as the excipients in certain formulations are not explicitly stated. Examples of excipient syndromes are shown in Table 3–7. Propylene glycol is used as a preservative and vehicle for both oral and parenteral drugs; it is metabolized to lactic acid.

Table 3–7. EXCIPIENT SYNDROMES

Syndrome	Agent	Predisposing Factors or Disease
Bronchospasm	Sodium metabisulfite	Asthma
Phenytoin toxicity	Phenytoin	Change in formulation
Myocardial depression–acute heart failure	Propylene glycol	—
Urticaria, asthma	Tartrazine	Aspirin sensitivity
Metabolic acidosis	Propylene glycol	—

Table 3–8. WITHDRAWAL SYNDROMES

Syndrome	Agent(s) Withdrawn
Central nervous system signs with agitation, confusion, delirium, seizures, and coma	Depressants, e.g., alcohol, barbiturates, and, to a lesser extent, benzodiazepines
Addisonian crisis (acute adrenal insufficiency)	Corticosteroids, e.g., cortisone, prednisone
Opioid withdrawal syndrome	Opioids (e.g., morphine, codeine, heroin), and opiate-like drugs (e.g., pentazocine, propoxyphene)
Headache	Caffeine, clonidine, ergot alkaloids, methysergide

In certain hospitalized patients, the amount of propylene glycol in certain products is sufficient to cause lactate acidosis.[22]

Many patients may suffer withdrawal symptoms when certain drugs are withdrawn. Shown in Table 3–8 are several very common withdrawal syndromes. For example, patients who chronically take barbiturates (e.g., more than 0.4 to 0.6 grams per day of secobarbital or pentobarbital) may undergo a withdrawal syndrome (e.g., seizures and delirium) if the drugs are suddenly stopped. Similarly, in patients who drink enough caffeine (e.g., eight or more cups of coffee a day, each containing approximately 100 mg of caffeine), withdrawal headache may occur when the patient abruptly stops drinking coffee. The mechanism is probably cerebral vasodilation following prolonged caffeine-induced vasoconstriction.

Many drugs have been associated with teratogenic characteristics in humans. Well-documented examples are shown in Table 3–9. In most cases the mechanism is not known.

Table 3–9. TERATOGENIC DRUGS

Syndrome	Agents
Fetal malformations	Antineoplastic drugs, e.g., methotrexate, aminopterin, cyclophosphamide
Phocomelia	Thalidomide
Virilizing effects and other congenital defects	Androgenic steroids
Adenocarcinoma of vagina	Diethylstilbesterol
Fetal warfarin syndrome	Warfarin
Fetal alcohol syndrome	Ethanol

Drugs can cause or simulate many of the disease-induced syndromes seen in humans. For example, in the cardiovascular system it is ironic that many of the drugs used to treat cardiac disorders can, in fact, cause significant and life-threatening cardiovascular syndromes. Other organ systems are also occasionally compromised by cardiovascular drugs. Examples are shown in Table 3–10. Many of these syndromes are recognized only if there is a high index of suspicion. In most cases these syndromes disappear when the drug is stopped. An example is the complication called torsade de pointes, which is a type of atypical ventricular tachycardia in which the QRS baseline undulates.[14] This syndrome can be caused by many cardiac drugs (see Table 3–10). Torsade de pointes should not be treated in the same way as idiopathic ventricular fibrillation, but rather requires treatment with isoproterenol and pacing for successful maintenance of cardiac output while the patient metabolizes the drug.

A series of respiratory syndromes due to drugs is shown in Table 3–11. Many of these syndromes are well described and can be expected in certain patients. For example, in hospitalized patients, approximately 1 percent of patients who receive opioid analgesics suffer significant respiratory depression at

Table 3–10. CARDIOVASCULAR SYNDROMES

Syndrome	Agents
Arrhythmias	
Ventricular tachycardia and fibrillation, and/or torsade de pointes	Digitalis,* quinidine, procainamide, intravenous contrast agents, sympatheticomimetic drugs
Bradycardia	Digitalis,* β-blockers
Heart block	Digitalis,* β-blockers
Supraventricular tachycardia	Digitalis,* antidepressants, hydralazine
Depression of cardiac output	β-blockers, quinidine, procainamide, disopyramide, alcohol, verapamil
Cardiac damage	Alcohol, emetine, daunorubicin, doxorubicin
Cardiac ischemia	Birth control pills (rare), ergot alkaloids, aspirin
Hypertension	Phenylpropanolamine and other sympatheticomimetics; withdrawal of antihypertensives (e.g., clonidine), birth control pills
Hypotension	Antihypertensive drugs, tricyclic antidepressants, nitrates
Peripheral vasoconstriction	Ergot alkaloids, dopamine, β-blockers
Thromboembolism	Oral contraceptives

*Approximately 9% of hospitalized patients suffer significant electrical cardiac toxicity (arrhythmias or heart block) from digitalis; in 2%, the toxicity is life threatening.

Table 3–11. RESPIRATORY SYNDROMES

Syndrome	Agents
Respiratory depression	Narcotics, barbiturates, anesthetics; drugs that cause muscle weakness
Bronchospasm	
Allergic and/or chemical	Penicillin, aspirin, morphine, excipients (e.g., tartrazine)
Receptor agonists and antagonists	β-blockers; cholinergic drugs
Pulmonary edema	Salicylates, opioids, β-blockers and other drugs that cause myocardial depression
Pneumonitis	
Lupus-type	Procainamide, hydralazine
Diffuse	Sulfonamides, nitrofurantoin
Pulmonary fibrosis	Nitrofurantoin, antineoplastic drugs (e.g., busulfan, bleomycin)
Pulmonary granulomatosis	Pentazocine (after intravenous injection of tablets)

standard doses of these drugs. In many respiratory syndromes, the mechanism of the toxicity is unclear; however, in some cases, the mechanism is apparent. For example, bleomycin is toxic to the lung because the degrading enzyme is present in the lung at very low concentrations.

Gastrointestinal and hepatic syndromes due to drugs are shown in Tables 3–12 and 3–13. Hepatic syndromes, especially with elevation of serum en-

Table 3–12. GASTROINTESTINAL SYNDROMES

Syndrome	Agents
Esophageal ulceration	Doxycycline, tetracycline, ferrous salts
Nausea/vomiting	Digitalis, opioids (e.g., morphine), estrogens, levodopa, theophylline, bromocriptine, ferrous sulfate, tetracycline, quinidine
Diarrhea	Antibacterial drugs (e.g., ampicillin), magnesium salts, digitalis, cathartic abuse
Colitis	Antibacterial agents, methyldopa
Constipation	Opioids, anticholinergic drugs, phenothiazines, aluminum hydroxide, ferrous salts
Gastritis and gastric ulcerations	Aspirin, nonsteroidal anti-inflammatory drugs
Pancreatitis	Azathioprine, sulfonamides, methyldopa

Table 3–13. HEPATIC SYNDROMES

Syndrome	Agents
Cholestasis	Anabolic steroids, oral contraceptives
Cholelithiasis	Clofibrate, oral contraceptives
Hepatitis (dose-dependent) that may lead to cirrhosis	Antineoplastic agents (e.g., azathioprine, methotrexate)
Hepatitis (dose-independent)	
Diffuse	Isoniazid, methyldopa, halothane, valproic acid
Cholestatic and mixed	Phenothiazines (e.g., chlorpromazine), nonsteroidal anti-inflammatory drugs, sulfonylureas (e.g., chlorpropamide), rifampicin, sulfonamides
Liver tumors	Synthetic androgens, oral contraceptives

zymes due to diffuse disease, or cholestatic syndromes with elevation of bilirubin and alkaline phosphatase, are commonly seen with use of certain drugs. In some cases (e.g., after halothane or valproic acid), fatal hepatitis has occurred.

Drugs can cause renal damage of various types (Table 3–14). One of the difficult problems with the treatment of serious infections has been renal damage due to aminoglycoside antibiotics and amphotericin, one of the few drugs

Table 3–14. RENAL SYNDROMES

Syndrome	Agents
Acute renal failure	
Urinary obstruction	Anticholinergics; tricyclic antidepressants; methysergide; warfarin, heparin; sulfonamides; drug-induced hemolysis
Vascular occlusion	Thiazide diuretics
Interstitial nephritis	Antibiotics (e.g., methicillin), sulfonamides; nonsteroidal anti-inflammatory agents
Tubular necrosis	Amphotericin, aminoglycoside antibiotics (e.g., gentamicin), furosemide, intravenous contrast agents, *cis*-platinum
Diabetes insipidus–like syndrome	Lithium, methoxyflurane
Nephritis and nephrotic syndrome	Gold salts, penicillamine, captopril
Lupus nephritis	Hydralazine, procainamide

effective against systemic fungal infections. The adverse reactions to these drugs make therapy with these drugs difficult.

Drugs can also cause significant hematological (Table 3–15), endocrine, metabolic, muscle, bone, connective tissue, and, of course, dermatological syndromes (Table 3–16).

In this section, several common drug-produced syndromes (by organ systems) have been discussed. The reader, however, should recognize that this is an extremely incomplete discussion of these syndromes; the examples given are only some of the more common and well documented. The reader needs to review the standard textbooks and literature[14–16, 20, 21] and, if necessary, contact the drug manufacturers for specific questions.

Table 3–15. HEMATOLOGICAL SYNDROMES

Syndrome	Agents
Pancytopenia (aplastic anemia)	Chloramphenicol, phenytoin, trimethadione, phenylbutazone, gold salts, quinacrine, sulfonamides, cytotoxic agents
Agranulocytosis (see also Pancytopenia)	Chloramphenicol, sulfonamides, phenylbutazone, gold salts, indomethacin, propylthiouracil, methimazole, carbimazole, phenothiazines, cytotoxic agents, tolbutamide, trimethoprim-sulfamethoxazole, tricyclic antidepressants, captopril, zidovudine (Azidothymidine, AZT)
Thrombocytopenia (see also Pancytopenia)	Quinidine, quinine, furosemide, chlorthalidone, thiazides, gold salts, trimethoprim-sulfamethoxazole, indomethacin, phenylbutazone, chlorpropamide, phenytoin and other hydantoins, methyldopa, carbamazepine, digitoxin, novobiocin, heparin
Megaloblastic anemia	Folate antagonists (methotrexate, trimethoprim, trimethoprim-sulfamethoxazole), phenytoin, primidone, phenobarbital, triamterene, oral contraceptives, zidovudine (Azidothymidine, AZT)
Hemolytic anemia	Methyldopa, levodopa, mefenamic acid, melphalan, isoniazid, rifampin, sulfonamides, penicillins, cephalosporins, insulin, quinidine, chlorpromazine, para-aminosalicylic acid, dapsone, procainamide
Leukocytosis	Lithium, corticosteroids

Adapted from Braunwald E, et al: Harrison's Principles of Internal Medicine, ed 11. McGraw-Hill, New York, 1987, p 356.

Table 3-16. DERMATOLOGICAL SYNDROMES

Syndrome	Agents
Exfoliative dermatitis (diffuse erythematous rash with scaling)	Penicillins, sulfonamides, barbiturates, phenytoin, phenylbutazone, gold salts, quinidine
Toxic epidermal necrolysis (bullous) (erythema with desquamation of sheets of epidermis, resulting in "scalded" appearance of skin)	Barbiturates, phenylbutazone, phenytoin, sulfonamides, phenolphthalein, penicillins, allopurinol, iodides, bromides, nalidixic acid
Erythema multiforme (symmetric eruption characterized by iris (target, bull's-eye) lesions as well as erythematous macules and papules, purpura, and vesiculobullous lesions); *or* Stevens-Johnson syndrome (severe form of erythema multiforme with involvement of eyes, mucous membranes, and viscera)	Sulfonamides, barbiturates, phenylbutazone, chlorpropamide, thiazides, sulfones, phenytoin, ethosuximide, salicylates, tetracyclines, codeine, penicillins
Erythema nodosum (erythematous tender nodules, usually on anterior surface of lower legs)	Penicillins, sulfonamides, oral contraceptives
Fixed drug eruptions (skin lesions that recur at same site(s) due to drug hypersensitivity)	Phenolphthalein, barbiturates, sulfonamides, salicylates, phenylbutazone, quinine, captopril
Photodermatitis (sunburn or chronic sun-damaged skin in exposed areas due to increased sensitivity to sunlight)	Tetracyclines (particularly demeclocycline), griseofulvin, sulfonamides, sulfonylureas, thiazides, furosemide, phenothiazines, nalidixic acid, oral contraceptives, chlordiazepoxide
Urticaria (hives)	Aspirin, penicillins, sulfonamides, barbiturates
Nonspecific rashes	Ampicillin, barbiturates, allopurinol, phenytoin, methyldopa
Hyperpigmentation	Busulfan, phenothiazines, vitamin A (toxic doses), oral contraceptives, gold salts, chloroquine and other antimalarials, cyclophosphamide, bleomycin
Purpura (see also Table 3–15, thrombocytopenia)	Corticosteroids, aspirin
Contact dermatitis	Topical antimicrobials, topical local anesthetics, topical antihistamines, cream and lotion preservatives, lanolin
Acne	Anabolic and androgenic steroids, corticosteroids, bromides, iodides, oral contraceptives, isoniazid, trimethadione

Adapted from Braunwald E, et al: Harrison's Principles of Internal Medicine, ed 11. McGraw-Hill, New York, 1987, pp 355–356.

ADVERSE DRUG INTERACTIONS

As noted earlier, approximately 5 to 10 percent of ADR in hospitalized patients are due to ADI. Although drug interactions are relatively infrequent causes of significant adverse drug reactions, potentially lethal reactions may occur. For example, drug interactions with anticoagulants, hypoglycemic agents, chemotherapeutic agents, nephrotoxic agents, digitalis glycosides, and others are well known. If anticipated, these adverse interactions are often predictable and preventable.

Classification

A classification of drug interactions by mechanism is shown in Table 3–17.[23, 24] There are three main categories of interactions. First, drugs may interact pharmacokinetically to alter the absorption, distribution and plasma binding, metabolism, or excretion of a second drug. Second, pharmacological interactions may occur at receptors or enzymes involved in the mechanism of action of the drug, or by other pharmacological mechanisms. Finally, there are a series of miscellaneous, but in many cases important, drug interactions. For example, food, especially protein, in the diet may interfere with the absorption of some drugs (e.g., levodopa). This is because levodopa and amino acids are transported by the same transport system in the GI tract.

A large number of factors help determine the severity and occurrence of certain adverse drug interactions. These factors were discussed in Chapter 2

Table 3–17. CLASSIFICATION OF DRUG INTERACTIONS BY MECHANISM

1. Pharmacokinetic Interactions
    A. Absorption
    B. Distribution and plasma binding
    C. Metabolism
    D. Excretion
2. Pharmacological Interactions
    A. Additive or synergistic
    B. Antagonistic
3. Miscellaneous
    A. Pharmaceutical
    B. Other (e.g., food, environmental agents, substances of abuse)
    C. Laboratory tests

(see Table 2–2). For example, if a patient's renal function or hepatic function is markedly altered, the metabolism and/or excretion of certain drugs may be altered in such a way as to increase the chance of ADI. Muscle weakness caused by interaction of aminoglycoside antibiotics and relaxing agents used in surgery (e.g., curare) may be aggravated in patients with renal failure.

Examples

Pharmacokinetic

Several examples of important pharmacokinetic drug interactions are shown in Table 3–18 with the probable mechanism.[14, 23, 24] As noted, drugs can interfere with the absorption of other drugs. One example is antacids, which may chelate tetracyclines and substantially decrease their absorption when taken concurrently. Another would be excipients in the formulation of certain drugs (e.g., phenytoin), which have markedly altered the absorption characteristics of phenytoin and have been associated with a severe epidemic of phenytoin toxicity in Australia.[25] Many drugs can interfere with either the rate or the extent of the absorption of other drugs. For example, cholestyramine can interfere with the absorption of many drugs and certain fat-soluble vitamins. Bleeding states have been associated with depletion of vitamin K due to the ingestion of cholestyramine. Drugs can interfere with plasma protein binding. A traditional example is phenylbutazone, which displaces warfarin from its binding sites in the plasma. This in fact does occur, but whether this explains the increased prothrombin time in patients on warfarin given phenylbutazone or whether there is interference with warfarin metabolism (by phenylbutazone in the liver) remains to be established. Probably altered binding and metabolism of warfarin by phenylbutazone are important and related to an increased prothrombin time and an increased risk of bleeding.[24, 25] Many drugs increase the metabolism of other substances. An excellent example is phenobarbital, which induces the metabolism of cortisol, testosterone, and warfarin. On the other hand, other drugs interfere with metabolism. For example, allopurinol and cimetidine decrease the metabolism of many drugs.[26] Still other drugs (e.g., the weak acid probenecid) interfere with the excretion of other weak acids. Moreover, thiazides interfere with the excretion of lithium. On the average, the introduction of thiazides in a patient taking lithium will decrease the lithium clearance by 30 to 40 percent. Thus, a patient with a therapeutic plasma concentration of lithium may develop a toxic concentration if given thiazides.[24, 25] Similarly, in a patient receiving therapeutic doses of a salicylate (e.g., aspirin), alkalinization of the urine with either antacids or sodium bicarbonate may increase salicylate excretion sufficiently to render salicylate therapy ineffective.

Table 3–18. PHARMACOKINETIC INTERACTIONS—
EXAMPLES

Process Altered (Direction)	Modifying Drug(s)	Drug(s) Affected	Mechanism
Absorption ($\downarrow$)	Antacids containing Mg^{2+}, Ca^{2+}, Al^{3+}, Fe^{2+}	Tetracyclines	Chelation
Absorption ($\downarrow$, $\uparrow$)	Excipients	Phenytoin, chloramphenicol tetracycline	Alteration of bioavailability
Absorption rate ($\downarrow$)	Anticholinergics, opioids	Acetaminophen	Slow gastric emptying
Absorption rate ($\uparrow$)	Metoclopramide	Acetaminophen	Increase gastric emptying
Absorption ($\downarrow$)	Cholestyramine	Warfarin; thyroxine; vitamins A, D, K	Binding
Plasma binding ($\downarrow$)	Phenylbutazone	Warfarin	Increase concentration of free drug secondary to drug displacement
Metabolism ($\uparrow$)	Barbiturates	Cortisol, testosterone, warfarin	Induce enzymes
Metabolism ($\downarrow$)	Allopurinol	Azathioprine, mercaptopurine	Inhibits xanthine oxidase
Metabolism ($\downarrow$)	Chloramphenicol, phenylbutazone	Tolbutamide	Reduced rate of drug metabolism
Metabolism ($\downarrow$)	Cimetidine	Theophylline, diazepam, warfarin	Reduced rate of drug metabolism
Excretion ($\downarrow$)	Thiazides	Lithium	Decreased lithium clearance
Excretion ($\downarrow$)	Salicylates, probenecid, sulfonamides	Methotrexate	Reduced renal secretion
Excretion ($\downarrow$)	Probenecid	Penicillins (some), cephalosporins	Reduced renal secretion
Excretion ($\uparrow$)	Isoniazid	Vitamin B_6	Isoniazid complexes with pyridoxal
Excretion ($\uparrow$)	Acidification of urine	Phencyclidine, amphetamines, quinidine	Ionic trapping
Excretion ($\uparrow$)	Alkalinization of urine	Salicylates and other weak organic acids	Ionic trapping

Pharmacological

Examples of pharmacological interactions are shown in Table 3–19.[14, 24, 25] Drugs may interact synergistically with each other to produce adverse side effects. For example, in patients taking benzodiazepines, barbiturates, or sedative-hypnotic drugs, the addition of alcohol, certain antihypertensive agents, or antihistamines may cause excessive sedation. Diuretics and ampho-

Table 3–19. PHARMACOLOGICAL INTERACTIONS—
EXAMPLES

Modifying Drug(s)	Drugs Affected	Clinical Effect	Probable Mechanism
Drug Synergism			
Alcohol, reserpine, antihistamines, and other depressant drugs	Benzodiazepines, barbiturates, and other sedative-hypnotic drugs	Excessive sedation	Potentiation of central depression
Ethacrynic acid, furosemide	Aminoglycosides	Ototoxicity	
Aminoglycosides, quinidine	Pancuronium, curare	Excessive paralysis	Act on different sites in neuromuscular transmission
Diuretics, amphotericin B	Digitalis	Digitalis toxicity	Hypokalemia
Drug Antagonism			
Antihistamines, anticholinergics, β-blockers	Physiological transmitters or mimetic agonists	Reversal of drug or transmitter action	Competitive inhibition generally
Naloxone	Narcotics	Reversal of drug action	Competitive inhibition generally
Anticholinergics	Physostigmine	Reversal of drug or transmitter action	Competitive inhibition generally
Vitamin K	Warfarin	Ineffective anticoagulation	Increased synthesis of clotting factors
Tricyclic antidepressants	Guanethidine	Ineffective blood pressure control	Blockade of uptake into neurons
Drugs that cause hypokalemia, e.g., diuretics	Antiarrhythmics	Ineffective arrhythmia control	Hypokalemic induction of arrhythmias

Table 3–20. MISCELLANEOUS PHARMACEUTICAL INTERACTIONS—EXAMPLES

Drug	Modifying Agents	Clinical Effect	Probable Mechanism
Penicillin G for intravenous use	Amino acids, vitamin E, gentamicin, heparin, phenytoin, tetracycline, chlorpromazine, chloramphenicol, promethazine	Decreased active penicillin injected	Degradation or binding or precipitation of penicillin
NaHCO$_3$	Ca^{2+} salts, hydrocortisone, streptomycin	Lack of drug effect, precipitation in intravenous bags	Binding, precipitation or inactivation
Levodopa	Protein in diet	Loss of effect of levodopa	Competition by amino acids for levodopa absorption sites in intestine
Griseofulvin	Fat in diet	Increased absorption	Fat increases remarkably absorption of several lipid-soluble drugs
Barbiturates, warfarin, corticosteroids	Pesticides	Decreased effect	Metabolizing enzyme induction
Theophylline	Smoking cigarettes	Decreased effect	Metabolizing enzyme induction
Birth control pills	Smoking cigarettes	Increased risk of ischemic heart disease	

tericin B, by causing an increased excretion of potassium, may, in fact, cause digitalis toxicity, as hypokalemia predisposes the patient to digitalis toxicity. On the other hand, some drugs may antagonize the effects of other drugs. For example, eating foods with large amounts of vitamin K or taking vitamins containing vitamin K may adversely affect anticoagulation with warfarin, as warfarin interferes with coagulation factor synthesis and vitamin K reverses that. Not all drug interactions are harmful, however. One of the most useful is the interaction of naloxone with opioids. This interaction is used in the treatment of patients who overdose with traditional opioid analgesics (e.g., morphine) and newer synthetic compounds (e.g., pentazocine or propoxyphene).

Miscellaneous

A group of miscellaneous drug interactions is shown in Table 3–20.[14, 24, 25] Pharmaceutical interactions can be very important. For example, penicillin G for intravenous use, when mixed with many other compounds, including amino acids and many other drugs (see Table 3–20), results in decreased amounts of active penicillin injected because of degradation, binding, or precipitation of the penicillin. Sodium bicarbonate causes binding or precipitation or inactivation of calcium salts and other drugs. Many other types of miscellaneous interactions occur. For example, large amounts of fat in the diet cause remarkable increases in the bioavailability (absorption) of griseofulvin. Exposure to pesticides, which induces many drug-metabolizing enzymes, may cause a decreased effect in patients given barbiturates, warfarin, or corticosteroids. It has been clearly shown that smoking cigarettes increases the clearance of theophylline by approximately 30 to 40 percent.[14] In initial studies of theophylline pharmacokinetics, subjects who smoked were used. When pharmacokinetic data on the metabolism of theophylline in smoking subjects were incorrectly extrapolated to nonsmoking subjects, many of the nonsmoking subjects and patients with other diseases (who clear theophylline much less quickly than smoking subjects) suffered toxicity. Thus, miscellaneous external factors (e.g., fat or beef in the diet, and smoking) may have profound effects on drug therapy. A final example includes the effects of smoking on the healing of peptic ulcers and on the relief of angina. Patients with ulcers treated with cimetidine or ranitidine and patients with angina treated with nitrates, propranolol, or both are much more refractory to these drugs if they continue smoking than if they stop. The mechanism for these adverse effects of smoking is unknown.

DRUG EFFECTS ON LABORATORY TESTS

Many drugs can alter standard laboratory tests. This is a large and important subject and the reader is referred to standard textbooks for further reading on the subject.[14, 24, 25] Several examples, though, are illustrative. For example, ethanol, clofibrate in patients with renal failure, and intramuscular injections of some drugs (e.g., digoxin) can raise serum aldolase and creatinine phosphokinase levels. Drugs that cause pancreatitis (e.g., azathioprine, thiazides, and ethanol) can raise the serum amylase. Many drugs can decrease the serum potassium, including amphotericin B, diuretics, and corticosteroids. Other drugs can affect hormone levels. For example, nicotine, estrogens, and adrenergic agents can increase serum cortisol. Carbidopa, phenothiazines, haloperidol, methyldopa, and metoclopramide can block dopamine release in the brain and increase serum prolactin. On the other hand, bromocriptine and L-dopa may decrease serum prolactin because they are agonists at dopamine receptors. Finally, many drugs can alter urine color. For example, rifampin colors the urine red.

CONCLUSION

Adverse drug reactions and interactions are, unfortunately, important factors in drug therapy at present. Until better drugs are designed and become available, pharmacologists, physicians, and other health care professionals must be aware of these factors because the risks of ADR and ADI, many of which can be avoided or minimized, must be balanced against the potential benefit to the patient for successful drug therapy.

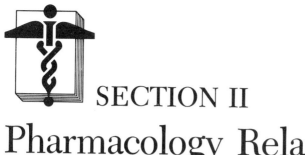

SECTION II
Pharmacology Related to the Nervous System

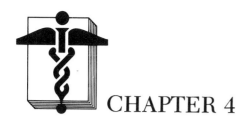

CHAPTER 4

Drugs Acting on the Peripheral Nervous System

J. P. LONG, Ph.D.

Drugs Acting on the Adrenergic Nervous System Effector Sites
(Postjunctional)
  Adrenoceptor Agonists—Postjunctional
    Major Catecholamines
    Other Adrenergic-Receptor Agonists
  Adrenoceptor Antagonists—Postjunctional
    α_1-Adrenergic Antagonists
      Noncompetitive Antagonists
      Competitive Antagonists
    β-Adrenergic Antagonists
Drugs Acting on the Adrenergic Nerve Terminal
(Prejunctional)
  Facilitation of Adrenergic Transmission—Prejunctional
    Inhibitors of Amine I Transport
    α_2-Adrenoceptor Blocking Agents
    Dopamine (DA_2) Adrenoceptor Blocking Agents
    Norepinephrine Releasing Agents
  Inhibition of Adrenergic Transmission—Prejunctional
    α_2-Adrenoceptor Agonists
    Norepinephrine Depleting Agents in Adrenergic
      Nerve Terminals

The peripheral nervous system is divided into afferent and efferent systems. Afferent neurons transmit information from sensory receptors in the periphery (e.g., skin, skeletal muscles, arterioles, internal organs) to the central nervous system (CNS). In contrast, the efferent system, which is divided into somatic and autonomic branches, transmits information from the CNS to the periphery. The somatic branch is under voluntary control and consists of motor neurons innervating skeletal muscles. The autonomic branch, which is primarily involuntary and includes parasympathetic and sympathetic divisions, supplies motor neurons to cardiac muscle, smooth muscle, exocrine glands, some endocrine glands (e.g., endocrine pancreas), and specialized effector sites (e.g., sinoatrial and atrioventricular nodes).

Drugs acting on the peripheral nervous system are classified according to the receptors with which they interact. **Neurotransmitter chemicals** (Table 4–1) are released from nerve terminals by depolarizing stimuli. **Acetylcholine** is the neurotransmitter at autonomic ganglia (sympathetic and parasympathetic), postganglionic parasympathetic sites (smooth and cross-striated muscle and glands), and the neuromuscular junction (skeletal muscle), and at specific sympathetic sites, such as sweat glands and certain blood vessels. **Norepinephrine** is the neurotransmitter at the postganglionic sympathetic site inner-

Table 4–1. NEUROTRANSMITTERS

Neuro-transmitter	Structure	Major Site of Action	Receptors
Acetyl-choline	$(CH_3)_3\text{—}\overset{+}{N}\text{—}CH_2\text{—}CH_2\text{—}O\text{—}\underset{O}{\overset{\parallel}{C}}\text{—}CH_3$	ganglionic neuromuscular postganglionic parasym- pathetic	nicotinic nicotinic muscarinic
Norepine-phrine (Levophed)		postganglionic sympathetic	$\alpha_1,\ \alpha_2,\ \beta_1$
Epinephrine (Adrenaline)		postganglionic sympathetic	$\alpha_1,\ \alpha_2,\ \beta_1,\ \beta_2$
Dopamine		postganglionic sympathetic	$\alpha_1,\ \beta_1,\ DA_1$

vating smooth and cross-striated muscle and glands. **Epinephrine** is released from the adrenal medulla into the systemic circulation following stimulation of the sympathetic nervous system. Purines and norepinephrine are released by sympathetic nerves at genitourinary sites. Neurotransmitters and drugs interact with receptors to alter ionic gradients across membranes (depolarize or hyperpolarize) or exert actions through second messenger molecules.

ANATOMY OF THE PERIPHERAL NERVOUS SYSTEM

Autonomic Nervous System (Involuntary)

Parasympathetic neurons exit from the central nervous system at cranial and sacral regions, and **sympathetic neurons** exit from the central nervous system in thoracolumbar regions. Figure 4–1 summarizes major anatomical features of autonomic neuronal innervation and lists whether responses of target organs are excitatory (E) or inhibitory (I). Some functions of the autonomic nervous system relate to anatomical features and these are outlined below.

Parasympathetic Division

The parasympathetic division of the autonomic nervous system is highly localized in function. Usually only one part is activated at a given time. For example, vagal nerve fibers (Xth cranial) to the heart may produce cardiac slowing (bradycardia) and decrease in force of contraction, and these responses are not accompanied by an increase in intestinal motility. The major function of parasympathetic autonomic nerves is to serve as efferent pathways in many reflex arcs. Also contributing to their restricted function is the absence of

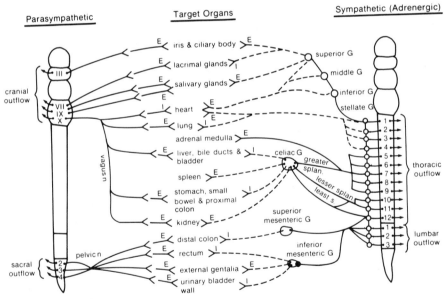

Figure 4–1. Anatomy of autonomic (parasympathetic and sympathetic) nervous system. Preganglionic fibers are myelinated and postganglionic fibers are nonmyelinated. In the thorax and abdomen, parasympathetic ganglia are located within innervated organs; while in the head and neck, ganglia are slightly removed from the target organ. Sympathetic ganglia are not adjacent to the target organ (except the adrenal medulla). E = excitatory; I = inhibitory; solid line = cholinergic (acetylcholine is neurotransmitter); broken line = adrenergic (norepinephrine is neurotransmitter).

branching of nerves. Parasympathetic ganglia (cell bodies) are located either within organs innervated (thorax and abdomen) or adjacent (head and neck).

Sympathetic (Adrenergic) Division

In contrast, the sympathetic division of the autonomic nervous system functions in a coordinated manner. Most sympathetic neuronal fibers synapse within the thoracolumbar chain of paraganglia, but distal ganglia are present in the abdomen. Thus several target organs may be innervated by postganglionic fibers emerging from a single ganglion. In most cases the postganglionic fibers are long and ramifying. This also helps explain the functional observation; when one part of the sympathetic nervous system is activated, all parts may be affected.

Anatomical Features

There are anatomical features common to both branches (sympathetic and parasympathetic) of the autonomic nervous system:

1. All preganglionic fibers are myelinated.
2. All postganglionic fibers are nonmyelinated.
3. The number of postganglionic fibers is higher than the number of preganglionic fibers. The ratio is about 1:50 for the sympathetic nervous system and about 1:2 for the parasympathetic nervous system.
4. Clusters of cell bodies (ganglia) characterize both branches of the autonomic nervous system; drugs show little or no selectivity for ganglia in the two branches of the autonomic nervous system.
5. After removal of ganglia, and allowing time for denervation of postganglionic nerve fibers, **postganglionic receptors exhibit denervation supersensitivity** to their respective neurotransmitters (acetylcholine for parasympathetic and epinephrine or norepinephrine for the sympathetic nervous system). Neither smooth nor cardiac muscle atrophy following denervation.

Somatic Nervous System (Voluntary)

Motor (somatic) nerves innervating skeletal muscle are myelinated and their cell bodies are within the CNS. The motor nerve terminals innervate regions near the middle of skeletal muscle and are known as end-plate regions. Sectioning motor nerves produces **denervation supersensitivity** to acetylcholine, which is accompanied by atrophy of skeletal muscle.

PHYSIOLOGY OF THE PERIPHERAL NERVOUS SYSTEM

Autonomic Nervous System

The **autonomic nervous system** helps maintain homeostasis by regulating primarily involuntary functions such as heart rate, blood pressure, gastrointestinal motility, bladder tone, body temperature (*via* regulation of sweating and cutaneous vascular tone), metabolism, and glandular secretions. In general, the **parasympathetic nervous system**, which functions in a localized way (as previously mentioned), acts to conserve energy and maintain vegetative functions. For example, parasympathetic effects include miosis, accommodation for near vision, bradycardia, hypotension, salivation, increased gastrointestinal motility and secretions, stimulation of urination and defecation, and generalized sweating (mediated by sympathetic cholinergic fibers). In contrast, the **sympathetic nervous system** acts in concert and is mainly involved in preparing a person for stressful situations. (Nevertheless, there is a constant basal sympathetic outflow.) Generalized sympathetic discharge results in the "fight-or-flight" response: mydriasis, increased heart rate and myocardial contractility, increased blood pressure, sweating of the hands and feet, vasodilation of skeletal muscle arterioles and vasoconstriction of cutaneous and visceral arterioles and veins, contraction of the anal and bladder sphincters, decreased gastrointestinal motility, and increased glycogenolysis and lipolysis, resulting in increased blood glucose and free fatty acids for energy expenditure.

Most organs have dual innervation by parasympathetic and sympathetic fibers, which usually have antagonistic effects (Table 4–2). For example, gastrointestinal secretions and peristalsis are stimulated by parasympathetic fibers, and peristalsis is inhibited by sympathetic fibers. Similarly, heart rate increases with sympathetic stimulation and decreases with parasympathetic stimulation. However, at some effector sites, the parasympathetic and sympathetic branches have similar effects; for instance, both increase salivary gland secretion. Parasympathetic neuronal stimulation increases saliva production, which is large volume and low viscosity. Sympathetic neuronal stimulation produces low saliva volume, but it is viscous and enzyme rich.

Somatic Nervous System

The somatic nervous system, consisting of motor neurons projecting from the CNS to skeletal muscle, allows voluntary control of movement. Acetylcholine release from motor neurons results in receptor-mediated depolarization of the motor end-plate producing contracture of skeletal muscle.

**Table 4–2. ACTIONS OF THE AUTONOMIC NERVOUS
SYSTEM ON VARIOUS EFFECTORS**

Organ	Sympathetic (Thoracolumbar)	Parasympathetic (Craniosacral)
Eye		
Iris	Dilation	Constriction
Intraocular pressure	Decreased	Decreased
Tear gland secretion	—	Increased
Glands		
Salivary	Viscous secretion	Watery secretion
Sweat	Secretion, palms	Generalized secretion*
Piloerectors	Contraction	—
Bronchioles		
Secretions	Mixed response	Increased
Smooth muscle	Relaxation	Contraction
Heart		
Rate	Acceleration	Deceleration
Force	Increased	Decreased
GI Tract		
Muscle wall (motility)	Relaxation	Contraction
Sphincters	Contraction	Relaxation
Secretion	—	Increased secretion
Spleen	Contraction	—
Urinary Bladder		
Fundus	Relaxation	Contraction
Trigone and sphincter	Contraction	Relaxation
Blood Vessels (arterioles)		
Skeletal Muscle	Dilation	Dilation†
Coronary	Dilation (β_2)	Dilation
Skin, viscera	Constriction	—

*Many sweat glands have receptors that are stimulated by acetylcholine-like drugs and blocked by atropine-like drugs. The anatomical origin of these nerves is sympathetic and they are often called "cholinergic sympathetic."

†Parasympathetic neurons do not innervate vascular beds found in skeletal muscle, but muscarinic receptors are on the vascular smooth muscle, and when stimulated, dilation will result.

Sites of Drug Action

Figure 4–2 lists major drugs that stimulate or inhibit the peripheral somatic and autonomic nervous systems. Note that the anatomical sites for drug action involve synapses (junctions). None of the agents discussed in this chapter stabilize membranes and block neuronal conduction (local anesthetic

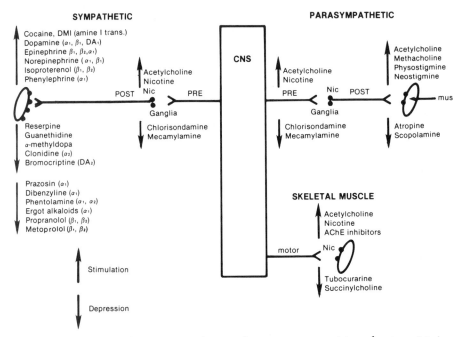

Figure 4–2. Sites for drug action and major drug receptor agonists and antagonists involving the peripheral nervous system. Acetylcholinesterase is found at all sites where acetylcholine is a neurotransmitter and terminates its action by hydrolysis of the ester linkage. Norepinephrine's action is terminated by various mechanisms: (1) diffusion from synapse into the systemic circulation, (2) reuptake into the nerve terminal, and (3) metabolism by two enzymes, monoamine oxidase and catechol-O-methyltransferase.

activity). Also shown in Figure 4–2 are locations of cholinergic receptors (nicotinic-Nic and muscarinic-Mus) where the neurotransmitter acetylcholine binds, or of adrenergic receptors (α_1, α_2, β_1, β_2, DA_1, and DA_2) where catecholamine neurotransmitters bind. These receptor types, biological responses resulting from receptor activation or inhibition, and drugs that stimulate or inhibit receptors will be discussed later under Cholinergic Nervous System and Adrenergic Nervous System, respectively.

A major pharmacological goal has been the development of drugs that are specific agonists or antagonists for the aforementioned receptors. Much of our knowledge concerning the physiology of the autonomic nervous system has resulted from studies using these agents.

Table 4–3 lists various terminologies used to classify and define sites of action for these agents. Initially the many terminologies used can be confusing for beginning students, but with time they will become integrated into one's working vocabulary.

Table 4–3. TERMS USED TO DESCRIBE DRUG ACTION*

Site of Action	Receptor Agonist	Receptor Antagonist
Autonomic ganglia	Nicotinic	Antinicotinic
	Ganglionic stimulant	Ganglionic depressant
	Preganglionic stimulant	Preganglionic depressant
Postganglionic parasympathetic neuroeffector junction	Muscarinic agonist	Muscarinic depressant
	Cholinergic	Anticholinergic
	Muscarinic	Antimuscarinic
	Parasympathetic stimulant	Parasympathetic inhibitor
	Parasympathomimetic	Parasympatholytic
Postganglionic sympathetic neuroeffector junction	Adrenergic stimulant	Adrenergic blocker
	Sympathetic stimulant	Sympathetic inhibition
	Sympathomimetic	Sympatholytic
	α_1, β_1, etc., receptor agonist	α_1, β_1, etc., receptor antagonist
Myoneural junction	Myoneural stimulant	Myoneural depressant
	Neuromuscular agonist	Muscle relaxant
		Neuromuscular blocking agent

*Note that the terms agonist, -mimetic, and stimulant are interchangeable and likewise the terms antagonist, depressant, inhibitor, and blocking agent are often substituted for each other.

CHOLINERGIC NERVOUS SYSTEM

Chemical neurotransmission was first shown by O. Loewi in 1921 in frog hearts, and he termed the bradycardia-inducing material "vagalstoff." He and others during the next decade established that acetylcholine was the chemical agent, and thus Loewi's classical research launched the search for neurotransmitters and their reactive sites (receptors).

Cholinergic Synapses: Acetylcholine Biosynthesis and Degradation

Figure 4–3 illustrates a **cholinergic synapse.** It is believed that mechanisms are the same for synthesis, storage, and release of **acetylcholine (ACh)** at all cholinergic nerve terminals in both the peripheral and central nervous systems. Acetylcholine is synthesized by the enzyme **cholineacetyltransferase,** which is on the outer membrane of **synaptic vesicles.** ACh is stored within synaptic vesicles. Neuronal impulses induce synaptic vesicles to mi-

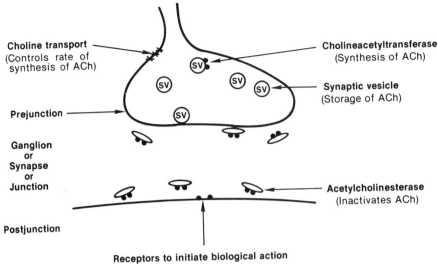

Choline transport
(Controls rate of synthesis of ACh)

Cholineacetyltransferase
(Synthesis of ACh)

Synaptic vesicle
(Storage of ACh)

Prejunction

**Ganglion
or
Synapse
or
Junction**

Acetylcholinesterase
(Inactivates ACh)

Postjunction

Receptors to initiate biological action

Figure 4–3. Outline of the major components involved in cholinergic transmission. Acetylcholine (ACh) is synthesized (choline acetyltransferase) and stored within synaptic vesicles found within the cholinergic nerve terminal (prejunction). Neuronal impulses release acetylcholine into the synapse (ganglion, junction), and following interaction with postjunctional receptors (muscarinic [MUS] or nicotinic [NIC]), which initiate biological activity, ACh then combines with receptors on acetylcholinesterase (AChE) and is inactivated by hydrolysis of the ester linkage. A portion of the resulting choline reenters the nerve terminal by the choline transport system and serves as the precursor for synthesis of ACh. Activity of the choline transport system controls the synthetic rate of ACh.

grate to nerve terminals where fusion of membranes occurs (exocytosis) and contents of synaptic vesicles, including ACh, are released into the junction. Following interaction with postjunctional receptors (muscarinic or nicotinic) to induce biological responses, ACh then combines with receptors on the enzyme **acetylcholinesterase,** and ACh is inactivated by hydrolysis of the ester linkage to form choline and acetic acid. Acetylcholine is at least 10,000 times more active than choline as an agonist at nicotinic and muscarinic receptors. Table 4–4 shows synthesis and degradation of ACh.

Rate of synthesis of ACh in cholinergic nerve terminals is controlled by activity of the choline transport system. An increase in neuronal activity will facilitate transport of choline (precursor for ACh synthesis) and stimulate synthesis of acetylcholine. The transport system is sodium-dependent, high affinity (active-nondiffusion), and competitively inhibited by the experimental compound hemicholinium (HC-3). Mechanisms by which neuronal impulses control activity of the choline transport system are unknown.

Table 4–4. SYNTHESIS AND INACTIVATION OF ACETYLCHOLINE

Synthesis

$$(CH_3)_3 \overset{+}{-} N - CH_2 - CH_2 - OH + -\overset{\overset{\displaystyle O}{\|}}{O}C - CH_3 \xrightarrow[\text{Mg}^{++}]{\text{cholineacetyltransferase}} (CH_3)_3 \overset{+}{-} N - CH_2 - CH_2 - O - \overset{\overset{\displaystyle O}{\|}}{C} - CH_3$$

$$\text{choline} \qquad\qquad \text{acetyl CoA} \qquad\qquad\qquad\qquad \text{acetylcholine}$$

Inactivation (Degradation)

$$(CH_3)_3 \overset{+}{-} N - CH_2 - CH_2 - O - \overset{\overset{\displaystyle O}{\|}}{O}C - CH_3 \xrightarrow[\text{H}_2\text{O}]{\text{cholinesterase (acetyl or plasma)}} (CH_3)_3 \overset{+}{-} N - CH_2 - CH_2 - OH + HO\overset{\overset{\displaystyle O}{\|}}{C} - CH_3$$

$$\text{acetylcholine} \qquad\qquad\qquad\qquad\qquad\qquad \text{choline} \qquad\qquad \text{acetic acid}$$

Cholinergic Receptors (Muscarinic and Nicotinic)

Acetylcholine stimulates cholinergic receptors which are divided into two groups: muscarinic and nicotinic (Table 4–5). **Muscarinic receptors,** which can be excitatory or inhibitory, are located on parasympathetic effector organs (M_2) (and a few sympathetic effector organs, e.g., sweat glands), parasympathetic nerve terminals (M_1), as well as in the CNS. **Nicotinic receptors** are usually excitatory and are located at ganglia, both parasympathetic and sympathetic, at the adrenal medulla, at the junction of the motor (somatic) nerves and skeletal muscle (neuromuscular junction), and in the CNS. Nicotinic receptors at the ganglia and neuromuscular junction are of different subtypes, N_1 and N_2, respectively. Consequently, some drugs, such as ganglionic blockers and neuromuscular blockers, are site-specific even though their actions are both mediated *via* nicotinic receptors and antagonism of acetylcholine. Reasons for this selectivity are unknown.

Drugs Acting on the Cholinergic Nervous System

There are two mechanisms by which drugs may mimic the parasympathetic nervous system. These are (1) drugs that directly stimulate muscarinic receptors and (2) drugs that inhibit acetylcholinesterase, thus increasing the concentration of ACh within a cholinergic synapse.

Table 4–5. CHOLINERGIC RECEPTORS FOR ACETYLCHOLINE

	Muscarinic	Nicotinic
Effects (excitatory vs. inhibitory)	Excitatory (usually) or inhibitory (heart and cholinergic nerve terminals)	Excitatory (including cholinergic and adrenergic nerve terminals)
Receptor subtypes	M_1-cholinergic nerve terminals M_2-post junctional	N_1-ganglia N_2-neuromuscular junction
Agonists	Acetylcholine, etc. Muscarine	Acetylcholine, nicotine (low dose—ganglia)
Antagonists	Atropine, etc.	Curare (neuromuscular) Nicotine (high dose—ganglia)
Location	Parasympathetic effector organs, some sympathetic effector organs (e.g., sweat glands) CNS*	Ganglia (sympathetic and parasympathetic), neuromuscular junction (skeletal muscle) CNS*

*Muscarinic receptors predominate in the CNS. It has been estimated that 95% of the cholinergic receptors are muscarinic and 5% are nicotinic receptors.

Muscarinic Receptor Agonists (Cholinergic Stimulants)

Drugs that directly stimulate muscarinic receptors involve the same molecular mechanisms as acetylcholine. These agents induce responses similar to stimulation of the parasympathetic nervous system (i.e., miosis, accommodation for near vision, salivation, sweating, increased bronchial secretions, bronchoconstriction, bradycardia, hypotension, increased gastrointestinal motility, increased secretions of glands, and urinary incontinence). Agents include **acetylcholine, methacholine** (Mecholyl), **carbachol, pilocarpine,** and **bethanechol** (Urecholine). Structures and major biological properties of these agents are shown in Table 4–6. A major difference among the drugs is their duration of action, and agents hydrolyzed by cholinesterase have a short duration. These drugs have been used in therapy of peripheral vascular disease, paroxysmal tachycardia, and urinary bladder retention. Solutions of pilocarpine and carbachol are applied topically to the cornea for therapy of acute-angle glaucoma.

Acetylcholinesterase Inhibitors

There are two major types of esterases involved with the pharmacology of cholinergic transmission: acetylcholinesterase (AChE) and plasma (pseudo) cholinesterase. ACh is an excellent substrate for both enzymes.

Acetylcholinesterase is found in very high concentrations at all cholinergic synapses in both the central and peripheral nervous systems. Its function is to inactivate ACh and prevent accumulation of excess ACh within cholinergic synapses. At the neuromuscular junction (skeletal) excess ACh can lead to persistent depolarization of the end-plate region, resulting in failure of transmission and respiratory failure. Excess ACh at muscarinic receptors (parasympathetic) does not produce persistent depolarization of smooth muscle, but marked "cholinergic" symptoms are noted, i.e., sweating, intestinal cramps, salivation, miosis, tearing, and so on. Centrally the respiratory center is depressed by excess acetylcholine. High concentrations of AChE are found in red blood cells, and its function is unknown.

Pseudocholinesterase (plasma cholinesterase) is found in plasma and is widely distributed in many tissues, including brain. This enzyme may serve to inactivate any acetylcholine that may "escape" from a cholinergic synapse.

There are two types of **inhibitors of cholinesterase,** termed **reversible** and **irreversible.** Reversible inhibitors, e.g., **neostigmine, edrophonium, physostigmine,** have a duration of action of approximately 1 hour or less. Edrophonium is an effective inhibitor for only about 10 minutes. Irreversible organophosphate inhibitors, e.g., diisopropylfluorophosphate (DFP), may have a duration of action corresponding to the turnover rate of the cholinesterase enzyme—2 to 3 weeks. Administration of either reversible or irreversible inhibitors of cholinesterase increases the concentration of ACh at cholinergic synapses, resulting in excess parasympathetic and somatic neuronal stimulation.

Table 4–6. MUSCARINIC RECEPTOR AGONISTS

Compound	Structure	Substrate for Cholinesterase Acetyl-	Substrate for Cholinesterase Pseudo-	Decrease Arterial Pressure	Stimulate Gastrointestinal	Contract Urinary Bladder	Used Topically In Eye	Antagonism by Atropine	Nicotinic Receptor Agonist	Duration of Action (Min)
Acetylcholine	$(CH_3)_3\overset{+}{N}-CH_2CH_2-O\overset{\;\;O}{\overset{\|}{C}}-CH_3$	+++	+++	+++	++	+	–*	+++	++	5
Methacholine	$(CH_3)_3\overset{+}{N}-\underset{CH_3}{\overset{H}{\underset{\|}{\overset{\|}{C}}}}H-O\overset{\;\;O}{\overset{\|}{C}}-CH_3$	+++	–	+++	++	+	+*	+++	–	10–15
Carbachol	$(CH_3)_3\overset{+}{N}-CH_2-CH_2-O\overset{\;\;O}{\overset{\|}{C}}-NH_2$	–	–	++	+++	+++	+++	++	++	60–90
Bethanechol	$(CH_3)_3\overset{+}{N}-CH_2-\underset{CH_3}{\overset{H}{\underset{\|}{\overset{\|}{C}}}}-O\overset{\;\;O}{\overset{\|}{C}}-NH_2$	–	–	++	+++	+++	+	++	–	60–90
Pilocarpine	(imidazole-lactone structure, CH_3-N ... CH_2 ... C_2H_5 lactone ring)	–	–	+	+	+	++	+	+	>120

*Agents induce miosis and lower intraocular pressure, if injected into anterior chamber, but fail to penetrate cornea following topical application.

+ = active.

– = inactive.

Two binding sites for ACh constitute a receptor, and only one receptor is found on a unit of cholinesterase (MW 35,000); a combination of four units forms the enzyme structure. The binding sites for acetylcholine are designated "cationic" where the positively charged nitrogen of ACh binds and "esteratic" where the ester group of ACh binds. Acetylcholine, carbamate inhibitors of acetylcholinesterase (e.g., neostigmine), and organophosphate molecules all alkylate the esteratic site. Acetylcholine is very reversible and probably binds to the esteratic site for no more than a microsecond. Neostigmine competes with ACh for binding sites on acetylcholinesterase. Organophosphates do not compete with ACh for the esteratic sites and have a duration of action of weeks, which corresponds to the synthesis of new enzyme (2 to 3 weeks). Molecular mechanisms involved in alkylation and reactivation of cholinesterase receptors are shown in Table 4–7.

Reversible Inhibitors. Drugs include **physostigmine** (eserine), **neostigmine** (Prostigmin), and **edrophonium** (Tensilon). Structures and major biological properties are shown in Table 4–8.

Physostigmine (Eserine) is a unique drug: (1) It is approximately equally effective as an inhibitor of both acetylcholinesterase and pseudocholinesterase, and (2) being a tertiary amine, it readily crosses membranes, including the blood-brain barrier. Its major clinical use is topical application to the cornea for therapy of acute-angle glaucoma. Physostigmine is also being used for therapy of cholinergic hypofunction involving the central nervous system, i.e., Alzheimer's disease. Unfortunately, the compound readily undergoes oxidation, and several of the metabolic products (e.g., eseroline) produce untoward stimulation of the CNS. An agent that is more stable and more selective for inhibition of acetylcholinesterase within the CNS is needed for possible therapy of Alzheimer's disease.

Neostigmine (Prostigmin) is a quaternary amine and does not cross the blood-brain barrier or corneal membranes. For many years it has been the prototype drug for inhibition of AChE, thus increasing the concentration of ACh at muscarinic receptors, resulting in parasympathetic nervous system stimulation. It is also the prototype drug for therapy of myasthenia gravis (deficient functional acetylcholine at the neuromuscular junction). Its clinical use for this disease results from inhibition of AChE as well as direct stimulation of nicotinic receptors on skeletal muscle. Neostigmine is also widely used to reverse inhibition induced by competitive inhibitors at the neuromuscular junction (e.g., curare).

Edrophonium (Tensilon) is widely used to reverse neuromuscular inhibition induced by competitive neuromuscular blocking agents such as curare. The duration of action of edrophonium is brief, approximately 10 minutes. The short duration of action makes edrophonium a useful test agent to determine if there is a deficiency in cholinergic transmission. The mechanisms of action to facilitate cholinergic transmission are (1) inhibition of AChE and (2) direct stimulation of nicotinic receptors at skeletal muscle.

Table 4–7. MOLECULAR MECHANISMS FOR
ALKYLATION OF CHOLINESTERASE

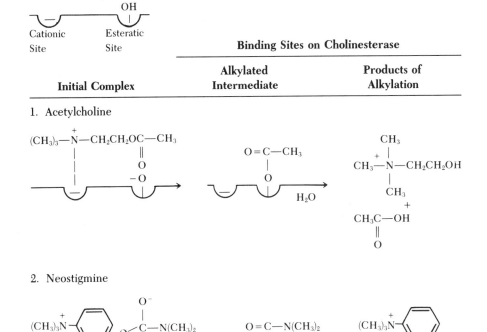

Initial Complex	Alkylated Intermediate	Products of Alkylation

1. Acetylcholine

2. Neostigmine

3. DFP

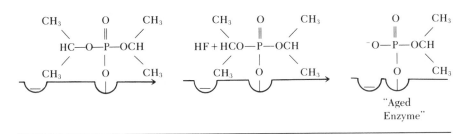

Irreversible Inhibitors. The use of organophosphate derivatives for inhibition of cholinesterase was developed in Germany during World War II. A major effort was directed toward development of "nerve gas" (soman, tabun, sarin) and by the end of the war they had stockpiled 10,000 tons of soman.

Fortunately for the Allied armies, the material was never used. The Germans also conducted extensive field experimentation with several organophosphate derivatives, e.g., parathion, and demonstrated the usefulness of these agents as insecticides. They also demonstrated that organophosphate molecules are not retained by animals following ingestion. Structures of representative compounds and biological properties are shown in Table 4–8. Irreversible inhibitors of cholinesterase include diisopropylfluorophosphate (DFP), tetraethyl pyrophosphate (TEPP), malathion, parathion (Paroxon), and hundreds of analogs. Derivatives of organophosphates are no longer used in clinical medicine to produce inhibition of cholinesterase. Chronic application to the cornea may damage the lens and increase incidence of detached retinas.

Intoxication with organophosphate insecticides presents difficult therapeutic problems. Symptoms include cholinergic hyperactivity, and in severe intoxication failure of respiration and/or cardiovascular collapse may occur. Therapy includes initial large doses of atropine (5 mg or more) followed by additional dosage when cholinergic symptoms reappear. These large doses of atropine are required to block the parasympathetic nervous system and to stimulate the respiratory center. **Pralidoxine** (2-PAM) may also be used in therapy of severe intoxication to reactivate receptors of acetylcholinesterase. Table 4–9 shows how the organophosphate molecule is transferred from the esteratic site of the enzyme to 2-PAM. If 2-PAM is used, administration of the agent must not be delayed. All organophosphate inhibitors of cholinesterase undergo molecular rearrangements following their attachment to the "esteratic site" of the receptor on cholinesterase. This process is known as "aging," and 2-PAM is ineffective after aging occurs. Fortunately the aging process with organophosphate insecticides may require 24 hours or more for completion, thus allowing time for evaluation of the severity of intoxication. Aging with nerve gases will occur within minutes.

Plasma cholinesterase is more sensitive than acetylcholinesterase for inhibition by organophosphate insecticides. Plasma cholinesterase may be 50 to 75 percent inhibited before inhibition of AChE is observed. Thus, individuals who are chronically exposed to these agents (e.g., commercial applicators) should have the activity of their plasma cholinesterase determined before exposure and weekly thereafter. When inhibition of their plasma cholinesterase approximates 50 percent, these individuals should be removed from exposure to these agents for 2 to 3 weeks and should not show symptoms of cholinergic stimulation and intoxication.

Muscarinic-Receptor Antagonists (Anticholinergic Drugs)

Many **antimuscarinic drugs** were derived from *Solanaceae* plants and have been used throughout history for both medicinal and nefarious purposes. The plant *Atropa belladonna* (deadly nightshade) contains mainly **atropine** and was used during the Middle Ages to poison people. Belladonna (beautiful lady), an extract from this plant, was used by ladies of Spanish royalty to dilate

Table 4-8. INHIBITORS OF CHOLINESTERASE

1. Reversible Inhibitors

Compound	Structure	Inhibition of Cholinesterase		Increase ACh in Brain	Topical Use—Eye	Major Uses
		Acetyl	Plasma			
Physostigmine		+ +	+	+ + +	+ + +	Glaucoma, CNS cholinergic
Neostigmine		+ + +	−	−	−	Cholinergic agonist, antag. curare
Edrophonium		+ +	−	−	−	Antag. curare

2. Irreversible Inhibitors (Organophosphates)

Compound	Structure				
DFP		+	+++	++	++* None
TEPP		+	+++	++	++* None
Malathion		+	++	++	+* Insecticide

*Irreversible inhibitors are no longer used in ocular pharmacology, because of damage to the lens and increased frequency of detached retinas.

+ = active.
− = inactive.

Table 4-9. MECHANISM OF ACTION OF 2-PAM

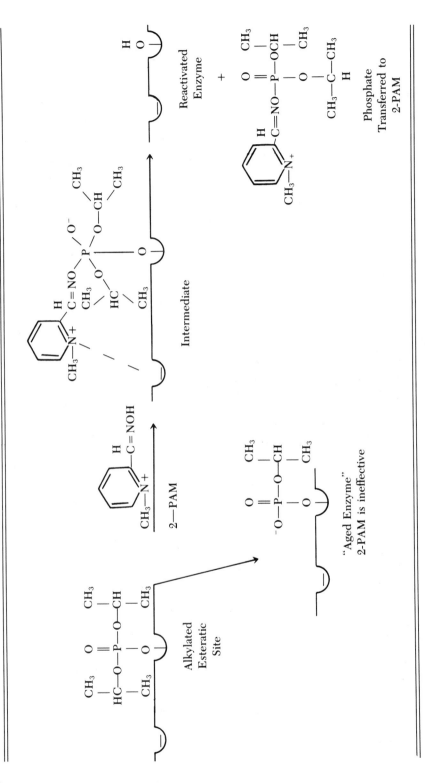

their pupils, since a dilated pupil was considered a sign of beauty. It was not until the 19th century that atropine was first used clinically to induce mydriasis and thus facilitate ophthalmologic examination.

Anticholinergic agents compete with acetylcholine for receptor sites (**muscarinic**) at the postganglionic parasympathetic neuroeffector junction and thus decrease activity of the parasympathetic nervous system. These drugs do **not** antagonize acetylcholine at nicotinic receptors (autonomic ganglia and neuromuscular junction). Reasons for this fortunate selectivity are unknown.

Tertiary amine derivatives (e.g., atropine, scopolamine, homatropine, and trihexyphenidyl) readily penetrate the CNS, while quaternary amine derivatives (e.g., methscopolamine) do not. Likewise, quaternary amine derivatives have erratic and incomplete absorption following oral administration. Scopolamine is a unique anticholinergic agent and is used primarily for its central effects; it produces **amnesia,** especially when combined with morphine, barbiturates, and a wide range of analgesic or CNS-depressant drugs. Scopolamine is also a potent peripheral anticholinergic agent that is about twice as active as atropine. Atropine and numerous other cholinergic blocking agents relieve spasm of smooth muscle. They may be useful in therapy of gastric hypermotility, spasticity of small intestines or colon, and pylorospasm. Anticholinergic agents slightly diminish gastric HCl production, and they have been replaced by H_2-receptor antagonists to diminish HCl production in ulcer therapy. Atropine will also tend to relax spasticity of the ureter and bile ducts. Atropine is used in urinary incontinence. Anticholinergic agents have minimal cardiovascular effects unless some clinical procedure (e.g., cardiac catheterization) or drug (e.g., muscarinic-receptor agonist) activates vagal neuronal transmission to the heart. Salivation and tearing are readily blocked by all anticholinergic agents. Atropine, homatropine, and tropicamide are widely used to inhibit third cranial (parasympathetic) neuronal innervation to the circular muscles of the iris, resulting in dilation of the pupil (mydriasis) and loss of accommodation for near vision (cycloplegia). **Atropine, scopolamine,** and **trihexyphenidyl** are sometimes useful for therapy of postencephalitic parkinsonism (CNS action). Dopamine-receptor agonists (levodopa and bromocriptine) are now the drugs of choice, but anticholinergic agents may be useful adjuncts to help control uncoordinated motor movements and saliva production. All agents will decrease sweating by inhibiting muscarinic receptors innervated by cholinergic sympathetic neurons, and thus increase skin temperature. **Atropine** (large dose, 5 mg or more) is the drug of choice for treatment of poisoning by irreversible organophosphate cholinesterase inhibitors. A summary of anticholinergic agents is given in Table 4–10.

Anticholinergic drugs (with possible exception of tropicamide) will elevate intraocular pressure in an individual with glaucoma. Individuals past 40 years of age should have their intraocular pressure checked before administration of these agents.

Table 4-10. ANTICHOLINERGIC AGENTS

Drug	Structure	Muscarinic Recep. Inhibition	Eye-Mydriasis and Cycloplegia (Topical)	Inhibit Secretions of Respiratory Tract	CNS—Amnesia	CNS—Anti-parkinson	Duration of Action (Hours)
Atropine	(phenyl)–CH(CH₂OH)–C(=O)–O– tropane (N–CH₃)	+++	+++	+++	–	++	5–10
Scopolamine	(phenyl)–CH(CH₂OH)–C(=O)–O– scopine (epoxide, N–CH₃)	++++	+++	+++	++++	+	5–10
Methscopol-amine	(phenyl)–CH(CH₂OH)–C(=O)–O– scopine (epoxide, CH₃–N⁺–CH₃)	++++	+	+++	–	–	5–10

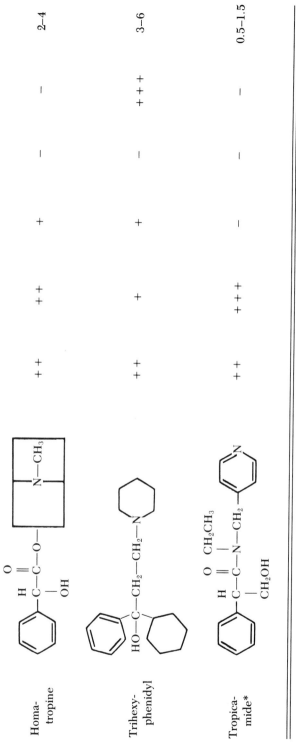

Homa-tropine	++	++	+	–	–	2–4
Trihexy-phenidyl	++	+	+	–	+++	3–6
Tropica-mide*	++	+++	–	–	–	0.5–1.5

*Tropicamide is used only for topical corneal application.

+ = active.

– = inactive or not relevant for clinical use.

Overdose with tertiary amine anticholinergic agents (**scopolamine, atropine, homatropine,** and **trihexyphenidyl**) will produce peripheral muscarinic-receptor blockade and induce various CNS reactions. With overdose hallucinations and amnesia may be present (especially with scopolamine) and the individual may appear either depressed or stimulated. Overdose with all of the postganglionic parasympathetic blocking agents will produce marked mydriasis, urinary retention, dry mouth, diminished sweating, and so on. These signs and symptoms inspired the classic description of atropine poisoning, "red as a beet, blind as a bat, dry as a bone, mad as a hatter, and dead as a doornail!" As a rule, the patient will recover from overdose without resorting to any supportive therapy. Cardiovascular and respiratory functions should be monitored, and patients with CNS toxicity must be observed closely. As a rule, CNS effects will disappear after 8 to 12 hours, depending on dosage. **Quaternary amine derivatives** do not cross the blood-brain barrier and have only peripheral anticholinergic action (such as dry mouth).

Nicotinic-Receptor Agonists (Ganglionic Stimulants)

None of these agents is used clinically, although **nicotine** is extensively consumed in tobacco products. **Ganglionic stimulants** are valuable experimental tools and are used to define sites of action of other agents. The most readily observed biological response of these agents is stimulation of sympathetic ganglia, producing an elevation in arterial pressure and heart rate. Plasma concentrations of epinephrine from the adrenal medulla and norepinephrine from adrenergic nerve terminals are elevated. Cigarette smoking is a major public health concern, in its association with such conditions as bronchial carcinoma and cardiovascular disease. Nearly 2000 different chemicals have been identified in cigarette smoke, including nicotine, carbon monoxide, various nitrosoamines, and aldehydes, and it is difficult to correlate various "risk factors" with a particular chemical. The smoke of American cigarettes is acidic; thus, smokers tend to inhale to neutralize the smoke and promote systemic absorption of nicotine. Cigar smoke is alkaline, and sufficient nicotine is absorbed from the oral cavity, which is why cigar smokers rarely inhale. The very high concentration of nicotine (50 mg) in a cigar may also be a factor, as even confirmed smokers may have difficulties with this quantity of nicotine. Nicotinic-receptor agonists are equally effective at parasympathetic and sympathetic ganglia and at the myoneural junction. Examples of this class of agents include **acetylcholine** (large dose), **nicotine** (low concentrations), and **tetramethylammonium** (TMA).

Nicotinic-Receptor Antagonists (Ganglionic Blocking Agents)

These agents **inhibit neuronal transmission at both sympathetic and parasympathetic ganglia** by blocking receptor sites (nicotinic) with which acetylcholine combines. Pharmacological responses to these drugs relate to dominance of either sympathetic or parasympathetic neuronal innervation of target organs (Table 4–11). Interrupting sympathetic ganglionic neurotransmission inhibits cardiovascular reflexes, and orthostatic hypotension is particularly noticeable when a patient changes from a supine to an upright position. Orthostatic hypotension results from pooling of blood in veins and arteries of lower extremities and is accompanied by tachycardia, decreased cardiac output, decreased total peripheral resistance, and fainting. Inhibition of parasympathetic ganglionic transmission produces dry mouth, constipation, mydriasis, impaired sexual functions, and so on.

Examples of ganglionic blocking agents include **hexamethonium** (C-6), **chlorisondamine** (Ecolid), **mecamylamine** (Inversine), and high concentrations of **nicotine**. Ganglionic blocking agents are no longer regarded as "first choice" to lower arterial pressure in hypertension, because of numerous side effects that result from inhibition of ganglionic transmission in both the sympathetic

Table 4–11. BIOLOGICAL RESPONSES RESULTING
FROM INHIBITION OF GANGLIONIC TRANSMISSION

Site	Ganglionic Inhibition of Parasympathetic/Sympathetic		Clinical Response
Sweat glands	—	I*	Decreased sweating
Secretory glands (salivary, tear)	I	—	Decreased secretions
Urinary bladder	I	I	Urinary retention
Gastrointestinal	I	I	Decreased motility and constipation
Eye			
Iris	I	I	Mydriasis, cycloplegia—failure to
Ciliary muscle	I	I	accommodate for near-vision
Heart	I	I	Tachycardia† and decrease in cardiac output
Arterioles	—	I	Vasodilation, decrease in mean arterial pressure
Veins	—	I	Venodilation, diminished return of blood to the heart resulting in decreased cardiac output and tachycardia

*I = inhibition of autonomic innervation, which relates to clinical response.

†Tachycardia is also related to incomplete inhibition of sympathetic ganglia and thus failure to inhibit reflex activation of the sympathetic nervous system following decrease in mean arterial pressure.

and parasympathetic nervous systems. Untoward responses are numerous and often severe (e.g., mydriasis, blurring of vision and photophobia, dryness of mouth, constipation, decreased sweating, dizziness, and fainting). Ganglionic blocking agents may be useful to help diagnose pheochromocytoma tumors. These agents also produce a marked fall in arterial pressure by inhibiting sympathetic ganglionic innervation of the adrenal medulla and the gland's ability to release epinephrine into the systemic circulation. Ganglionic blocking agents are sometimes used for therapy of peripheral vascular disease and may be used as adjunct agents for therapy of severe hypertension. With these diseases, vasodilation and decreased peripheral resistance are desired. Establishing a proper and successful maintenance dose for these drugs requires close physician-patient cooperation.

Neuromuscular Blocking Agents

These agents diminish the ability of **skeletal muscle** to contract in response to neuronal impulses passing over **somatic nerves**. Nondepolarizing agents (e.g., curare) act as competitive antagonists and compete with acetylcholine for receptor sites. In contrast, depolarizing agents (e.g., succinylcholine) act as acetylcholine receptor agonists and produce persistent depolarization of the end-plate region, thereby preventing repolarization of the muscle membrane and inhibiting the ability of muscle to contract. Succinylcholine and ACh are both depolarizing agents and are additive for inhibition of transmission. Succinylcholine is not a substrate for acetylcholinesterase but is an excellent substrate for plasma cholinesterase. Either mechanism (nondepolarizing–competitive or depolarizing–noncompetitive) results in loss of skeletal muscle tone and, ultimately, flaccid muscle paralysis. **Tubocurarine chloride** (curare), **gallamine** (Flaxedil), **pancuronium**, and **succinylcholine** are muscle relaxants used primarily as adjuncts in general anesthesia. Comparison of the pharmacological properties of major neuromuscular blocking agents appears in Table 4–12.

Curare, which is obtained from various plants, particularly *Strychnos* species, was used for hundreds of years by Indians near the Amazon River as arrow poison for hunting or warfare. It causes skeletal muscle paralysis, resulting in death from asphyxiation. Curare must be used with care in patients with myasthenia gravis (decreased functional acetylcholine at skeletal muscle) or liver and renal dysfunction (impaired metabolism and excretion of curare).

Inhibition of acetylcholinesterase with drugs (e.g., neostigmine, edrophonium) will readily reverse neuromuscular blockade produced by competitive blocking agents, and reversal of neuromuscular inhibition should be complete within minutes. Curare may decrease arterial pressure by release of histamine from mast cells and is a weak ganglionic blocking agent.

There are no agents clinically available to antagonize neuromuscular inhi-

Table 4–12. COMPARISON OF NEUROMUSCULAR
BLOCKING AGENTS

Drug	Type of Inhibition	Reversal of Inhibition by Inhibition of Cholinesterase	Hydrolysis by Plasma Cholinesterase	Ganglionic Inhibition and Release of Histamine	Duration (Min)
Curare	Competitive	Yes	No	Yes	30–40
Gallamine	Competitive	Yes	No	No	25–30
Pancuronium	Competitive	Yes	No	No	15–25
Succinylcholine	Depolarize end-plate	No—inhibition increased	Yes	No	5–8

Initial depolarization of skeletal muscle will produce fasciculations (contracture of skeletal muscle), possibly causing (1) increase in intraocular pressure by contracting extraocular skeletal muscles, and (2) release of potassium into the systemic circulation, which on rare occasions may depress cardiac muscle.

bition produced by succinylcholine; however, this does not limit its use because it is usually short acting because of rapid hydrolysis and inactivation by pseudocholinesterase. Liver disease, genetic defects (resulting in low plasma levels of pseudocholinesterase), or prior exposure to organophosphate inhibitors of pseudocholinesterase cause functional plasma cholinesterase levels to be low. With low functional pseudocholinesterase, the duration of action and potency of succinylcholine are increased.

ADRENERGIC NERVOUS SYSTEM

Adrenergic Synapses

Norepinephrine (levarterenol) is the neurotransmitter synthesized, stored in synaptic vesicles, and released into the junction by adrenergic neuronal impulses at the postganglionic adrenergic site. At the postjunctional site, norepinephrine interacts with β_1 or α_1 adrenoceptors.

About 40 percent of the norepinephrine molecules released from the adrenergic nerve terminal are actively transported (amine I transport) back into the nerve terminal to be recycled for transmission. The majority, 60 percent of the molecules, diffuses into the systemic circulation and can be assayed in plasma (1 to 4 $\mu g/l$) or urine.

Epinephrine is synthesized, stored, and released into the venous circulation by adrenergic neuronal impulses originating from the greater splanchnic (sympathetic) nerves. As shown in Figure 4–1, there are no postganglionic fibers innervating the adrenal medulla. Neuronal innervation is ganglionic, and nicotinic-receptor agonists will release epinephrine into the venous circulation; ganglionic blocking agents will inhibit release of epinephrine. Epinephrine was the first neurohormone to be isolated (1909) by both Abel and Takamine. It is not a neurotransmitter, but epinephrine's potent pharmacological properties relate directly to the adrenergic nervous system.

Catecholamine Biosynthesis

Synthetic pathways for norepinephrine, epinephrine, and dopamine are outlined in Figure 4–4. Tyrosine is the amino acid precursor. Tyrosine hydroxylase is the rate-limiting enzyme in the synthetic sequence and its activity is controlled by negative feedback inhibition. Rate of synthesis of catecholamine neurotransmitters is regulated by frequency of neuronal firing, the higher the frequency (demand) the more rapidly the compounds are synthesized.

Catecholamine Metabolism

Most norepinephrine, epinephrine, and dopamine molecules are metabolized by monoamine oxidase and/or catechol-O-methyltransferase (see Figure 4–4). Monoamine oxidase is found in adrenergic nerve terminals and many tissues—primarily the liver. Large concentrations of the enzyme are found in the brain at sites where catecholamines are neurotransmitters. Monoamine oxidase deaminates catecholamines, thus rendering them inactive. Catechol-O-methyltransferase, found in many tissues and especially the liver, replaces the hydrogen of the 3-OH of catecholamines with a methyl group, markedly reducing the biological activity of catecholamines. Thus, several different metabolic products of catecholamines may be detected in plasma and urine.

During the past decade several sensitive and specific analytical procedures have been developed to quantify the concentration of catecholamines and their metabolic products in plasma and urine, i.e., high-performance liquid chromatography using electrochemical detection. A tumor of the adrenal medulla (pheochromocytoma) will greatly elevate plasma and urine concentrations of epinephrine and its metabolic products. Analytical assays for these compounds are used to facilitate diagnosis of the tumor.

Adrenergic Receptors

Adrenergic receptors (adrenoceptors), which are located presynaptically or postsynaptically, mediate the actions of the catecholamines: norepinephrine, epinephrine, dopamine, and a large number of synthetic analogs. **Postsynaptic receptor subtypes** include α_1, β_1, β_2, and the dopamine receptor

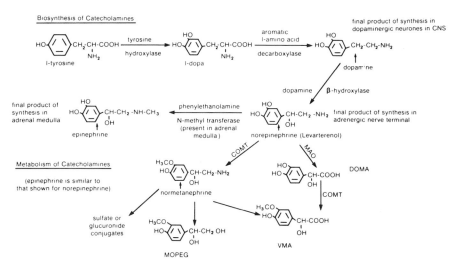

Figure 4–4. Pathways for synthesis and metabolism of catecholamines (norepinephrine, epinephrine, and dopamine).

Synthesis: Tyrosine is the major precursor amino acid for synthesis of catecholamines. Tyrosine hydroxylase appears to be the rate-limiting enzyme involved with synthesis. Rate of synthesis of L-dopa by tyrosine hydroxylase is controlled by the concentration of L-dopa and subsequent compounds in the synthetic sequence (negative feedback inhibition). Calcium ions appear to play a major role in regulation of tyrosine hydroxylase activity.

Metabolism: Epinephrine and norepinephrine undergo similar enzymatic alterations in structure. Both compounds are substrates for (1) MAO (monoamine oxidase), which is found in adrenergic nerve terminals, most postjunctional sites, and tissues throughout the body. Most compounds (including epinephrine, norepinephrine, and dopamine) that are not branched on the carbon (α) adjacent to the amino group undergo deamination and oxidation, yielding an acid analog that may or may not be reduced to the alcohol and (2) COMT (catechol-O-methyltransferase), which is found primarily in liver, methylates 3-OH of catecholamines. 3-Methoxy analogs of epinephrine, dopamine, and norepinephrine are much less active than parent compounds.

Since either or both enzymes may interact with a given molecule, several metabolic products (and nonmetabolized compounds) are found in plasma and urine. Chemical assay procedures have been developed to determine concentrations of cathecholamines and their metabolic products in plasma and urine.

COMT = Cathechol-O-methyltransferase (inhibited by pyrogallol or tropolone—not in clinical use); MAO = monoamine oxidase (inhibited by tranylcypromine, pargyline, and so forth); DOMA = 3,4-dihydroxymandelic acid; VMA = 3-methoxy-4-hydroxymandelic acid; MOPEG = 3-methoxy-4-hydroxyphenylethylglycol.

DA_1. α_1 Adrenoceptors are found on most smooth muscle, and stimulation of these receptors will cause vasoconstriction, among other effects. Although α_1 adrenoceptors have an excitatory action at most effector sites, they inhibit gastrointestinal motility. β_1 Adrenoceptors, which are excitatory, are located in heart and adipose tissue. By increasing the firing rate of the sinoatrial node, β_1-adrenoceptor stimulation increases heart rate. Other β_1-adrenoceptor–mediated effects include enhanced cardiac contractility and stimulation of lipolysis. β_2 Adrenoceptors, which are inhibitory, are widely distributed throughout the body and relax smooth muscle of bronchioles, intestines, uterus, and coronary and skeletal muscle arterioles. The dopamine receptor (DA_1) is inhibitory and causes vasodilation of renal and mesenteric arteries, resulting in increased blood flow to these organs.

While postsynaptic receptors directly mediate effects at specific organs or tissues, **presynaptic receptors** such as α_2 and the dopamine receptor DA_2 have an inhibitory modulating role on the ability of adrenergic neurons to release norepinephrine. These inhibitory receptors are located on sympathetic presynaptic nerve terminals and when stimulated, inhibit release of norepinephrine (negative feedback). Postsynaptic as well as presynaptic α_2 and D_2 receptors (dopamine) are present in brain. Central dopamine receptors, D_1 and D_2, appear to be the same as the peripheral dopamine receptors DA_1 and DA_2, respectively. The effects mediated by the adrenergic receptors are summarized in Table 4–13.

Drugs Acting on the Adrenergic Nervous System Effector Sites (Postjunctional)

Adrenoceptor Agonists—Postjunctional

This class of agents is widely used in clinical medicine, and their biological effects are often quite varied. In general, responses tend to mimic those of generalized sympathetic neuronal discharge: mydriasis; sweating; tachycardia; and increases in arterial pressure, skeletal muscle blood flow, blood glucose, and free fatty acids ("fight-or-flight" response).

Major Catecholamines. As **norepinephrine, epinephrine, dopamine,** and **isoproterenol** are widely used in clinical medicine, Table 4–14 is included for comparison of their pharmacological properties.

Receptor selectivity and anatomical distribution of adrenergic receptors determine biological responses of drugs. Following is a listing of receptors with which these catecholamines interact.

Drug	Receptors			
Epinephrine	α_1,	α_2,	β_1,	β_2
Norepinephrine	α_1,	α_2,	β_1	
Dopamine	α_1,	—,	β_1,	—, DA_1, DA_2*
Isoproterenol	—,	—,	β_1,	β_2

*Dopamine stimulates DA_2-receptors and inhibits adrenergic transmission only if the amine I transport system is inhibited with agents such as cocaine or tricyclic antidepressants. The reasons for this selectivity are unknown.

Table 4–13. ADRENERGIC RECEPTORS

α_1 **Adrenoceptor** (excitatory,* postsynaptic)
  Vasoconstriction (cutaneous, renal, etc.)
  Myocardial ectopic excitation
  Myometrial contraction
  Iris dilator contraction (mydriasis)
  Intestinal relaxation
  Pilomotor contraction
  Glycogenolysis (liver)
  Splenic contraction
  Ejaculation
α_2 **Adrenoceptor** (inhibitory, presynaptic†)
  Sympathetic nerve terminal—agonists decrease release of NE
β_1 **Adrenoceptor** (excitatory, postsynaptic)
  Increase heart rate (positive chronotropic action)
  Increase heart contractile force (positive inotropic action)
  Increase lipolysis
β_2 **Adrenoceptor** (inhibitory, postsynaptic)
  Skeletal muscle vasodilation ⎫
  Coronary vasodilation   ⎪
  Myometrium relaxation   ⎬ smooth muscle relaxation
  Bronchial relaxation   ⎪
  Intestinal relaxation   ⎪
  Ureter relaxation   ⎭
  Lower intraocular pressure
  Increase tremor associated with highly coordinated muscle movements
  Increased glycogenolysis (liver, skeletal muscle)
Dopamine (DA$_1$) Adrenoceptors** (inhibitory, postsynaptic)
  Vasodilation (renal, mesenteric)
Dopamine (DA$_2$) Adrenoceptors** (inhibitory, presynaptic)
  Sympathetic nerve terminal—agonists decrease release of NE

---

  *α_1 Receptors are inhibitory in the gastrointestinal tract, except for the sphincters.
  †Postsynaptic α_2 receptors are present in the CNS and some other sites.
  **Dopamine receptors are widely distributed in the CNS. DA$_1$ receptors and D$_1$ receptors (central) are similar; DA$_2$ receptors and D$_2$ receptors (central) appear to be the same.

Norepinephrine is primarily an α_1- and β_1-adrenoceptor agonist. The only clinical use, a very important one, is therapy of **shock**. Elevation of mean arterial pressure results from constriction of small arteries and veins (α_1), which is accompanied by an increase in peripheral resistance. Norepinephrine also increases force of cardiac contraction, resulting in increased cardiac output (β_1). Both physiological responses (increases in peripheral resistance and cardiac output) are the reasons for use of norepinephrine to treat shock. Norepi-

Table 4–14. COMPARISON OF PHARMACOLOGICAL
PROPERTIES OF EPINEPHRINE, NOREPINEPHRINE,
DOPAMINE, AND ISOPROTERENOL

	Epinephrine	Norepinephrine	Dopamine	Isoproterenol
Cardiac				
Heart rate	↑	↓,—	↑	↑↑↑
Stroke volume	↑↑	—,↓ (↑↑ shock)	—,↑	↑↑
Cardiac output	↑↑↑	—,↓ (↑↑ shock)	↑	↑
Arrhythmias	↑↑↑↑	↑↑↑	—	↑
Coronary flow	↑↑	↑↑↑ (↓ after β block)	↑↑	↑
Arterial Pressure				
Systolic arterial	↑↑↑	↑↑↑	↑↑	↓
Mean arterial	↑	↑↑	↑↑	↓
Diastolic arterial	↑,—,↓	↑↑	↑↑	↓↓
Peripheral Circulation				
Total peripheral resistance	↓	↑↑	↑↑	↓↓
Cerebral blood flow	↑	—,↓	—,↑	—
Skeletal muscle blood flow	↑↑	—,↓	—,↓	↑↑↑
Cutaneous blood flow	↓↓	↑,—,↓	—	—
Renal blood flow	↓↓	↑,—,↓	↑↑↑	—
Splanchnic blood flow	↑↑,—,↓	—,↑	↑↑	↑
Metabolic Effects				
O₂ consumption	↑↑	—,↑	—	↑
Blood sugar	↑↑↑	—,↑	—	↑
Blood lactic acid	↑↑↑	—,↑	—	↑
Central Nervous System				
Subjective sensation	↑	—,↑	—	—

↑ = increase.
— = no change.
↓ = decrease.

nephrine is the most active vasopressor for therapy of severe shock. Heart rate will show little change because the increase in mean arterial pressure triggers the baroreceptor reflex. Norepinephrine is compatible with a wide range of intravenous fluids. It is administered **only** by intravenous infusion following dilution (approximately 4 mg/l of fluid). The rate of infusion is adjusted according to response of arterial pressure. Great care must be exercised with catheter placement or removal to prevent the solution containing norepinephrine from coming into contact with nonvascular tissue and inducing intense local vasoconstriction and tissue anoxia. Catheters should be placed in large veins and moved every 2 to 3 days to prevent damage to the vessels.

Epinephrine is a very potent drug, and biological responses are complex but relate directly to sensitivity and anatomical location of adrenoceptors. β₁ and β_2 adrenoceptors are extremely sensitive to epinephrine. Very low concentrations of this drug will increase force of cardiac contractions and induce tachycardia (β_1), resulting in increased cardiac output, relaxing various smooth muscles (β_2), and increasing blood flow to skeletal muscle (vasodilation—β_2).

Epinephrine is ineffective when administered orally but may be administered by parenteral routes and inhalation. Great care must be exercised with intravenous administration. The compound must be diluted and administered very slowly. A common formulation of epinephrine is a 1 ml vial containing a 1:1000 dilution (1 mg). For intravenous injection 0.2 to 0.3 ml are diluted to 10 ml and this diluted solution is injected slowly intravenously. Do not forget that injection of 1 ml of epinephrine (1 mg) would be expected to be fatal.

Important therapeutic applications for epinephrine involving β-adrenoceptors would include relaxation of bronchial smooth muscle in therapy of asthma (usually administered by inhalation) and cardiac stimulant for reintroducing heart beat. Epinephrine is the drug of choice for therapy of anaphylactic shock. When the concentration of epinephrine is increased approximately 10-fold, α_1 adrenoceptors are also stimulated. Epinephrine is a very potent vasoconstrictor agent (α_1) and is often added to solutions of local anesthetic agents (administered subcutaneously or intramuscularly) to increase their duration of action and decrease their rate of absorption into the systemic circulation, thus diminishing the chance of cardiac or central nervous system toxicity. Epinephrine is often applied to surface wounds to decrease oozing of blood. Even though epinephrine increases cardiac output and constricts arteries and veins, it is not useful for therapy of shock (other than anaphylactic) owing to the intense constriction of renal arteries and diminished renal function. For therapy of shock, dopamine and norepinephrine have pharmacological properties that are superior to those of epinephrine.

Isoproterenol (Isuprel) stimulates only β_1 and β_2 adrenoceptors. Its major therapeutic use is relaxation of bronchial smooth muscle (β_2) in asthma. Even though the compound is normally administered by inhalation of a mist, systemic absorption occurs and tachycardia is often observed (same for epinephrine). The compound is a potent cardiac stimulant and sometimes is used in therapy of heart block (impaired A-V conduction).

Dopamine stimulates α_1 and β_1 adrenoceptors and elevates arterial pressure and is widely used for therapy of many types of shock. The compound is not as active as norepinephrine as a vasopressor agent. Dopamine stimulates α_1 and β_1 adrenoceptors by two mechanisms: (1) direct stimulation of the aforementioned receptors and (2) release of norepinephrine from adrenergic nerve terminals, which then stimulates α_1 and β_1 adrenoceptors. In addition, dopamine dilates renal blood vessels (DA_1) and increases renal blood flow. Enhanced renal blood flow facilitates elimination of metabolic products and diminishes the likelihood of acidosis. Dopamine is administered by intravenous infusion. Since the compound is about one-twentieth as active as norepinephrine, larger quantities of the drug must be used to support arterial pressure.

Dopamine is the only available vasopressor agent that dilates renal arteries and by this mechanism facilitates renal blood flow.

Other Adrenergic-Receptor Agonists. Many analogs of the catecholamines have been introduced into clinical medicine. Major drugs and significant clinical uses are shown in Table 4–15. Orally effective agents are available for therapy of asthma, i.e., **albuterol, terbutaline, metaproterenol,** and **ephedrine** (see Chapter 13). Long-acting vasopressor agents (**metaraminol, methoxamine,** and **mephentermine**) are often administered prior to spinal anesthesia to prevent hypotension resulting from inhibition of adrenergic neuronal outflow from the spinal cord. The use of these agents for therapy of shock is restricted because their major action is vasoconstriction and they have minimal or no efficacy to increase cardiac output.

Dobutamine is administered by intravenous infusion to increase cardiac output and function. Little or no tachycardia is observed. Thus, the compound is quite selective for stimulating β_1 adrenoceptors associated with cardiac contractility. Dobutamine is used to increase cardiac output in patients with congestive heart failure.

Amphetamine is a potent stimulant of the CNS. The compound is a vasopressor resulting from direct stimulation of α_1 and β_1 adrenoceptors. The compound also releases norepinephrine from adrenergic nerve terminals. The agent has been used to treat chronic hypotension and enhance pain relief when used in conjunction with analgesic agents such as morphine. There is no evidence that amphetamine effectively controls weight when used over a period of a few months. Because amphetamine impairs judgment and coordination, its administration in patients who will operate machinery (e.g., automobiles) is dangerous. In the CNS, amphetamine releases norepinephrine and dopamine from their respective neurons.

Ephedrine was isolated in 1925 from the Chinese herb Ma Huang and is quite a unique drug. It produces considerable increase in cardiac output, elevates arterial pressure, and is a mild stimulant of the CNS. It stimulates β_1, β_2, and α_1 adrenoceptors by direct action and also by releasing norepinephrine from adrenergic nerve terminals. Ephedrine is effective orally and is a mild dilator of bronchial smooth muscle (β_2), but it is much less active than isoproterenol, epinephrine, or terbutaline. **Ephedrine** may be less effective with repeated administration, an occurrence that is known as **tachyphylaxis.** One explanation for tachyphylaxis is that ephedrine and a number of similar compounds replace norepinephrine within synaptic vesicles (adrenergic nerve terminals), and when released into the junction, ephedrine and similar compounds are less effective at postjunctional receptors than is norepinephrine. These chemicals have been termed "**false transmitters.**" Another mechanism to produce a false transmitter is to introduce a chemical into the synthetic sequence of norepinephrine (see Fig. 4–4), for example, α-methyldopa (Aldomet) in place of dopa, resulting in synthesis of α-methylnorepinephrine, which is about one-tenth as active as norepinephrine at α_1 and β_1 adrenoceptors.

Adrenoceptor Antagonists—Postjunctional

Therapeutic agents have now been developed that inhibit α_1, β_1, and β_2 adrenoceptors. Specific drugs are outlined in the following sections.

α_1-**Adrenergic Antagonists.** There are a variety of adrenergic blocking agents, and their therapeutic applications depend on site of action, receptor selectivity, and mechanism of action. Most therapeutic applications of these agents relate to inhibition of α_1 adrenoceptors, resulting in vasodilation and diminished mean arterial pressure.

Noncompetitive Antagonists. Agents such as **phenoxybenzamine** alkylate α_1 adrenoceptors and inhibit amine I transport following formation of an intermediate cyclic derivative. The duration of action is approximately 24 hours. The compound may be administered orally or intravenously. Like most α_1-adrenoceptor blockers, phenoxybenzamine is prone to induce tachycardia, which results from reflex activation of the adrenergic nervous system (owing to decrease in mean arterial pressure) and the compound's failure to inhibit β_1 adrenoceptors in the heart. Noncompetitive α_1-adrenoceptor antagonists are not widely used in clinical medicine, but may be used as an adjunct drug in therapy of severe hypertension.

Competitive Antagonists. These drugs may be specific inhibitors of α_1 adrenoceptors (e.g., **prazosin**) or they may inhibit both α_1 and α_2 adrenoceptors (e.g., **phentolamine** and **tolazoline**). Prazosin was recently introduced for therapy of hypertension (see Chapter 9) and represents a definite advance for therapeutic application. One important reason is that patients receiving prazosin will have little or no tachycardia. The site involved for inhibition of the expected reflex tachycardia is unknown, but prazosin does not inhibit cardiac β_1 adrenoceptors. The compound is effective orally and has considerable duration of action (12 hours). **Phentolamine** (Regitine) and **tolazoline** (Priscoline) inhibit α_1 and α_2 adrenoceptors with approximately the same efficacy. Therapeutic use relates to α_1-adrenoceptor inhibition. These agents are relatively short acting (1 to 2 hours) and are administered parenterally. Phentolamine (Regitine) is more active than tolazoline and has virtually replaced tolazoline as the therapeutic agent of choice.

Phentolamine (Regitine) is also used as an aid in the diagnosis of pheochromocytoma tumor of the adrenal medulla. This tumor is associated with very high plasma concentrations of epinephrine, which produce tachycardia and elevated arterial pressure. With administration of phentolamine, α_1 adrenoceptors (vasoconstrictors) are promptly inhibited, resulting in marked hypotension. In addition, circulating epinephrine stimulates β_2 adrenoceptors in the vascular beds of skeletal muscle (vasodilator), causing an additive hypoten-

Table 4–15. ADRENERGIC RECEPTOR AGONISTS

Phenyl ring (positions 3, 2 / 4, 5) — $C_\beta(H)(OH)$ — $C_\alpha(H)$ — $N(H)(R)$

Drug	3,2 / 4,5	β	α	R	Receptors	Routes of Administration	Major Clinical Usage
Epinephrine	3,4 *di*-OH	OH	H	CH$_3$	β_1, β_2, α_1	IV infusion, parenteral, aerosol	Anaphylactic shock, relax bronchial smooth muscle, local vasoconstriction, mydriatic
Norepinephrine	3,4 *di*-OH	OH	H	H	β_1, α_1	IV infusion	Vasopressor
Dopamine	3,4 *di*-OH	H	H	H	β_1, α_1, DA$_1$	IV infusion	Vasopressor
Dobutamine	3,4 *di*-OH	H	H	R*	β_1	IV infusion	↑ force cardiac contraction, ↑ cardiac output
Isoproterenol	3,4 *di*-OH	OH	H	—HC(CH$_3$)CH$_3$	β_1, β_2	Aerosol, parenteral	Relax bronchial smooth muscle, cardiac stimulant (A-V block)
Metaproterenol	3,5 *di* OH	OH	H	—HC(CH$_3$)CH$_3$	β_1, β_2	Aerosol (powder), oral	Relax bronchial smooth muscle

Name					Receptor	Route	Use
Terbutaline	3,5 *di* OH	OH	H	—C(CH$_3$)$_3$	β$_1$, β$_2$	Parenteral, oral, aerosol	Relax bronchial smooth muscle
Metaraminol	3-OH	OH	CH$_3$	H	α$_1$, β$_1$	Parenteral, oral, IV infusion	Vasopressor
Phenylephrine	3-OH	OH	H	CH$_3$	α$_1$	Nasal, ophthalmic, parenteral	Nasal decongestant, vasopressor, local vasoconstrictor, mydriatic
Tyramine	4-OH	H	H	H	†	IV infusion	No clinical use
Methoxamine	2,5 *di* OCH$_3$	OH	CH$_3$	H	α$_1$	IM, IV infusion	Vasopressor
Albuterol	3—CH$_2$OH, 4—OH	OH	H	—C(CH$_3$)$_3$	β$_2$	Oral, aerosol	Relax bronchial smooth muscle
Amphetamine	—	H	CH$_3$	CH$_3$	α$_1$, β$_1$**	Oral	CNS stimulant, narcolepsy
Ephedrine	—	OH	CH$_3$	CH$_3$	α$_1$, β$_1$, β$_2$**	Ophthalmic, oral, parenteral, nasal	Vasopressor, mydriatic, nasal decongestant, relax bronchial smooth muscle, CNS stimulant
Mephentermine	—	OH	CH$_3$	H	α$_1$**	Parenteral	Vasopressor

$$*R = -\overset{\text{H}}{\underset{\text{CH}_3}{\overset{|}{\underset{|}{C}}}} -(CH_2)_2- \text{—OH}$$

†Tyramine releases norepinephrine from adrenergic nerve terminals, thus indirectly stimulating α$_1$ and β$_1$ adrenoceptors.

**Also releases norepinephrine from adrenergic nerve terminals.

sive response. Thus, hypotension induced by phentolamine is much more severe in patients with a tumor of the adrenal medulla than in patients with essential hypertension. This clinical procedure is known as the "Regitine test."

Ergot alkaloids (derivatives of **lysergic acid**) were originally derived from a fungus (*Claviceps purpurea*) that grows on rye. Throughout history, numerous outbreaks of ergot poisoning have resulted from people eating bread made from contaminated grain. Ancient Greek writings from 400 to 300 B.C., in a probable reference to ergot-induced abortion, mention "noxious grasses that cause pregnant women to drop the womb."[27] In later epidemics, appropriately named St. Anthony's fire, additional manifestations of ergot poisoning were noted, including CNS stimulation, convulsions, burning sensations, and blackening of the extremities, as if the limbs were on fire. Actually, the blackening was gangrene secondary to intense vasoconstriction induced by the ergot alkaloids. Poisoning by these agents is called "ergotism" and is now extremely rare owing to modern milling of grain. Many biologically active alkaloids have been isolated from fungus-contaminated rye, and a number of these complex chemical structures serve as intermediates for synthetic derivatives. Parent alkaloids or synthetic derivatives may be potent stimulants or inhibitors of serotonin receptors, dopamine-receptor agonists (e.g., **pergolide** and **bromocriptine**), α_1-adrenoceptor antagonists (e.g., **ergonovine** and **ergotamine**), direct smooth muscle stimulants (musculotropic) (e.g., ergonovine and ergotamine), and agents that stimulate the CNS or are hallucinogens that are synthetic derivatives of lysergic acid (**LSD-25**). **Histamine** was first isolated from contaminated rye, and its original name was ergamine.

Table 4–16 shows the structures, major biological properties, and clinical utilities of some derivatives of lysergic acid. Note the wide variation in pharmacological properties. Even though **ergonovine** and **ergotamine** are α_1-adrenoceptor antagonists and vasodilation would be expected, direct vascular smooth muscle stimulation (musculotropic) predominates, resulting in vasoconstriction. Thus, clinical use of these two drugs relates to their ability to stimulate smooth muscle. **Ergonovine** is used to prevent postpartum bleeding by contracting uterine smooth muscle (**oxytocic**). **Ergotamine,** usually combined with caffeine, has been used for decades to abort onset of migraine headaches. It is believed that the use of ergotamine relates to vasoconstrictor action of distended cerebral blood vessels. Dosage of ergotamine must not exceed the recommended amount, because of possible damage to entima of blood vessels resulting in increased frequency of clot formation.

β-Adrenoceptor Antagonists. The discovery of **propranolol** by Sir James Black in England allowed several major therapeutic advances. The compound was originally introduced into therapy as an antiarrhythmic agent in the early 1960s. In 1966 Dr. Franz Gross in Germany first reported that propranolol lowered arterial pressure in **hypertensive** individuals. The compound re-

Table 4–16. DERIVATIVES OF LYSERGIC ACID
(ERGOT DERIVATIVES)

Compound		Major Biological Response	Major Clinical Application
Lysergic acid	R = —COOH	None	None
LSD-25	$R = -\overset{\overset{O}{\|\|}}{C}-N(C_2H_5)_2$	Hallucinogenic, inhibits serotonin receptors (peripheral), stimulates serotonin receptors (central)	None
Ergonovine	$R = -\overset{O}{\underset{}{C}}-\overset{H}{\underset{}{N}}-\overset{H}{\underset{CH_3}{C}}-CH_2OH$	Stimulates smooth muscle (uterine), inhibits α_1 adrenoceptors	Prevents postpartum bleeding
Metergoline	$R = -CH_2-\overset{H}{N}-\overset{O}{\underset{}{C}}-OCH_2-\bigcirc$	Inhibits serotonin receptors (S_1 and S_2)	Experimental
Ergotamine	$R = -\overset{O}{\underset{}{C}}-\overset{}{\underset{H}{N}} \cdots$ (ergotamine structure) $R'\,CH_3;\ R'' = -CH_2-\bigcirc$	Stimulates smooth muscle, inhibits α_1 adrenoceptors	Migraine headaches
Bromocriptine	R = Same as ergotamine $R' = -CH(CH_3)_2$ $R'' = -CH_2CH(CH_3)_2$ 2-BR	Dopamine-receptor (D_2, DA_2) agonist, inhibits D_1 receptors	Parkinson's disease, hypotensive, lowers intraocular pressure

103

ceived final FDA approval as an antihypertensive drug in December 1976, and its use as an antihypertensive agent soon became widespread (see Chapter 9).

Dr. Al Lands and coworkers reported in 1967 that β adrenoceptors existed in different functional forms, which they designated as β_1 and β_2 adrenoceptors. (For biological responses of these receptors, see Table 4–13.) With the demonstration that propranolol was equally effective as an inhibitor of both β_1 and β_2 adrenoceptors, research efforts were then directed toward development of agents that were selective inhibitors of β_1 adrenoceptors and also agents with longer duration of action. Agents that are selective inhibitors of β_1 adrenoceptors are (1) effective hypotensive agents and (2) less prone to induce constriction of bronchial smooth muscle in patients with asthma. For comparisons of major β-adrenoceptor antagonists, see Table 4–17.

Several β-adrenoceptor antagonists (e.g., **timolol, metoprolol,** and **propranolol**) have been shown to be effective prophylactic agents to prevent recurrence of **myocardial infarction.** Timolol was the original agent to be evaluated in an extensive study in Norway involving 5000 patients. β-Adrenoceptor blocking agents **lower intraocular pressure** following corneal application, and timolol (Timoptic) is widely used for therapy of glaucoma. Whether the mechanism of action is related to β-receptor inhibition is unknown because the *d*-isomer, which is nearly inactive as a β-adrenoceptor antagonist, is an effective agent to lower intraocular pressure in experimental animals.

Frequency of adverse reactions varies considerably from patient to patient. Several agents such as propranolol and metoprolol have definite involvements of the CNS. **Ataxia** and **dizziness** are quite common with these agents, especially with initial therapy. Patients must be alerted to these possibilities. **Nadolol** and **atenolol** produce few CNS side effects, which is probably related to their diminished ability to cross the blood-brain barrier. β-Adrenoceptor antagonists must be used with caution in patients with cardiac insufficiency. The possibility of inducing cardiac failure must be considered. Inhibition of cardiac β_1 adrenoceptors will decrease heart rate, decrease force of cardiac contraction, and cause some decrease in cardiac output.

β-Adrenoceptor inhibitors are widely used for **therapy of hypertension.** They may be used in conjunction with diuretics or with a number of other antihypertensive agents. Chapter 9 outlines physiological factors involved in hypertension and therapeutic responses of β-receptor blocking agents.

Drugs Acting on the Adrenergic Nerve Terminal (Prejunctional)

Drugs may increase or inhibit adrenergic neurotransmission by several mechanisms, which are outlined here.

Facilitation of Adrenergic Transmission—Prejunctional

Several mechanisms have been identified that may stimulate transmission. These are shown in Figure 4–5.

Inhibitors of Amine I Transport. Active transport (amine I) of norepinephrine into nerve terminals helps remove the neurotransmitter from the synapse. Agents such as cocaine or tricyclic antidepressants that inhibit amine I transport increase the concentration of norepinephrine within the junction, which enhances responses associated with adrenergic transmission (vasoconstriction, tachycardia, mydriases, and so on). Cocaine and tricyclic antidepressants inhibit entry of all compounds actively transported into the adrenergic nerve terminal, such as ephedrine, dopamine, norepinephrine, epinephrine, and tyramine. Inhibition of amine I transport in the adrenergic nerve terminal is of no therapeutic value but may be a major consideration for drug interactions and is of toxicological importance. In the CNS, antidepressant activity of tricyclic derivatives is associated with inhibition of reuptake of serotonin, norepinephrine, and dopamine into their respective neurons, which increases the concentrations of the neurotransmitters within their respective synapses.

α_2-**Adrenoceptor Blocking Agents.** There are no approved drugs that are selective inhibitors for prejunctional α_2 adrenoceptors. Since α_2-adrenoceptor activation by norepinephrine decreases the release of norepinephrine into the junction and thus serves as the final control system involved in regulation of the adrenergic nervous system, inhibition of α_2 adrenoceptors (autoreceptors) will facilitate release of norepinephrine from adrenergic nerve terminals. The alkaloid **yohimbine** is widely used in the experimental laboratory, but unfortunately humans have many adverse reactions to yohimbine involving the CNS. Selective α_2-receptor antagonists, when they become available, may be useful in therapy of shock by facilitating adrenergic neuronal transmission.

Dopamine (DA$_2$) Adrenoceptor Blocking Agents. Dopamine adrenoceptors (DA$_2$) are found on adrenergic nerve terminals (see Fig. 4–5). Stimulation of DA$_2$ receptors produces functional responses that are very similar to stimulation of α_2 adrenoceptors, e.g., stimulation of either receptor produces inhibition of norepinephrine release. Sensitivity of both α_2 and DA$_2$ adrenoceptors to their respective agonists depends heavily on frequency of neuronal firing; at lower frequencies the agonists are more active. Haloperidol, chlorpromazine, and related antipsychotic agents facilitate release of norepinephrine in the peripheral nervous system by inhibiting DA$_2$ adrenoceptors, but they are also α_1-adrenoceptor antagonists which diminish adrenergic-induced responses.

Dopamine is not an agonist of DA$_2$ adrenoceptors unless the amine I transport system is inhibited by agents such as cocaine or tricyclic antidepressants. These transport inhibitors do not alter DA$_2$-receptor agonist activity of synthetic derivatives, such as apomorphine, bromocriptine, and pergolide.

Norepinephrine Releasing Agents. Many phenylethylamine derivatives,

Table 4–17. β-ADRENERGIC ANTAGONISTS

Compound	Structure	Relative Potency	Daily Dosage Frequency for Hypertension (No. of Doses per Day)	Major Clinical Use
1. Inhibitors of β$_1$ and β$_2$ Adrenoceptors (Nonselective)				
Propranolol		1.0	2–3	Antihypertensive, antiarrhythmic, angina pectoris, migraine headache
Nadolol		0.5	1	Antihypertensive
Pindolol		7.0	2–3	Antihypertensive

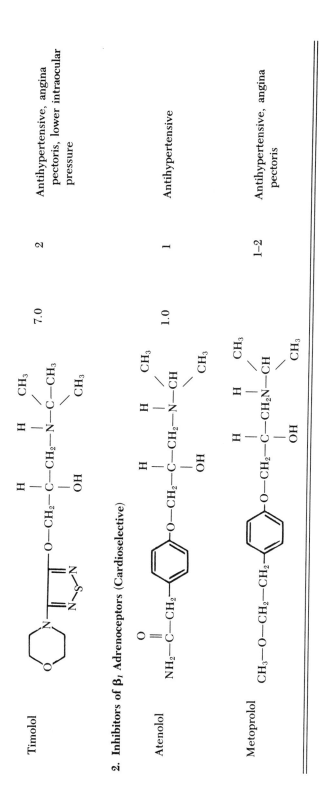

Timolol   7.0   2   Antihypertensive, angina pectoris, lower intraocular pressure

2. Inhibitors of β_1 Adrenoceptors (Cardioselective)

Atenolol   1.0   1   Antihypertensive

Metoprolol   1-2   Antihypertensive, angina pectoris

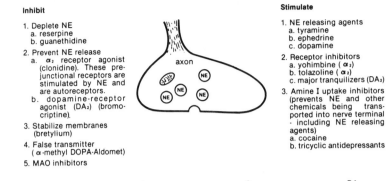

Inhibit

1. Deplete NE
   a. reserpine
   b. guanethidine
2. Prevent NE release
   a. α_2 receptor agonist (clonidine). These pre-junctional receptors are stimulated by NE and are autoreceptors.
   b. dopamine-receptor agonist (DA$_2$) (bromo-criptine).
3. Stabilize membranes (bretylium)
4. False transmitter (α -methyl DOPA-Aldomet)
5. MAO inhibitors

Stimulate

1. NE releasing agents
   a. tyramine
   b. ephedrine
   c. dopamine
2. Receptor inhibitors
   a. yohimbine (α_2)
   b. tolazoline (α_2)
   c. major tranquilizers (DA$_2$)
3. Amine I uptake inhibitors (prevents NE and other chemicals being transported into nerve terminal - including NE releasing agents)
   a. cocaine
   b. tricyclic antidepressants

α_1		β_1		β_2		DA$_1$	
Stimulate	Inhibit	Stimulate	Inhibit	Stimulate	Inhibit	Stimulate	Inhibit
NE	tolazoline	Epi	propranolol	Epi	propranolol	dopamine	experimental
EPI (Hi conc)	prazosin	NE	metoprolol	Isu	metoprolol		compounds only
phenylephrine		Isu		terbutaline			
dopamine		dopamine					
many long							
acting compds.							

Figure 4–5. Summary of major drugs that facilitate (stimulate) or inhibit adrenergic neuronal transmission.

Nerve terminal (Prejunctional): Drugs that stimulate will increase the concentration of norepinephrine within the junction. Mechanisms involve (a) norepinephrine releasing agents, e.g., tyramine; (b) inhibition of α_2-adrenoceptors, thus preventing negative feedback stimulation by norepinephrine; (c) inhibition of amine I transport system, which removes a major mechanism by which norepinephrine is removed from the junction; and (d) inhibition of dopamine (DA$_2$)-adrenoceptors.

Drugs may inhibit the adrenergic nerve terminal by several mechanisms, including (a) "false-transmitters;" (b) lowering norepinephrine concentrations within synaptic vesicles by depleting agents, e.g., reserpine; (c) stimulating α_2-adrenoceptors, e.g., clonidine, or DA$_2$-adrenoceptors, e.g., bromocriptine. Activation of either receptor will decrease the amount of norepinephrine released into the junction.

Postjunctional: Receptors include α_1, β_1, β_2, and DA$_1$. Stimulation of these receptors by specific drugs will induce physiological responses corresponding to those outlined in Table 4–13. Inhibition of receptors by their respective blockers has wide applications in therapeutics.

NE = norepinephrine (levarterenol); Epi = epinephrine; Isu = Isuprel (isoproterenol).

e.g., **tyramine, dopamine,** and **ephedrine,** are transported into the adrenergic nerve terminal by the amine I transport system. These agents displace norepinephrine from its storage sites and increase the concentration of norepinephrine at adrenergic transmission sites. Thus, these agents are known as "releasing" agents. **Tyramine** is not used clinically but is widely used experimentally and acts only as a releasing agent. It has been estimated that 85 percent of the sympathomimetic effects of **ephedrine** results from its ability to release norepinephrine. Tricyclic anti-depressants and cocaine will antagonize ephedrine and dopamine or completely inhibit biological responses of tyramine.

Inhibition of Adrenergic Transmission—Prejunctional

Development of agents that inhibit adrenergic neuronal transmission has led to the introduction of several classes of drugs that are useful for therapy of hypertension; the more widely used drugs are shown in Figure 4–5. Mechanisms of action include (1) α_2-adrenoceptor agonists (e.g., clonidine), (2) depletion of norepinephrine stored within synaptic vesicles (e.g., reserpine), (3) DA_2-receptor agonists (e.g., bromocriptine), and (4) false transmitters (e.g., α-methyldopa).

α_2-**Adrenoceptor Agonists. Clonidine** and **guanabenz** are potent agonists of α_2 adrenoceptors on adrenergic nerve terminals and inhibit the ability of adrenergic neuronal impulses to release norepinephrine. However, most investigators believe that the site for hypotensive action of these agents is the CNS (see Chapter 9). Since the compounds are hypotensive following depletion of norepinephrine stores by reserpine or destruction of adrenergic neurons by the neurotoxin 6-hydroxydopamine, α_2 adrenoceptors involved with the control of arterial pressure and site of action for these agents may be postjunctional within the CNS. The exact site is unknown but may involve nucleus tractus solitarius.

Clonidine and guanabenz decrease mean arterial pressure and atrial rate, which is consistent with decreased frequency of adrenergic neuronal action potentials. Plasma levels of norepinephrine are reduced. There is little or no alteration of plasma renin activity. Postural hypotension is rare and probably relates to neuronal frequency specificity, which these drugs exhibit. When an individual changes from a supine to an upright position, the frequency of adrenergic neuronal action potentials increases (counteracting pooling of blood in lower extremities), and with higher frequency of neuronal firing the compounds will be less effective as agonists of α_2 adrenoceptors, thereby promoting redistribution of blood.

Adverse reactions to these agents are frequent and include sedation; xerostomia; anorexia; fluid retention, which may be prevented with simultaneous use of diuretics; vivid dreams; and stimulation of the CNS. Many adverse reactions will diminish or disappear after 2 to 4 weeks of therapy. Drugs should be withdrawn slowly to prevent hypertensive crisis and various CNS-related responses.

α-**Methyldopa** is an antihypertensive agent that enters adrenergic neurons both centrally and peripherally. The compound partially replaces **dopa** in the synthetic sequence leading to synthesis of norepinephrine (see Fig. 4–4). α-**Methylnorepinephrine (MNE)**, instead of norepinephrine, is synthesized and stored in synaptic vesicles. MNE has been termed a "false transmitter," as it is released from adrenergic neurons and has less efficacy than norepinephrine as an agonist of α_1 and β_1 adrenoceptors. However, MNE is also a potent agonist of α_2 adrenoceptors, and the preponderance of evidence indicates that the hypotensive action of MNE results from stimulation of α_2 adrenoceptors within the CNS, resulting in decreased frequency of adrenergic neuronal impulses. This is consistent with an observed decrease in peripheral resistance and some decrease in heart rate. Reductions in mean arterial pressure are more pronounced in an individual who is standing than in one who is supine.

Side effects may include sedation, postural hypotension, dizziness, sleep disturbances, impotence, dry mouth, and nasal congestion. After 1 to 2 weeks of therapy many of these side effects diminish. Chronic therapy may result in a positive Coombs' test result (10 to 20 percent), hemolytic anemia, leukopenia, hepatitis, lupus-like responses, and many other adverse responses. Patients receiving α-methyldopa must be monitored closely.

Norepinephrine-Depleting Agents in Adrenergic Nerve Terminals. Reserpine and **guanethidine** reduce concentrations of norepinephrine in synaptic vesicles (see Fig. 4–5), thus decreasing the amount of norepinephrine released into the synapse. Decreased peripheral resistance and bradycardia are observed.

Reserpine was introduced into Western medicine more than 30 years ago. The alkaloid was isolated from *Rauwolfia serpentina*, a plant that grows in India. Roots of this plant have been used in herbal medicine for thousands of years.

Reserpine depletes stores of biogenic amines (epinephrine, norepinephrine, dopamine, and serotonin) in both the central and peripheral nervous systems. Reserpine is a very potent, orally effective drug that has a long duration of action. With parenteral administration, reserpine initially releases norepinephrine from adrenergic nerve terminals, but after 5 to 6 hours reduction in norepinephrine concentrations can be detected, with maximal reduction occurring within 24 hours. Following oral administration, reserpine does not release norepinephrine, and only reductions in plasma norepinephrine and epinephrine concentrations are observed. Several weeks may be required to produce maximal hypotensive response. Reserpine lowers mean arterial pressure, and bradycardia may be marked.

Adverse effects of reserpine usually relate to the CNS. Sedation is observed, possibly accompanied by depression: Patients receiving reserpine have an increased incidence of suicide. Because reserpine decreases the threshold for electroshock, the drug must be withdrawn for 2 weeks prior to administering electroshock therapy. Reserpine stimulates gastrointestinal motility (resulting from elevated tissue concentration of ACh), which increases the incidence of ulcers.

Guanethidine (Ismelin) is an orally effective antihypertensive agent that is usually reserved for therapy of more severely elevated arterial pressures.

The compound is transported into adrenergic neurons by amine I transport; thus, the hypotensive activity can be antagonized by agents that inhibit transport, i.e., cocaine or tricyclic antidepressants. Neuronal inhibition results from

1. Stabilization of neuronal membranes that interfere with release of norepinephrine (this response occurs within a few minutes following exposure of the membrane to guanethidine)
2. Chronic administration of guanethidine, which decreases the concentration of norepinephrine within synaptic vesicles of adrenergic nerve terminals

Minimal effects are observed involving other biogenic amines, i.e., epinephrine and dopamine. Guanethidine has minimal effects involving the CNS. The compound does not readily pass the blood-brain barrier.

The past 30 years have seen the development of numerous drugs, acting by different mechanisms, that decrease biological functions associated with the adrenergic nervous system. Prior to the development of these drugs there were no effective agents for therapy of hypertension. Introductions of these agents for therapy of hypertension represent dramatic advances in science and clinical medicine.

CHAPTER 5

Drugs Acting on the Central Nervous System (CNS)

R. K. BHATNAGAR, Ph.D.,

G. R. DUTTON, Ph.D., and

G. F. GEBHART, Ph.D.

ANTIANXIETY AND SEDATIVE-HYPNOTIC DRUGS

These drugs are used to alleviate the effects of anxiety and sleep disorders, as adjuncts to anesthesia, as preoperative aids, in the treatment of alcohol withdrawal, in epilepsy and other seizure disorders, and as muscle relaxants in specific neuromuscular disorders (Table 5–1). Benzodiazepines are the most commonly prescribed drugs for anxiety and insomnia, largely be-

Table 5-1. ELIMINATION HALF-LIVES AND THERAPEUTIC
USES OF SOME COMMON BENZODIAZEPINES

Name	Elimination Half-Life* (Hours)	Active Metabolites	Therapeutic Uses
Diazepam (Valium)	50-90 (Long)	nordiazepam oxazepam	anxiolytic preoperative cardioversion endoscopy status epilepticus skeletal muscle spasms hallucinogen toxicity acute alcohol withdrawal
Flurazepam (Dalmane)	50-100 (Long)	hydroxyethyl-flurazepam desalkylflurazepam hydroxyflurazepam	hypnotic
Chlordiazepoxide (Librium)	7-100 (Long)	desmethylchlordiaz-epoxide demoxepam oxazepam	acute alcohol withdrawal anxiolytic
Clonazepam (Clonopin)	20-30 (Long)	none (7-amino-clonazepam is inactive)	seizures (petit mal, myo-clonic, akinetic) status epilepticus
Oxazepam (Serax)	6-24 (Intermediate)	none, directly glucuronidated	hypnotic anxiolytic
Lorazepam (Ativan)	10-20 (Short)	none, directly glucuronidated	hypnotic preoperative anxiolytic
Temazepam (Restoril)	10-20 (Short)	oxazepam	hypnotic
Triazolam (Halcion)	2-4 (Short)	hydroxytriazolam	hypnotic

*Ranges include active metabolite half-lives.

cause of their relative safety. They have a **high therapeutic index,** low risk of physical dependence, low incidence of interaction with other drugs, and lack of life-threatening withdrawal symptoms. The barbiturates and other classes of sedative-hypnotics are also used for these purposes, albeit less frequently.

While operating *via* different mechanisms of action, antianxiety and sedative-hypnotic agents have the same four major, dose-dependent pharmacological properties: sedative-hypnotic, anxiolytic, anticonvulsant, and muscle relaxant. Not all agents are equally desirable for clinical use in all of these situations, because of liabilities associated with their CNS depressant effects. The benzodiazepines, barbiturates, and other minor groups (the piperidinediones, carbamates, quinazolines and cyclic ethers) are considered here.

As discussed in Chapter 4, the central nervous system (CNS), comprising the brain and spinal cord, receives sensory information from the peripheral nervous system *via* afferent neurons, and returns both voluntary and involuntary commands to muscles and organs *via* efferent neurons. Disorders of the central nervous system can impair the workings both of the body (seizures, movement disorders such as parkinsonism) and of the mind (psychoses, affective disorders, anxiety). Many of these disorders can be effectively treated or controlled by drugs that work directly on various receptors in the CNS. In addition, analgesics affecting central nervous system receptors are useful in controlling pain.

This chapter includes discussion of drugs affecting the central nervous system primarily in relation to their therapeutic goals. Unfortunately many of these substances are used for their "pleasurable" effects. Chapter 6 focuses on those substances such as narcotics that are readily abused, while Chapter 18 includes a discussion of alcohol.

The Benzodiazepines

The benzodiazepines derive their name from the fusion of a seven-member diazepine ring with a six-member benzene ring. In general, benzodiazepines are highly lipid soluble, extensively bound to plasma proteins (>90 percent), and completely absorbed following oral administration. The benzodiazepines are not **general CNS depressants** but act at specific receptor sites in the brain and spinal cord intimately associated with inhibitory gamma-aminobutyric acid (GABA) neurotransmitter receptors. Benzodiazepines enhance the inhibitory effects of GABA, and their affinity parallels their therapeutic potency. The benzodiazepine receptor is in physical proximity to the GABA receptor and the Cl^- ionophore (channel), where agonist binding enhances the probability of Cl^- channel opening in response to activation of the GABA receptor (Fig. 5–1). This regulation may occur through an allosteric mechanism, and it takes place only in the presence of GABA. GABA-mediated Cl^- channel function can be modulated by three types of ligands acting at the benzodiazepine receptor: agonists, antagonists, and **inverse agonists**. Whereas agonists are anxiolytic, hypnotic, muscle relaxant, and anticonvulsant and enhance GABA-receptor function, inverse agonists are anxiogenic and convulsant and reduce GABA function; on the other hand, antagonists block the effects of both agonists and inverse agonists but have no pharmacological ef-

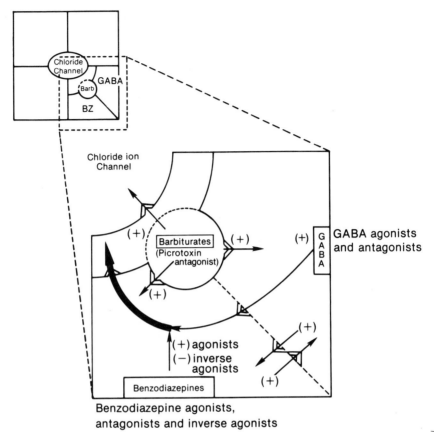

Figure 5–1. Schematic representation of a model of the GABA-benzodiazepine Cl⁻ channel complex emphasizing its possible tetrameric form.

fects in and of themselves. The Cl^- channel portion of this macromolecular complex also contains a binding site for convulsants (e.g., picrotoxin) and barbiturates. It is not yet clear whether the benzodiazepine receptor is composed of several physically separable subclasses of receptors, or if there is only one binding site that exists in different conformations. However, this complex may exist in tetrameric form.

With increasing drug-induced depression of the CNS, one observes sedation, hypnosis, anesthesia, and finally death. This dose-dependent continuum does not strictly hold true for the benzodiazepines, in that stupor, but not true anesthesia, is produced at high concentrations. Sedation produced at lower effective concentrations results in diminished response to stimuli without general CNS depression. At even lower doses most benzodiazepines produce their muscle relaxant and antianxiety effects, largely without sedation. The efficacy of the benzodiazepines as sleep aids is realized at higher concentrations where hypnosis is produced. Sleep latency and REM sleep time are decreased and the threshold to awakening is increased. While the time spent in stage 2 sleep (major non-REM sleep) is increased, stages 3 and 4 (slow-wave sleep) are markedly decreased. Tolerance is fairly quickly established to changes in sleep patterns, and abrupt withdrawal of the shorter half-life drugs may lead to a "rebound" effect of increased insomnia. Benzodiazepines are used in preoperative and preanesthetic procedures in which the anterograde amnesia they produce is useful. **Diazepam (Valium)** (Fig. 5–2) and **midazolam** are frequently used for this purpose because their rapid absorption and large volume of distribution result in an easily controlled rapid onset and short duration of action. The effects of benzodiazepines on respiration are minimal even at preanesthetic levels. Likewise, cardiovascular effects are mild, except in cases of extreme intoxication where peripheral vascular resistance and cardiac output decrease. The muscle relaxant effects of the benzodiazepines occur as a result of enhanced presynaptic inhibition of spinal afferents involving the internuncial neurons. Only at very high doses is neuromuscular blockade achieved.

Side Effects

Common side effects include ataxia, confusion, drowsiness, impairment of thought, anterograde amnesia, weakness, nausea, and diarrhea. Concurrent use with other CNS depressants (especially alcohol) should be avoided because of their additive effects (see Chapter 3).

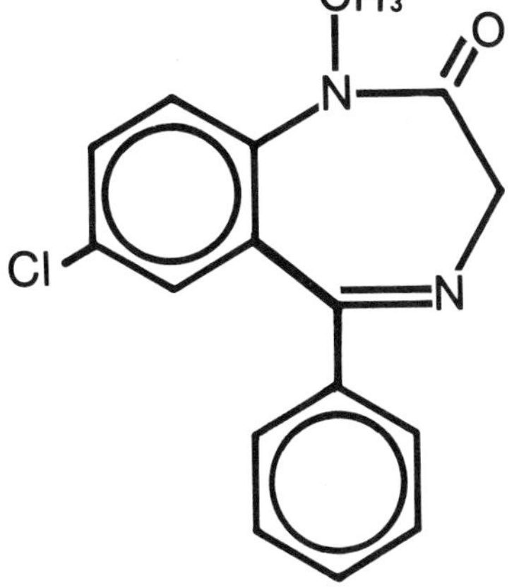

Figure 5–2. Chemical structure of diazepam.

Tolerance

Tolerance (metabolic and functional) and both physical and psychological dependence are produced by the benzodiazepines. **Metabolic (dispositional) tolerance** is minimal because little induction of liver metabolizing enzymes occurs, an important factor contributing to the safety of these drugs. **Functional tolerance** can be related to the state of the tissue (**pharmacodynamic**) involved, to the behavior of the organism, or to both. Although the mechanism(s) remains obscure, some form of compensatory change in the level of CNS activity produced by the presence of the drug may be responsible. Upon withdrawal from the drug, the tissue and behavior return to normal, leaving no evidence of pathology. Tolerance to the pharmacological properties of the benzodiazepines occurs most readily for their anticonvulsant effects, and then to their sedative-hypnotic and muscle relaxant properties. Tolerance to antianxiety effects is less common. **Cross-tolerance** between the benzodiazepines and other CNS depressants is well known.

Toxicity and Withdrawal

Both physical and psychological dependence, and compulsive use of the drug for its pharmacological effects (addiction), can occur with extended use of the benzodiazepines. Abrupt withdrawal can produce anxiety, agitation, and insomnia, and in extreme cases convulsions may be precipitated. The severity of symptoms is inversely related to the duration of action of the drug in question; thus, the shorter-acting benzodiazepines produce more severe withdrawal symptoms than the longer-acting members of this class. Even though benzodiazepines are frequently implicated in toxicity cases because of intentional overdosage, serious results are uncommon unless other depressants, notably alcohol, are involved. Treatment of toxic overdose includes the support of respiration and cardiovascular function.

Clinical Applications

All marketed benzodiazepines are qualitatively similar in their pharmacological properties; however, since their metabolism and distribution vary, specific members of this family are targeted for different clinical uses (see Table 5–1).

The benzodiazepines vary in their lipid solubility over a 50-fold range. They also differ in their duration of action, which is partly a function of the redistribution of the parent compound and its metabolites from the CNS to the periphery. However, many benzodiazepines, while rapidly absorbed, undergo hepatic biotransformation to metabolites that are themselves active and may have very long half-lives (e.g., **flurazepam**). Thus, there may be little relationship between the half-life of the administered parent compound and the observed duration of action. The more rapidly metabolized drugs in this class (e.g., **triazolam**) have been targeted for use as hypnotics because they have rapid onset and short duration of action and do not produce daytime sedation following use. However, **"rebound" anxiety** and early morning insomnia have been reported with these drugs, and while not yet fully understood, these effects may result from the precipitation of withdrawal caused by rapid overnight clearance of metabolites from the body.

Miscellaneous Antianxiety Drugs

Recent progress has been made in developing drugs with selected pharmacological properties. Although not yet generally available, some are in clinical trials. The triazolopyridazines (e.g., Cl 218,872) possess anticonvulsant and antianxiety but no sedative-hypnotic or muscle relaxant properties. These drugs bind to the benzodiazepine receptor but do not facilitate GABA neurotransmission. Another group, the pyrazolopyridines (e.g., cartazolate), possess only antianxiety properties but do not bind to the benzodiazepine receptor site. Derivatives of quinoline (e.g., PK 8165) are also effective anxiolytics but also are without effect on GABA receptors. Finally, drugs of the class of azaspirodecanediones (e.g., **buspirone**; BuSpar) appear to be effective in treating anxiety in clinical trials. Buspirone, which has recently gained FDA approval for use in the treatment of general anxiety disorders, has few other pharmacological properties, does not potentiate other CNS depressants, and does not influence GABA or benzodiazepine binding sites.

The Barbiturates

The barbiturates are nonselective, general CNS depressants that have essentially the same pharmacological properties as the benzodiazepines. They were widely used previously, but their use is severely limited today because of liabilities associated with their toxicity and with their low therapeutic index, and because of the availability of the safer benzodiazepines.

Barbiturates are synthetic derivatives resulting from the condensation of thioureas or oxyureas and malonic acids. The thiobarbiturates are more lipid soluble than the oxybarbiturates, and thus have a more rapid onset and shorter duration of action. In addition, the thiobarbiturates are more rapidly metabolized, and the extent of their lipid solubility is directly related to the binding of plasma proteins. **Thiobarbiturates** (e.g., **thiopental**) are used as intravenous anesthetics (or as adjuncts thereto), whereas the longer-acting oxybarbiturates are best suited as sedative-hypnotics and anticonvulsants. The thiobarbiturates and other highly lipid-soluble barbiturates are rapidly redistributed from the brain to other tissues, and thus it is their redistribution and

not their metabolism that is responsible for their short duration of action. Whereas kidneys excrete the unmetabolized portion of the less lipid-soluble compounds (barbital and, to a lesser extent, phenobarbital), other compounds undergo biotransformation in the liver. Inactivation usually accompanies metabolism; these products appear in the urine either in free or glucuronidated form.

Barbiturates suppress neuronal activity in the brainstem reticular formation and cortex. Their effects on excitatory neurons include a slowing of conduction of the action potential, a decrease in the amount of Ca^{2+}-dependent neurotransmitter released, and perhaps a direct antagonism of the receptor for the excitatory neurotransmitter glutamate. Barbiturates also produce an enhancement of inhibition and prolongation of GABA effects by binding at or near the Cl^- channel, where they decrease the frequency of channel opening but increase the average open-channel lifetime (see Fig. 5–1). Benzodiazepines, on the other hand, increase only the frequency of Cl^- channel opening, with little effect on the lifetime of the open state. Barbiturates also produce a dose-dependent CNS depression that ranges from sedation, hypnosis, and anesthesia to coma and death. At sedative doses, some of the longer-acting barbiturates (e.g., **phenobarbital**) have been used as anxiolytics. However, because of the higher degree of sedation and euphoria (and therefore abuse) produced by barbiturates, the benzodiazepines are the drugs of choice. In cases in which pain is involved, barbiturates should be avoided because of the **hyperalgesia** or hyperexcitability, or both, that may be precipitated, especially in the young and elderly. Barbiturates are not analgesics and can attenuate some effects of opioid analgetics. Effects on sleep patterns include a decrease in sleep latency and REM activity, but tolerance to these effects occurs upon repeated nightly use.

The effect of barbiturates on respiration is not unlike natural sleep at hypnotic doses. However, with increasingly higher concentrations neurogenic, hypoxic, and chemoreceptor drives fail, resulting in severe respiratory depression that is life threatening. The levels of drug that produce severe respiratory depression are only 10- to 20-fold greater than those at which hypnosis occurs. This major liability is due to the fact that tolerance to the medullary-based suppression of respiration is represented largely by the induction of hepatic microsomal drug-metabolizing enzymes (**dispositional tolerance**) and is minimal.

Barbiturates induce hepatic drug-metabolizing enzymes and combine with the P-450 cytochrome to competitively inhibit transformations of barbiturates *per se* and other drug classes that are substrates for this enzyme. This may lead to alterations in the metabolic rates of different drugs, causing adverse reactions (e.g., potentiation of CNS depressants such as ethanol, antihistamines, monoamine oxidase inhibitors, phenothiazines, and antihypertensives). The level of enzyme induction by the barbiturates increases their metabolism about twofold in normal individuals and represents the dispositional component of the observed cross-tolerance with other CNS depressants.

Side Effects

Sedative-hypnotic doses have little effect on the cardiovascular system and result in only small decreases in blood pressure and heart rate. At larger doses ganglionic inhibition can cause hypotension, a condition frequently accompanied by decreased body temperature and respiration. Other unwanted side effects include a "hangover" feeling from residual CNS depression after use at hypnotic doses. In addition, motor skills and judgment are impaired. Additional aftereffects include nausea, vertigo, and irritability. Some individuals demonstrate allergic reactions, including facial edema and, in extreme cases, exfoliative dermatitis, which is life threatening. The use of barbiturates is absolutely contraindicated in individuals with intermittent porphyria.

Toxicity

Toxic doses produce severe CNS depression, and death may result from respiratory failure. The short- and intermediate-acting barbiturates are more toxic (and have more abuse potential) than the longer-acting compounds, and concomitant use with other CNS depressants exacerbates the problem. Comatose patients may have constricted pupils that react to light in the earlier stages of intoxication; however, later, when hypoxia sets in, the pupils may become dilated. Blood pressure may fall precipitously with the development of shock and renal failure. Treatment is usually to support respiration; hemodialysis is effective for the longer-acting barbiturates, which are less extensively bound to plasma proteins than the shorter-acting derivatives.

Withdrawal

The severity and time to onset of withdrawal symptoms vary according to the barbiturate in question, the level of use at cessation, and the abruptness of withdrawal. In general, the shorter the half-life and the greater the dose, the more rapid the onset and the more severe the withdrawal symptoms. This may range from rebound insomnia at hypnotic doses, to anxiety and nausea at higher doses, and to seizures and delirium at toxic levels. This latter stage may lead to cardiovascular collapse and death. Upon withdrawal, substitution with a longer-acting barbiturate may be necessary so that the drug can be slowly and carefully tapered off in order to reduce the severity of symptoms.

Tolerance

Tolerance to the barbiturates can result from the induction of hepatic drug-metabolizing enzymes (dispositional), from changes (adaptation) in the functional state of the tissue (pharmacodynamic), and via an unknown mechanism wherein a single dose (e.g., intravenous thiopental) of short-acting drug can cause acute tolerance that is neither dispositional nor pharmacodynamic.

Enhanced metabolic disposition may occur in just a few days and may account for a twofold increase in tolerance. Pharmacodynamic effects, however, may take weeks or months to reach maximum levels and may account for an additional twofold to threefold increase in tolerance. Since tolerance to the sedative-hypnotic effects of these drugs is much greater than that produced to their anticonvulsant properties or lethal respiratory depressant effects, the effective therapeutic index **decreases** with the development of increasing tolerance.

Abuse

The short-acting barbiturates **pentobarbital (Nembutal)** and **secobarbital (Seconal)** have a high incidence of abuse. The desired effects of addicted individuals include the alcohol-like intoxication and use with other drugs (e.g., amphetamines) in order to potentiate mood elevation.

Clinical Applications

Even though the use of barbiturates as sedative-hypnotics has largely been supplanted by the benzodiazepines, barbiturates still remain the drugs of choice in certain cases. Phenobarbital and mephobarbital are used chronically in the prophylactic treatment or management of grand mal and focal motor seizures. The side effects of phenobarbital when used chronically as an anticonvulsant include sedation, ataxia, nystagmus, rash, hypoprothrombinemia in newborns, megaloblastic anemia (due to folate antagonism), and osteomalacia (due to an increased rate of vitamin D metabolism and target organ resistance). Phenobarbital, pentobarbital, and thiopental are also used in the emergency treatment of convulsions associated with brain edema due to head trauma, tetanus, and cerebral hemorrhage.

Nonbenzodiazepine, Nonbarbiturate Sedative-Hypnotics

Several additional groups of drugs are also used as sedative-hypnotics, and although they in some cases replaced the use of the barbiturates, today they too are used to a lesser extent than the benzodiazepines. These include the carbamates, quinazolines, piperidinediones, cyclic ethers, and alcohols. In general, these drug classes have greater toxicity liabilities, lower therapeutic indices, and higher physical dependence and abuse potentials than the benzodiazepines.

The propanediol carbamates (e.g., **meprobamate; Miltown**) possess the same pharmacological properties as the barbiturates and benzodiazepines and are used in the treatment of anxiety and as sedative-hypnotics. Their mechanism of action is unknown, but this class does not appear to enhance GABA inhibitory neurotransmission. Of the quinazolines, **methaqualone (Quaalude)** is the most widely prescribed in this class. It is popularly abused for its alcohol-like intoxicating effects; may lead to physical dependence; and can produce coma, convulsions, and death with acute overdose. Two piperidinediones available as hypnotics are glutethimide and methyprylon. **Glutethimide (Doriden)** has the same qualitative, albeit weaker, pharmacological properties as the barbiturates and is a useful sedative-hypnotic; however, its margin of safety in acute poisoning is less than that of the barbiturates. Unexpected and sudden death, probably due to cardiac arrest, may occur in severe cases. **Methyprylon (Noludar)** is a very potent hypnotic for daytime and nighttime use by individuals who cannot tolerate barbiturates. Toxic doses may produce respiratory depression, persistent hypotension, or both. Precipitous withdrawal from this drug may induce irritability and convulsions. The cyclic ether **paraldehyde (Paral)** has very good hypnotic properties and is effective in the treatment of convulsive episodes precipitated by alcohol withdrawal, tetanus, status epilepticus, and convulsive drug toxicity. Its use and abuse is limited because of an undesirable odor it produces on the breath. Withdrawal effects include delirium tremens in severe cases. The alcohols considered here are chloral hydrate and ethchlorvynol. The pharmacology and toxicology of alcohol (ethanol) is discussed in Chapter 18. **Chloral hydrate (Noctec)** is a hypnotic whose action can be attributed to its metabolic product, trichloroethanol. It is especially useful in the elderly, infants, and children because it does not produce paradoxical excitability or hyperalgesia as can the barbiturates. **Ethchlorvynol (Placidyl)** is used as a daytime or nighttime sleep aid. Its pharmacological effects at therapeutic and higher doses are similar to those of barbiturates. It acts selectively on the CNS and does not appear to induce drug-metabolizing enzymes.

DRUGS USED IN THE TREATMENT OF SEIZURE DISORDERS

Seizures are caused by CNS dysfunction, are associated with the appearance of excessive and abnormal electrical brain activity, and are usually abrupt and transitory. Chronic disorders of this nature are referred to collectively as epilepsies and may be expressed as disturbances of convulsive (motor), autonomic, psychic, or sensory systems. Approximately 0.5 percent of the general population has some form of epilepsy, whose etiology may be unknown (**idiopathic**), or whose association with specific causal factors (**symptomatic**) can be identified (e.g., traumatic, toxic, infectious, neoplastic, developmental, or metabolic). About 50 percent of epilepsies are completely controlled with anticonvulsant therapy, with another 25 percent appreciably improved.

The accurate classification of seizure activity is the basis for appropriate drug selection and may be divided into two broad groups: generalized and focal (Table 5–2). Generalized seizures are designated as grand mal, petit mal, and minor motor, the last of which is further distinguished as akinetic, myoclonic, and massive seizures. Focal (partial) epilepsies include motor, sensory (both simple partial and jacksonian), and psychomotor (complex partial) seizures. Status epilepticus, a life-threatening form of epilepsy involving contin-

**Table 5–2. CLASSIFICATION AND DRUG TREATMENT
OF SEIZURE DISORDERS**

Seizure Type	Observations	Drugs
I. Generalized Seizures		
A. Grand Mal (tonic-clonic)	Tonic-clonic movements, loss of consciousness, post-ictal depression	phenobarbital (Luminal) phenytoin (Dilantin) primadone (Mysoline) valproic acid (Depakene)
B. Petit mal (absence)	Frequent, brief lapses of consciousness, with or without clonic motor activity, high frequency in children	ethosuximide (Zarontin) clonazepam (Clonopin) trimethadione (Tridione) valproic acid (Depakene)
C. Minor motor		
1. Akinetic (atonic)	Sudden and brief loss of postural muscle tone	valproic acid (Depakene)
2. Myoclonic	Clonic contractions of trunk muscles	clonazepam (Clonopin)
3. Massive (hypsarrhythmias)	Infantile motor spasms, progressive mental deterioration, not true epileptic seizures	corticotropin adrenocorticosteroids valproic acid (Depakene)
II. Focal (Partial) Seizures		
A. Motor (jacksonian) (simple partial)	Cortical lesion, single limb or muscle group convulsion	phenobarbital (Luminal) phenytoin (Dilantin) carbamazepine (Tegretol) primidone (Mysoline)
B. Sensory (jacksonian) (simple partial)	Cortical lesion sensory	
C. Psychomotor (complex partial)	Temporal lobe lesion, altered affect, perception or behavior, clouded consciousness	
III. Status Epilepticus	State of continual seizure activity, usually generalized tonic-clonic	diazepam (Valium) phenytoin (Dilantin)

ual seizure activity, can also be precipitated by drug withdrawal and requires emergency medical treatment. Current classification of epileptic seizures is based on the original concepts of John Hughlings Jackson, who proposed that seizures result from local discharges occurring in gray (neuronal) matter and become convulsive when they spread into surrounding normal tissue. It has since been established that the focal area of seizure activity consists of neuronal circuits that give rise to synchronous excitatory discharges, spread to adjacent neuronal loci, and extend the area of involvement. Under normal circumstances, it is thought that inhibitory neuronal networks may act to inhibit, *via* a feedback loop, this excitation, thus suppressing seizure activity. However, at a focus (or foci) of paroxysmal discharges, lower levels of inhibitory activity appear to exist, such that the storm of excitatory activity is not contained. In some cases, foci may discharge only infrequently, without the production of seizures, but seizures may be precipitated by various physiological changes (e.g., stress, fatigue, blood glucose level changes, electrolyte or endocrine imbalance), which by themselves in normal individuals are without consequence.

Mechanism of Action

Attempts to explain the therapeutic effects of anticonvulsants in terms of a unified mechanism of action have been only partially successful. Drugs used in the treatment of most seizures, perhaps with the exception of petit mal (absence) epilepsies, may have in common an interaction with GABA-mediated inhibitory neuronal networks. Drugs (convulsants) that antagonize this system (e.g., pentylenetetrazole, bicuculline, and picrotoxin) also induce epileptiform discharges in the CNS. Conversely, several classes of anticonvulsant drugs (e.g., barbiturates, benzodiazepines, valproic acid, and progabide) act to enhance or mimic GABA-mediated inhibitory neurotransmission by facilitating Cl^- conductance (see Fig. 5–1). Thus, it is possible that decreased or abnormal function of the GABA neurotransmitter system, in or near epileptic foci, may be involved in these types of seizure phenomena.

Anticonvulsants used to treat petit mal seizures present a much more complex picture. These include **ethosuximide (Zarontin)** and **trimethadione (Tridione)**, whose mechanisms of action are not well understood, but which do not appear to produce changes in neuronal membrane Ca^{2+}, Na^+, and K^+ fluxes as do the other anticonvulsants. The situation is further complicated in that both **valproic acid (Depakene)** and **clonazepam (Clonopin)**, used to treat many other seizure types, are also effective in petit mal seizure treatment. There is some evidence from animal studies that important neocortical noradrenergic pathways, whose activities are modified by presynaptic GABAergic neurons, may be involved.

Drug Selection

There is striking similarity in the chemical structures of drugs used in the treatment of seizure disorders (Table 5–3). The **barbiturates phenobarbital** and **methobarbital (Mebaral)** and the deoxy-derivative **primidone (Mysoline)** are beneficial in treating generalized tonic-clonic (grand mal) and focal (partial) seizures. Therapeutic doses are usually below those that normally produce sedation or hypnosis, and tolerance to their anticonvulsive effects is not marked. Primidone, whose major active metabolite is phenobarbital, is used in the same situations as are phenobarbital and methobarbital and frequently in conjunction with phenytoin. The pharmacological properties of the barbiturates, their mechanism of action, toxicity, and abuse potential are described in the preceding section on sedative-hypnotics.

Of the **hydantoins**, phenytoin, mephenytoin, and ethotoin are the most effective in treating all seizure types except absence seizures. Phenytoin is a diphenyl-substituted hydantoin and the most completely investigated of all anticonvulsant drugs. Its effectiveness lies in its ability to limit the spread of focal activity by nonspecifically stabilizing neuronal membranes, thus preventing the development of maximal seizure action. Unlike the barbiturates, however, phenytoin does not produce sedation, raise seizure thresholds, or act as a general CNS depressant. Its mechanism of action most likely includes reduction of Na^+ and Ca^{2+} fluxes during neuronal depolarizations, thus suppressing repetitive nerve firing.

Phenytoin (Dilantin) is very lipid soluble, is tightly bound to plasma proteins, is metabolized in the liver by para-hydroxylation, and is glucuronidated and excreted in the urine. Phenytoin has dose-dependent pharmacokinetics, where at low levels its metabolism is proportional to concentration, but at higher levels (in the therapeutic range) maximal liver metabolic capacity is reached. This can result in further small increases in dose, causing disproportionately larger elevations in drug plasma levels. Under these conditions, drug half-life rises dramatically, plasma levels continue to increase, and toxicity results. Differences in the bioavailability of commercial preparations compound this problem, such that phenytoin absorption may be variable and sometimes incomplete. Some of the toxic CNS effects of chronic phenytoin use are dose-related and involve the cerebellar-vestibular pathway, producing vertigo, nystagmus, and ataxia. In addition, behavioral changes reflecting CNS excitation, such as hyperactivity, hallucinations, and drowsiness may be seen. Other reactions include gingival hyperplasia, GI disturbances, hirsutism, megaloblastic anemia, and osteomalacia. Phenytoin is a suspected teratogen and is associated with fetal hydantoin syndrome; its use during pregnancy must be carefully evaluated. With excessive intravenous injection, cardiac arrhythmias can occur and may be accompanied by CNS depression and a fall in blood pressure. In general, however, the hydantoins have high therapeutic indices and are considered relatively safe drugs.

Table 5–3. DRUGS USED IN THE TREATMENT OF SEIZURE DISORDERS

Class	General Structure	Examples
Barbiturates		Phenobarbital (Luminal) Mephobarbital (Mebaral) Primidone (Mysoline)[+]
Hydantoins		Phenytoin (Dilantin) Ethotoin (Peganone) Mephenytoin (Mesantoin)
Succinimides		Ethosuximide (Zarontin) Methosuximide (Celontin) Phensuximide (Milontin)
Oxazolidinediones		Trimethadione (Tridione)
Miscellaneous		
Benzodiazepines		Clonazepam (Clonopin) Diazepam (Valium)
Iminostilbenes		Carbamazepine (Tegretol)
Newer Drugs	Valproic Acid	Valproic Acid (Depakene) Progabide (SL 76002)*

+ A deoxybarbiturate

*In clinical trials

Mephenytoin (**Mesantoin**) differs from phenytoin in that it produces sedation and raises seizure thresholds. The drug's minor side effects, when they occur, are less intense than those of phenytoin, but its more serious side effects are the ones that occur more frequently. Thus, mephenytoin is reserved for individuals who are unresponsive to the safer drugs. **Ethotoin** (**Peganone**) is of low potency and is used mainly in combination with other anticonvulsants. Both mephenytoin and ethotoin share with phenytoin the liability of being maximally metabolized by the liver at therapeutic doses.

The **succinimides** ethosuximide, methsuximide, and phensuximide are used to treat absence seizures. **Ethosuximide** (**Zarontin**) is the most selective for this class of epilepsy. Its mechanism of action is not known, but it does have the ability to increase presynaptic GABA release. Ethosuximide is completely absorbed orally, is uniformly distributed in body fluids, does not bind plasma proteins, is metabolized by hydroxylation, and its inactive metabolites are glucuronidated and excreted in the urine. Common side effects include GI problems, sedation, photophobia, and behavioral changes resembling CNS stimulation. More serious complaints such as skin rash (Stevens-Johnson syndrome), systemic lupus erythematosus (SLE), blood dyscrasias, and parkinsonism-like reactions have also been reported. Adverse side effects of **methsuximide** are common and include blood dyscrasias, depression, leukopenia, aplastic anemia, and hepatotoxicity. **Phensuximide** (**Milontin**) is less effective than ethosuximide and therefore is not widely used.

Trimethadione (**Tridione**) was the drug of choice for absence seizures before being replaced by the succinimides. It has been extensively investigated, although its mechanism of action remains unknown. Toxic effects include sedation, blurred vision, nausea, serious skin reactions, and blood dyscrasias. Because of the severity of the latter, it is used primarily in patients who cannot tolerate other effective agents. Owing to its teratogenic effects, it should not be used during pregnancy.

The **benzodiazepine clonazepam** (**Clonopin**) is used to treat absence and minor motor (myoclonic and akinetic) seizures. Intravenously administered, **diazepam** (**Valium**) is effective against status epilepticus. The benzodiazepines appear to act by reducing the spread of seizures from foci without inhibiting abnormal focal discharges. Two major disadvantages that limit their therapeutic effectiveness are that they produce considerable sedation and that tolerance to their anticonvulsant properties is achieved relatively quickly. Their pharmacological properties, mechanism of action, metabolism, and toxicity are discussed in the preceding section on sedative-hypnotics.

Carbamazepine (**Tegretol**), the prototype immunostilbene, is used extensively in the treatment of all epilepsies except absence seizures. Its mechanism of action is unknown, but in laboratory studies it increases the neuronal firing of noradrenergic neurons and may activate GABAergic inhibitory circuitry. Its more common side effects are ataxia, dizziness, diplopia, nausea, and skin disorders; the more serious include blood dyscrasias (agranulocytosis, aplastic anemia) and hepatic dysfunction. At toxic levels, carbamazepine produces respiratory depression, convulsions, and coma. Nonepileptic uses include the treatment of neuralgias—particularly trigeminal neuralgia—and some cases of manic-depression in which lithium is ineffective.

Valproic acid (n-dipropylacetic acid; **Depakene**), also called valproate, is effective against most generalized seizures, including some cases of infantile motor spasms. It suppresses seizures in a number of animal model systems and causes little sedation. Valproate's mechanism of action is not clearly understood; it produces small increases in brain GABA concentrations *via* weak inhibition of the GABA catabolic enzyme, GABA transaminase. However, its more important action may be directly on the Cl^- ionophore, where it may act by facilitating Cl^- conduction. Side effects include GI problems, ataxia, tremor, and anorexia. Infrequent hepatotoxicity (fulminant hepatitis), teratogenicity, alopecia, and acute pancreatitis have also been noted.

Progabide, currently undergoing clinical tests, has a demonstrated efficacy against both generalized and partial epilepsies. A GABA-receptor agonist, progabide has a low incidence of mild metabolic, sedative, GI, neurological, and endocrine side effects. It is devoid of teratogenic activity, and tolerance to its anticonvulsant properties does not appear to develop.

Therapy of Seizure Disorders

For the purpose of correctly identifying a specific type of seizure, and thus the most efficacious drug, three important diagnostic tools are employed. The first is a complete history, physical examination, and neurological examination. As a part of this procedure, a **computerized axial tomography (CAT)** or **magnetic resonance imaging (MRI)** scan of the brain is performed to establish a symptomatic or idiopathic etiology. More than 70 percent of all epilepsies are idiopathic. A thorough **electroencephalographic (EEG) examination** is necessary to evaluate accurately the location of epileptic foci and to classify the electrical characteristics of the seizure activity. In addition, continual assessment of EEG patterns, drug plasma levels (to check patient compliance), and toxic reactions is necessary.

Treatment is for the long term (years or a lifetime) and should begin with conservative levels of the most effective drug. Subsequent dosage increases should be slowly titrated (over weeks or months) until a balance of maximal therapeutic benefit with minimal toxicity is achieved. If adequate remission is not attained, a second drug may be initiated, or the first very slowly withdrawn (to prevent the precipitation of seizure activity) and then gradually replaced by the second. In some cases, when more than one type of epilepsy is present, or when conversion from one seizure type to another takes place, multiple drug use is necessary. However, the simultaneous use of large numbers of anticonvulsants should be minimized or avoided.

If the patient remains seizure-free for 2 to 3 years on the therapeutic doses provided, then, all other conditions (e.g., age, general health) and test results (e.g., EEG) being normal, the slow withdrawal of the anticonvulsant agent(s) may be considered. Although specific seizure types (e.g., absence) may disappear spontaneously, it should be remembered that anticonvulsant drug therapy is only prophylactic. The treatment of epilepsy during pregnancy poses special problems in light of the fact that, although many anticonvulsant drugs are teratogenic, fetal damage may result also from uncontrolled seizures.

ANTIPSYCHOTIC DRUGS

Antipsychotic (neuroleptic) agents provide symptomatic relief from psychoses associated with structural, metabolic, toxic, infectious or physical injury to the brain, schizophrenia, and isolated delusional psychoses or paranoia. Schizophrenias are characterized by severe disorders of perception (auditory hallucinations and illusions) and thought (delusions and illogical rambling), and of emotional withdrawal. Impairment of memory and disorientation are usually present in psychoses with the exception of schizophrenia, paranoia, and isolated delusions.

Central biogenic amines, particularly **dopamine,** have been implicated in the manifestation of psychoses, and **central dopamine receptors** appear to mediate the effects of antipsychotic drugs. Psychotic symptoms are hypothesized to be the consequence of **hyperactive central dopaminergic neurotransmission.** The evidence in support of this hypothesis is as follows:

1. The affinity of binding of antipsychotic drugs to the D_2 subtype of CNS dopamine receptor correlates well with their clinical potency.
2. As a consequence of binding of antipsychotic drugs to dopamine receptors, the turnover of dopamine increases during early treatment, and the spontaneous firing of dopaminergic neurons in the substantia nigra is enhanced.
3. Drugs that cause the release of dopamine (e.g., amphetamine) or that increase the synthesis of dopamine (e.g., dihydroxyphenylalanine; L-dopa) produce psychotic symptoms or worsen existing psychoses.
4. Small doses of antipsychotic drugs block the effects of dopaminergic agonists (e.g., apomorphine).

Dopaminergic systems in the **basal ganglia** (caudate, putamen, globus pallidus, and associated nuclei) are important in the control of posture and involuntary (extrapyramidal) movements, whereas dopaminergic systems in the **mesofrontal and limbic regions** of the cerebral cortex are implicated in psychoses. It is thought that **antipsychotic drug-induced antagonism of dopamine** systems in the basal ganglia leads to extrapyramidal effects, whereas antagonism of neurotransmission in the limbic, mesocortical, and perhaps hypothalamic dopamine systems leads to therapeutically useful antipsychotic effects. The major evidence against the dopamine hypothesis is that antipsychotic drug effects usually take 3 weeks to develop, reaching peak efficacy in 6 weeks to 6 months; these drugs, however, block dopamine receptors upon first administration. In addition, the early effects of antipsychotic drugs on dopamine receptors, at least in the basal ganglia, are opposite to those seen after prolonged use when D_2 dopamine receptor **super**sensitivity develops without any marked changes in therapeutic effect. Clearly, the long-term effects of antipsychotic drugs on dopamine and its receptors are complex. It may be that mesolimbic and mesocortical dopaminergic systems, often implicated in psychoses, respond differently from those in the basal ganglia. Indeed, it has been shown that increases in dopamine turnover induced by antipsychotic drugs are blocked by anticholinergic drugs in the basal ganglia but not in limbic areas.

Clinical Applications

Antipsychotic drugs are effective in all psychotic disorders, effecting changes in thought, perception, and mood associated with psychoses. However, because of their dopamine receptor antagonism, they produce neurological disorders similar to **parkinsonism**. In addition, antipsychotic drugs are also used as antipruritic (anti-itching) drugs; for dissociative anesthesia; in the control of nausea and vomiting caused by gastroenteritis, radiation sickness, pregnancy, chemotherapeutic agents, and uremia (but not that caused by motion sickness); in the control of intractable hiccups; and in the management of chronic alcoholism, Gilles de la Tourette's syndrome (tics, grunts, involuntary movements), and Huntington's disease. Antipsychotic drugs are classified into several major groups (Table 5–4).

In general, the clinical effectiveness of the prototype phenothiazine and that of the newer nonphenothiazine antipsychotic drugs are similar. These drugs are metabolized by liver microsomal drug-metabolizing enzymes and conjugated; most metabolites are inactive. Glucuronides and sulfoxides are excreted in the urine, and demethylated nonpolar metabolites are excreted *via* the bile and feces or reabsorbed. The elimination half-lives of these drugs is usually between 20 and 40 hours. Differences between drugs and the bases of selection for therapy lie in unwanted side effects and potency. Antipsychotic drugs with low potency tend to produce sedation, more α-adrenoceptor antagonism, and hypotensive effects and seizures, whereas those with greater potency produce less sedation and cardiovascular effects but prominent antiemetic and extrapyramidal effects. Combinations of antipsychotic drugs

Table 5-4. DRUGS USED IN THE TREATMENT OF PSYCHOSES

Class/Examples	Typical Structure	Dose* and Potency

Phenothiazines
  Chlorpromazine (Thorazine)
  Thioridazine (Mellaril)
  Mesoridazine (Serentil)
		300-800 mg, low
		200-600 mg, low
		75-300 mg, low

Thioxanthenes
  Chlorprothixene (Taractan)
  Thiothixene (Navane)
		50-400 mg, low
		6-30 mg, high

Butyrophenones Haloperidol (Haldol)		6-20 mg, high

Miscellaneous
  Loxapine (Loxitane)
  Molindone (Moban)
		60-100 mg, intermediate
		50-100 mg, intermediate

*usual daily dose range

do not seem to be more beneficial therapeutically than single agents. They are, however, sometimes combined with antidepressant drugs in the management of depressed psychotics or patients with agitated depression. Antipsychotic drugs are not curative, and symptoms return upon cessation of therapy. They are more effective in alleviating disorders of thought and perception than flat affect, apathy, behavior disturbances, and poor insight and judgment.

Pharmacological Properties

All antipsychotic drugs have similar efficacy and share several pharmacological effects (Table 5–5). **Chlorpromazine (Thorazine)** is the prototypical antipsychotic drug, producing prominent actions on the central nervous, autonomic nervous, cardiovascular, and endocrine systems. Chlorpromazine produces sedation and drowsiness from which patients can be easily aroused. A

Table 5–5. COMPARISON OF LOW-POTENCY AND HIGH-POTENCY ANTIPSYCHOTIC DRUGS

Effects	Low-potency (e.g., chlorpromazine) 300–800 mg[a]	High-potency (e.g., haloperidol) 6–20 mg[a]
1. Extrapyramidal effects (parkinsonism, akathisia, dystonia)	+ +	+ + +
2. Sedative effect	+ + +	+
3. α-Adrenergic antagonism (hypotension)	+ +	+
4. ↓ Cardiac contractility; prolonged QT interval	+ +[b]	uncommon
5. Anticholinergic effects (blurred vision, dry mouth, constipation, urinary retention)	+ +	least frequent
6. Antiemetic effects	+[c]	+ +
7. Endocrine effects (Gynecomastia)	+ +	+ +
8. ↓ Seizure threshold	+ +	less likely[d]
9. Allergic/hypersensitivity reactions (rash, cholestatic jaundice, blood dyscrasias)	+ +	+

[a]Usual daily oral dosage range.
[b]More common with thioridazine.
[c]Thioridazine has no antiemetic effect.
[d]Most high-potency drugs do not significantly reduce seizure threshold, but haloperidol has variable and unpredictable effect.

neurolept syndrome is produced, however, which is characterized by a decrease in spontaneous motor activity, relative lack of initiative and interest in one's surroundings, and a decrease in affect and emotion. There is also indifference to pain, but nociceptive responses are retained.

Antipsychotic drugs, particularly chlorpromazine, are **antagonists at multiple neurotransmitter receptors**. In decreasing order, they block α adrenoceptors > dopamine receptors > serotonin receptors > histamine-1 receptors > muscarinic receptors > bradykinin receptors. In addition, chlorpromazine decreases the neuronal release of norepinephrine, thus producing an antiadrenergic effect; conversely, chlorpromazine blocks the uptake of neuronally released amines. Because of multiple receptor involvement, autonomic nervous system effects are erratic, unpredictable, and complex. However, potent drugs like the piperazine phenothiazines (e.g., fluphenazine) and haloperidol, in clinically therapeutic doses, have little antiadrenergic activity. Chlorpromazine produces miosis, but **thioridazine (Melleril)**, the most potent muscarinic antagonist among the antipsychotic drugs, produces mydriasis. Constipation, decreases in gastric secretion and motility, and decreases in sweating (which can precipitate heat stroke and hyperthermia) and salivation are common. These anticholinergic actions are less prominent with the more potent antipsychotic drugs. Most of these drugs, except thioridazine, also have an antiemetic effect, owing to their interaction with dopamine receptors in the chemoreceptor trigger zone in the medulla.

Orthostatic hypotension and reflex tachycardia are prominent because of central actions and peripheral α-adrenoceptor antagonism. Tolerance to the hypotensive effect of antipsychotic drugs develops, but is never complete. Chlorpromazine and thioridazine are much more likely to produce cardiovascular effects than haloperidol, loxapine, molindone, or piperazine phenothiazines. Chlorpromazine also has a direct depressant action on the heart.

Chlorpromazine also exerts central effects on **hypothalamic neurons** and **pituitary mammotrophs**. Normal temperature regulation is disrupted and, depending on the environmental temperature, hypothermia or hyperthermia ensues. A relative hypothermia is typically observed, as body temperature is usually higher than room temperature. This is further complicated by peripheral vasodilation. Prolactin secretion from the pituitary is increased, and the urinary content of gonadotropins, estrogens, and progestins decreases. These effects can result in infertility and galactorrhea in females and gynecomastia in males. Chlorpromazine but not haloperidol produces an increase in appetite and subsequent weight gain.

Side Effects

Undesirable effects of antipsychotic drugs are an extension of therapeutic effects and their actions at multiple receptor sites. They depend on the drug, dose, and susceptibility of the patient. These agents, however, have a wide margin of safety, a **high therapeutic index,** and deaths from intoxication are rare with the exception of those caused by thioridazine and mesoridazine. Jaundice and blood dyscrasias are rare and are a risk only with low-potency antipsychotic drugs such as chlorpromazine. Dermatological reactions (e.g., hypersensitivity, contact dermatitis, and photosensitivity) are common with the use of phenothiazines. Opacity of the cornea and lens of the eye have been noted after long-term therapy with low-potency drugs (e.g., chlorpromazine). Thioridazine, another low-potency drug, may produce pigmentary retinopathy after high doses.

In high doses, antipsychotic drugs with a prominent anticholinergic action may produce confusion and delirium. The most common adverse effects (seen in 40 percent of patients), however, are extrapyramidal symptoms. They are more frequent with potent antipsychotic agents (e.g., piperazine-phenothiazines and butyrophenones), but are produced by all antipsychotic drugs.

Extrapyramidal symptoms include parkinsonism, acute dystonia, akathisia, and tardive dyskinesia. Parkinsonism is characterized by bradykinesia, rigidity and tremor at rest, masklike face, and a shuffling gait. It is seen early during treatment and can be treated with antiparkinsonism drugs, particularly of the anticholinergic class. **Acute dystonias** include facial grimacing and torticollis. **Akathisia** is characterized by aimless and uncontrollable restlessness. **Tardive dyskinesia,** however, remains the most troublesome complication of long-term therapy with antipsychotic agents because it is irreversible. After extended treatment (usually longer than 3 to 6 months), extrapyramidal disorders characterized by a variable mixture of orofacial dyskinesias, tics, choreas, dystonias, athetoses, or facial grimacing may appear. Collectively, these are sometimes referred to as a "bucco-linguo-masticatory" syndrome. The prevalence rates among patients exposed to treatment for at least 1 year ranges from 10 to 20 percent, but with increasing age the incidence, severity, and intractability increase. Tardive dyskinesia is **iatrogenic** and best explained by the postsynaptic supersensitivity that develops from chronic exposure of the nigro-striatal dopaminergic pathway to the dopamine receptor blocking action of antipsychotic agents. This interpretation is supported by the fact that L-dopa and anticholinergic drugs (e.g., **benztropine; Cogentin**) exacerbate, whereas drugs depleting (reserpine) or blocking (phenothiazines) dopamine activity attenuate, tardive dyskinesia. There is also some evidence that neurons responsible for modulating dopamine activity (e.g., GABAergic and cholinergic) may be injuriously affected. GABA-receptor agonists (e.g., valproate, muscimol, and baclofen) and cholinergic drugs (e.g., choline and lecithin) have been shown to be only mildly effective in reducing symptoms over the short term.

No treatment produces consistent relief from tardive dyskinesia, and fewer than half of treated patients show even moderate reduction in symptoms; thus, prevention must be emphasized. This can be attempted by early and repeated periods of withdrawal from the drug, accompanied by both psychiatric and movement disorder evaluation. Another approach is to use only those agents that offer a smaller risk for producing tardive dyskinesia (e.g., thioridazine). When tardive dyskinesia is already present, the best course is to withdraw treatment, when possible, for a long enough period to allow the disorder to dissipate. In cases in which the dyskinesia is severe and debilitating, reintroduction of a dopamine-receptor blocking agent may be required. However, increasing the dose of drug to suppress the dyskinesia may again exacerbate the movement disorder after continued use.

A rare but potentially fatal **neurolept malignant syndrome** may occur early during treatment. It is characterized by hyperthermia, skeletal muscle hypertonia, disturbance of consciousness, tachycardia, cardiac arrhythmias, fluctuations in blood pressure, and pallor. A decrease in dopaminergic function may lead to this syndrome as well as to akathisia, dystonia, and parkinsonism. This syndrome is best treated with **dantrolene (Dantrium),** a skeletal muscle relaxant; **bromocriptine (Parlodel)** is sometimes useful.

Tolerance

Tolerance develops to the sedative, hypotensive, and anticholinergic effects of antipsychotic drugs over a period of days to weeks; tolerance does not develop to their antipsychotic effects. Prolonged use of antipsychotic agents may result in disuse supersensitivity of dopaminergic systems and is reflected as a form of tolerance in certain behavioral and biochemical tests. Dopamine-containing neurons in brain areas implicated in psychoses (e.g., limbic and cortical forebrain) may not show as much tolerance as the basal ganglia dopaminergic system. Physical dependence, if any, is very mild and reflected by muscular discomfort and insomnia.

DRUGS USED IN THE TREATMENT OF MOVEMENT DISORDERS

Most movement disorders involve dysfunction of the brain's **extrapyramidal system**. Extrapyramidal structures are all those that affect bodily (somatic) movement, excluding the pyramidal tract, motor neurons, and motor cortex. The extrapyramidal system is made up of the **basal ganglia** (globus pallidus, putamen, and caudate nucleus), their associated structures (substantia nigra and subthalamic nuclei), and descending midbrain connections. Some of the anatomical relationships and functional neurotransmitters are diagrammed in Figure 5–3. Many lesions of the basal ganglia, thought to be responsible for movement (motor) disorders, appear to involve the loss of dopaminergic neurons or loss of inhibitory (GABAergic and/or dopaminergic) input control.

The major disorders of movement fall into four broad categories: choreic movements, tremors, dystonias, and tics. These may be caused by specific disease states or aging or may be drug-induced. **Choreic movements** are the actions of single, isolated muscles, resulting in uncoordinated short and rapid jerks. These usually involve the muscles of the face, trunk, or proximal portions of the limbs. The latter, in their more violent form, are termed ballismus. **Tremors** consist of involuntary rhythmic, repetitive movements, and may occur at rest (associated with parkinsonism), during movement (intention tremor), or when a certain posture is assumed (postural tremor). **Dystonias** are brought about by prolonged muscle spasms that usually distort body posture. The spasms may be sustained or repetitive and, if associated with a writhing motion, are termed athetoses. **Tics** are repetitive and coordinated sudden movements, usually involving the head and face. These may be multiple or single, chronic or transient.

Only those movement disorders that affect the basal ganglia and that are subject to drug therapy are considered here. These include parkinsonism, Huntington's chorea, Tourette's syndrome, and Wilson's disease. Tardive dyskinesia also falls into this category but was discussed previously in the section on antipsychotic drugs.

CORTEX

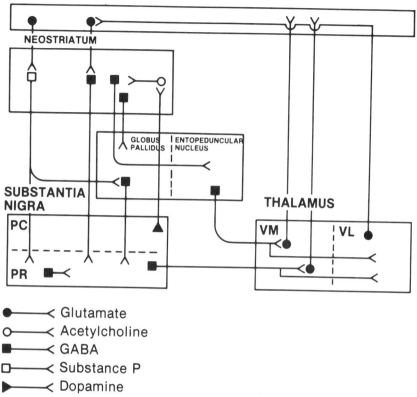

● ———< Glutamate
○ ———< Acetylcholine
■ ———< GABA
□ ———< Substance P
▲ ———< Dopamine

Figure 5–3. A diagrammatic representation of some of the major neuronal pathways within the basal ganglia, showing both cortical input and thalamic output. PC = pars compacta; PR = pars reticulata; VM = nucleus ventralis medialis; VL = nucleus ventralis lateralis.

Parkinsonism

Parkinsonism is an adult-onset, progressive **degenerative disorder** of the CNS involving loss of dopaminergic neurons in the substantia nigra and characterized by **bradykinesia, rigidity, resting tremor,** and, in late stages, by postural defects and impaired mental status. It can be broadly classified into two major groups: **primary** or **idiopathic,** and **secondary** or **symptomatic.** Primary Parkinson's disease is the most prevalent. The etiology remains unknown, but environmental influences appear to play a predominant role in its causation. Secondary Parkinson's disease could result from infections (postviral encephalitis), toxins (carbon monoxide, manganese, methylphenyltetrahydropyridine; MPTP), free radicals, atherosclerosis, drugs (antipsychotics), metabolic disorders (anoxia), tumors, head trauma, and some degenerative disorders. Secondary parkinsonism, except in few cases (e.g., MPTP-induced; see further on), is qualitatively different from primary parkinsonism. Moreover, levodopa (L-dopa), the drug highly effective in the therapy of primary parkinsonism, is only partially effective in secondary parkinsonism and, in addition, in fewer cases (25 percent). Exceptions are manganese- and MPTP-induced secondary parkinsonism, which **do** respond to L-dopa therapy. In contrast, anticholinergic drugs are more effective in the therapy of secondary parkinsonism than primary parkinsonism.

Parkinsonism is a disease of the **basal ganglia** and **dopamine,** where the latter is an inhibitory neurotransmitter acting on the excitatory cholinergic neurons in the striatum. It is believed that parkinsonism results from an **imbalance in dopamine and acetylcholine** neuronal functions following degeneration of dopamine-containing cells. A schematic representation of the relationships among the dopaminergic system, cholinergic neurons, and pathways of extrapyramidal motor output is depicted in Figure 5–3.

MPTP (1-methyl-4-phenyl-1,2,3,6-tetrahydropyridine), an intermediate in the synthesis of meperidine, has been established to **selectively damage dopamine-containing neurons** in the substantia nigra and produce an irreversible parkinsonism. MPTP binds to monoamine oxidase–type B (MAO-B) and is oxidized to 1-methyl-4-phenylpyridinium ion (MPP^+) extraneuronally. MPP^+ in turn is taken up and concentrated by dopamine-containing cells which gradually die. Inhibitors of MAO-B prevent this toxicity. Neuromelanin in neurons in the substantia nigra seems to be involved in the toxicity of MPTP because, in contrast to humans and monkeys, rats lack neuromelanin and are resistant to the toxic effects of MPTP. Thus, chronic exposure to small amounts of similar chemicals, in conjunction with aging, may precipitate secondary parkinsonism.

Although current evidence strongly supports the involvement of dopamine in Parkinson's disease, only approximately 75 percent of patients suffering from this disorder respond to therapy with drugs that increase dopaminergic function or content in the CNS; 25 percent respond to anticholinergic therapy. Manipulations of neurotransmitter systems other than dopamine or acetylcholine have no significant ameliorative effect. The etiology and optimal course of treatment of this disorder has yet to be established.

The most effective drug treatment for parkinsonism focuses on central dopaminergic activity; enhancing dopamine synthesis (L-dopa), decreasing dopamine catabolism (selegiline, an MAO-B inhibitor), enhancing dopamine release (amantadine), or administration of D_2 receptor agonists (bromocriptine) (Table 5–6).

Two types of **dopamine receptors** are known to be present in the CNS: D_1 and D_2. Interaction of dopamine with D_1 receptors results in activation of adenylate cyclase and accumulation of cyclic AMP. In the basal ganglia, D_1

Table 5-6. DRUGS USED IN THE TREATMENT
OF PARKINSON'S DISEASE

Drugs which enhance dopaminergic activity

Dihydroxyphenylalanine (Levodopa/L-DOPA)	Dopar, Larodopa
Carbidopa	Lodosyn
Levodopa + Carbidopa	Sinemet
Amantadine	Symmetrel
Selegilene (deprenyl)	
Bromocriptine	Parlodel

L-DOPA

Carbidopa

Anticholinergic Drugs

Benztropine	Cogentin
Trihexyphenidyl	Artane
Biperiden	Akineton
Procyclidine	Kemadrin
Ethopropazine	Parsidol

Benzotropine

Antihistamines

Diphenhydramine	Benadryl
Orphenadrine	Disipal

receptors are localized postsynaptically. The function of D_1 receptors in the CNS is unknown. Interaction of dopamine with D_2 receptors results in either the inhibition of or no change in adenylate cyclase activity. D_2 receptors are localized both postsynaptically and presynaptically. **Presynaptic D_2 receptors, or autoreceptors,** regulate the release of dopamine from the nerve terminal and modulate dopamine turnover *via* negative feedback. Activation of postsynaptic D_2 receptors on cholinergic neurons inhibits acetylcholine release, whereas activation of nigral D_2 receptors inhibits neuronal activity of dopamine neurons. Presynaptic and postsynaptic D_2 receptors are qualitatively different and can be distinguished on the basis of their relative affinities for dopamine agonists and antagonists. D_2 receptors are also present on the mammotrophs of the anterior pituitary, on neurons in the medullary chemosensitive trigger zone, and on noradrenergic nerve terminals. Their activation at these locales results in inhibition of prolactin release, emesis, and inhibition of norepinephrine release, respectively.

Levodopa

Apomorphine, the first dopamine-receptor agonist of beneficial use in parkinsonism, was withdrawn because of renal toxicity. Dopamine itself cannot be used, as it does not cross the blood-brain barrier. Therefore, L-dopa, **the immediate precursor of dopamine,** is used. Since 95 percent of orally administered L-dopa is decarboxylated in the periphery to form dopamine, and only 1 percent or less of administered L-dopa enters the brain, very high doses must be administered (maintenance levels of up to 6 to 8 g per day). Although biosynthetic enzymes for dopamine are drastically reduced in parkinsonism, the remaining intact neurons can synthesize dopamine. Moreover, because the decarboxylation of L-dopa is not the rate-limiting step, most of the L-dopa reaching the CNS is rapidly converted to dopamine. All primary neurological symptoms except tremor show improvement—particularly bradykinesia and rigidity. Posture, facial expressions, and other disturbances also show dramatic improvement. Mental status is improved such that there is a feeling of well-being, increase in self-esteem, and greater interest in self and family. The increase in dopamine peripherally following high doses of L-dopa produces orthostatic hypotension and cardiac stimulation, α- and β-adrenoceptor-mediated effects, respectively. The orthostatic hypotension is most likely due to accumulation of dopamine in norepinephrine nerve terminals where dopamine may act as a false transmitter with only partial agonist activity at α_1 receptors. Cardiac arrhythmias and transient tachycardia may occur. Tolerance to all of these cardiovascular effects over several weeks develops.

The most common (80 percent) unwanted effects of L-dopa therapy are nausea, vomiting, anorexia, and other elements of epigastric distress. Nausea and vomiting result from dopaminergic stimulation of the chemosensitive trigger zone in the medulla. Tolerance to the GI effects develops over 6 to 12 weeks. Behavioral effects of L-dopa include hallucinations, depression, anxiety, mania, insomnia and paranoia, particularly in the elderly. About 15 percent of patients develop severe depression, confusion, and delirium. Patients with a history of mental illness may develop psychotic reactions.

There are **four major problems** associated with long-term therapy with L-dopa:

1. **abnormal involuntary movements**
2. changes in drug efficacy characterized by "**on**" (drug is effective)–"**off**" (drug is ineffective) phenomenon during the course of daily drug therapy
3. **decreasing efficacy**
4. **impairment of mental status**

Abnormal involuntary movements are the most important limiting factor in establishing an optimal maintenance dose, since tolerance to this effect does not develop. A majority (90 percent) of patients develop faciolingual tics, grimacing, and a variety of rocking movements within about 1 year of therapy with L-dopa; in about 50 percent of patients they appear early (2 to 4 months). An increase in postsynaptic D_2 receptors and resultant receptor supersensitivity may contribute to the development of abnormal movements. After about 2 years of therapy, patients begin to develop swings between beneficial effects ("on") and akinesia ("off") during the daily course of oral doses. The "on" stage is often seen close to the time of peak plasma drug concentration of L-dopa, and the "off" stage close to that of low plasma concentration. Because of the short half-life (1 to 3 hours) of L-dopa (and therefore dopamine), it is difficult to maintain a stable ameliorative effect on bradykinesia and rigidity (and therefore mobility).

The decrease in efficacy of levodopa after 2 to 3 years of therapy may be due to the progressive, degenerative nature of the disease. In addition, D_2 receptors may become **subsensitive** with continuous exposure to dopamine, also reducing drug efficacy. Recommendation of "drug holidays" is based on the possible existence of receptor subsensitivity.

Inhibitors of decarboxylase (e.g., **carbidopa**) that do not cross the blood-brain barrier offer several advantages in the therapy of parkinsonism. When administered concurrently with **L-dopa,** the peripheral decarboxylation of L-dopa is prevented and plasma concentrations of L-dopa and its half-life increase; more L-dopa enters the CNS and less is metabolized to dopamine and norepinephrine in the periphery. A preparation of the combination of **carbidopa** and **L-dopa (Sinemet)** has several advantages over L-dopa administration alone: the dose of L-dopa can be reduced by 75 percent, the onset of action is faster, the incidence of nausea and vomiting is reduced, cardiac effects are diminished, and both the percent of people showing improvement and the degree of improvement seem to be greater. However, the incidence of abnormal involuntary movements and impaired mental status persists and is even exaggerated and appears sooner during therapy.

Other Agents Affecting Dopaminergic Activity

Amantadine (Symmetrel), an antiviral agent, **releases dopamine** from nerve terminals and also blocks the uptake of released dopamine. It has no anticholinergic actions. Although it has a long duration of action, amantadine loses its efficacy following 6 to 8 weeks of therapy. It is, therefore, used episodically for 2 to 3 weeks at a time. Amantadine is relatively free of side effects and may be effectively combined with L-dopa or used alone. It may also be combined with anticholinergic drugs.

Several **ergot derivatives** are also **dopamine-receptor agonists: bromocriptine,** lisuride, pergolide, and lergotrile. Because of toxicity, only **bromocriptine (Parlodel)** among the ergot derivatives is used extensively. It stimulates dopamine receptors in the CNS and periphery, has a preference for D_2 receptors, and inhibits the D_1 receptor. Bromocriptine, in high doses, is almost as effective as L-dopa. Often, subminimal doses of bromocriptine and L-dopa can be combined beneficially, particularly in patients manifesting an "on-off" sydnrome. Bromocriptine, however, is very expensive and produces severe CNS effects, such as auditory and visual hallucinations, delusions, and psychotic reactions.

Monoamine oxidase (MAO) is an enzyme important in the inactivation of monoamines and exists as two isoenzymes: MAO-A and MAO-B. MAO-A preferentially metabolizes norepinephrine and serotonin, whereas MAO-B metabolizes dopamine. Certain areas in the brain, such as dopamine-containing neurons, are rich in MAO-B. Selective inhibitors of MAO-B (e.g., selegiline) are useful not only in prolonging the beneficial effects of dopamine but also in preventing the hypertensive effects normally seen with the use of nonspecific MAO inhibitors such as phenelzine (Nardil).

Anticholinergic Drugs

Anticholinergic drugs were among the first to be used in the treatment of Parkinson's disease. These agents are not as effective as L-dopa, and at best, tremor is reduced, with only 25 percent of patients showing beneficial effects. L-dopa and carbidopa have since become the drugs of choice. Anticholinergic drugs still retain their usefulness in patients who do not respond to L-dopa or cannot tolerate its undesirable effects. Parkinsonism-like symptoms produced by antipsychotic drugs are better ameliorated with anticholinergic drugs. Tremor responds better than do bradykinesia and rigidity to this class of drugs. Trihexyphenidyl (Artane) is the prototype drug of this class, whose use is limited by peripheral (e.g., blurred vision, urinary retention, constipation) and central (confusion, delirium, hallucinations) anticholinergic effects. One of the anticholinergic effects—inhibition of salivation—is desirable because it ameliorates the sialorrhea of parkinsonism. The anticholinergics should be avoided in patients with narrow-angle glaucoma; they also worsen tardive dyskinesia and may produce hyperpyrexia because of reduced sweating.

Huntington's Chorea

Huntington's chorea is a genetically transmitted autosomal dominant disease characterized by progressive dementia and choreic movements. Its onset usually occurs after the third or fourth decade of life, with fatal outcome in 10 to 15 years. Choreic movements are the predominant motor dysfunction; however, both dystonias and the parkinsonian syndrome begin somewhat later in the illness and also become progressively worse.

Neuropathological changes observed in Huntington's chorea are neostriatal degeneration of cholinergic interneurons and loss of GABAergic neurons which project to the substantia nigra. Concentrations of the neuropeptides cholecystokinin, substance P, and methionine-enkephalin are also depleted, whereas that of somatostatin is elevated. A concomitant decrease in the activities of choline acetyltransferase and glutamic acid decarboxylase, the enzymes responsible for the synthesis of acetylcholine and GABA, respectively, is also seen. While the neuronal pathways involving dopamine and glutamate do not appear to be directly affected, the resulting imbalance of excess dopamine within the basal ganglia (in the absence of GABAergic inhibitory control) is probably responsible for the choreic movements. Similar dopaminergic overactivity in the mesolimbic system, where cell death also occurs, may also contribute to the psychiatric problems observed. The most useful drugs in containing the choreic movements are dopamine-receptor antagonists (e.g., phenothiazines and butyrophenones). Attempts to suppress the movement disorder by supplementing lost GABAergic and cholinergic activities with agonists or by inhibiting catabolism have met with little success.

Tourette's Syndrome

Gilles de la Tourette's (Tourette's) syndrome most commonly begins in childhood and usually consists of chronic tic movements of the face, eyes, and upper body. In severe cases, very complex motor (involving all types of movement disorders) and vocal tics and behavioral symptoms can occur. Those individuals who are most dramatically affected have the earliest onset of symptoms of the most severe kind. Both genetic and environmental factors appear to be important in the expression of this syndrome. The dopaminergic system appears to be important in Tourette's syndrome, and the butyrophenone **haloperidol (Haldol)** is the most effective drug used. There is some evidence that norepinephrine may also be involved because clonidine, an α_2-adrenoceptor agonist, is also effective in some cases.

Wilson's Disease

Wilson's disease is an autosomal recessive genetic disorder of copper metabolism, in which there is an abnormally low serum level of the copperbinding protein, ceruloplasmin. Copper accumulates in the liver, brain, and cornea. Neurological effects include dysarthria, progressing to dystonia and gait disorders. Treatment is aimed at removing excess copper by orally administering **penicillamine (dimethylcysteine)**, a chelating agent. Dietary measures are taken to avoid copper-containing foods such as chocolate, nuts, shellfish, liver, and cereals.

DRUGS USED IN THE TREATMENT OF AFFECTIVE DISORDERS

Drugs used in the treatment of depression (Table 5–7) are believed effective because of their ability to facilitate neurotransmission in central noradrenergic and/or serotonergic neurons. These drugs are not general CNS stimulants, however, and tricyclic and newer second-generation antidepressants produce little or no elevation of mood in normal individuals. These observations have led to the **biogenic amine hypothesis of depression**. The implication of the hypothesis is that depression is caused by hypoactivity of central adrenergic and perhaps serotonergic systems. In mania, these same neurotransmitter systems are believed to be hyperactive. Support for the hypothesis is provided by the effect of drugs, such as reserpine, which deplete biogenic amines, and produce a depression similar to endogenous depression. The hypothesis, however, is not entirely satisfactory, as blockage of amine

Table 5–7. DRUGS USED IN THE TREATMENT OF DEPRESSION

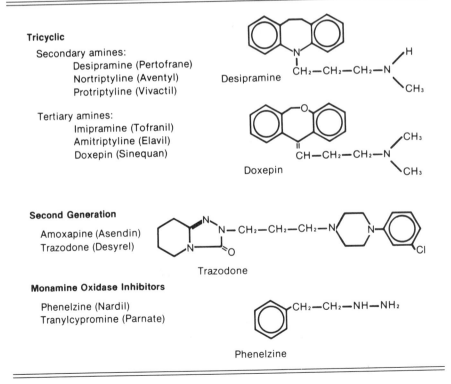

Tricyclic

Secondary amines:
Desipramine (Pertofrane)
Nortriptyline (Aventyl)
Protriptyline (Vivactil)

Desipramine

Tertiary amines:
Imipramine (Tofranil)
Amitriptyline (Elavil)
Doxepin (Sinequan)

Doxepin

Second Generation

Amoxapine (Asendin)
Trazodone (Desyrel)

Trazodone

Monamine Oxidase Inhibitors

Phenelzine (Nardil)
Tranylcypromine (Parnate)

Phenelzine

uptake by tricyclic and second-generation antidepressant drugs is prompt, whereas **clinical improvement is not manifest until after 2 to 3 weeks of therapy**. The action of tricyclic antidepressant drugs is further complicated in that their long-term effects on norepinephrine and serotonin metabolism, neuronal function, and presynaptic- and postsynaptic-receptor sensitivity are not the same as those observed after their initial administration. For example, after initial administration of a tricyclic antidepressant, neurotransmitter reuptake is inhibited; thus, more neurotransmitter is available to act at presynaptic autoreceptors, which **decrease** neurotransmitter release. With continuous treatment, both excitability and amine turnover return to normal or exceed normal while blockage of reuptake persists. After long-term treatment with tricyclic or monoamine oxidase inhibitor antidepressants, there is a decrease in postsynaptic β-adrenoceptor density, desensitization of cyclic nucleotide generating systems, **sub**sensitivity of presynaptic α_2-adrenoceptors to norepinephrine, and enhanced responses to α_1-adrenoceptor agonists and serotonin. Thus, the long-term effects of antidepressants on amine metabolism and receptor sensitivity are different and in opposition to those seen early during therapy. These observations have been employed to argue against a crucial role for biogenic amines in depression; however, they may reflect long-term adaptive changes in amine-containing neuronal function, as a consequence of the disease process or of chronic antidepressant drug therapy, or both.

Depression is associated with episodic and recurrent combinations of profound sadness, impairment of psychomotor function, pessimistic ideas, low self-esteem, feelings of worthlessness, guilt, loss of interest in sex and previously pleasurable activities, and somatic symptoms such as anorexia, weight loss, insomnia, fatigue, constipation, headaches, aches and pains, and bad taste in the mouth. Severe depression is characterized by suicidal thoughts and hopelessness. Three categories of depression have been established: **reactive, endogenous,** and **bipolar**. Reactive, or secondary, depression is most common and is usually associated with a loss in the family, illness (cancer), drug use (antihypertensives, contraceptives, corticosteroids, alcohol), organic causes (seizures, hypothyroidism), or other psychiatric illnesses (schizophrenia, anxiety, dementia). Endogenous depression (unipolar or major depression) is defined as biologically determined and is the next most common type of depression. In manic-depressive illness (bipolar depression), mania and depression alternate. Occasionally only depression, and rarely only mania, is present.

Tricyclic and Second-Generation Antidepressants

Despite claims to the contrary, there are no significant differences between the efficacy of tricyclic and second-generation antidepressants in the treatment of depression (see Table 5–7). Their most prominent actions are on central and autonomic nervous and cardiovascular systems. Tricyclic and second-generation antidepressants are not CNS stimulants and are not useful in organic or drug-induced depression. They are most useful in endogenous depression, but are not curative. Tricyclics tend to be most successful in patients who exhibit a distinctive quality of depressed mood (prominent and persistent dysphoria), diurnal variation in mood (with depression worst in morning), early morning awakening, poor appetite or weight loss, psychomotor agitation or retardation, lack of reactivity of depressed mood, and anhedonia.

The choice of antidepressant drug is individualized on the basis of past history of use and severity of depression. In order to minimize the occurrence of side effects, the initial dose should be low and increased over several days. Doses for elderly should be reduced. Tricyclic antidepressants are well absorbed orally, are highly lipophilic, bind extensively to plasma proteins, and have long plasma half-lives (15 to 78 hours). They are oxidized by hepatic microsomal drug-metabolizing enzymes. Mono-N-demethylation, N-demethylation, aliphatic hydroxylation, and aromatic hydroxylation, followed by conjugation with glucuronic acid, are the major paths of metabolism.

Acute CNS effects include sedation, unsteady gait, and anxiety. Tertiary amine tricyclics (e.g., amitriptyline, doxepin) elicit the highest incidence of sedation, whereas secondary amine tricyclics (e.g., desipramine, protriptyline) produce psychomotor activation and are less likely to produce sedation. Secondary amine tricyclics are therefore more useful in retarded depression. After repeated administration, mood elevation is apparent in depressed patients but not in normal healthy individuals. Therapeutic effects are not seen until after 2 to 3 weeks of therapy. All **tricyclics block the uptake of released serotonin and norepinephrine** into nerve terminals, the major mechanism for inactivation of neuronally released amines. The potency and selectivity of inhibition of amine uptake varies among individual drugs (Table 5–8). Tertiary amine tricyclics (e.g., amitriptyline) are more potent than secondary amine tricyclics (e.g., desipramine) in blocking serotonin uptake, whereas secondary amine tricyclics are more potent in blocking norepinephrine uptake. For example, desipramine is 100 to 1000 times less potent in blocking serotonin uptake than in blocking norepinephrine uptake. Trazodone, an atypical antidepressant, blocks only serotonin uptake. None of these drugs is effective in blocking dopamine uptake, as are the nonantidepressants cocaine and amphetamine.

Side Effects

Effects on the autonomic nervous system are a consequence of blockage of norepinephrine uptake peripherally and of **direct action at muscarinic cholinergic** and α_1 **adrenoceptors**. Dry mouth, blurred vision, urinary hesitancy,

Table 5–8. COMPARISON OF PHARMACOLOGIC
EFFECTS OF SEVERAL ANTIDEPRESSANT DRUGS*

Drug	Usual Range of Daily Dosage (mg)	Sedative Effects	Anticho-linergic Effects	Cardio-toxic Effects[†]	Inhibition of Reuptake of		
					NE	5-HT	DA
Tertiary Amines							
Imipramine	75–300	+ +	+ +	+ +	+ +	+ +	0
Amitriptyline	75–300	+ + +	+ + +	+ +	+	+ + +	0
Doxepin	75–300	+ + +	+ + +	+ +	+	+ +	0
Secondary Amines							
Desipramine	75–300	+	+	+ +	+ + +	0	0
Nortriptyline	40–150	+ +	+ +	+ +	+ +	+	0
Protriptyline	20–60	0	+ +	+ +	+ + +	uncertain	uncertain
Second Generation							
Amoxapine	75–400	+ +	+	minimal	+ +	+	+
Trazodone	75–400	+ + +	0	minimal	0	+	0

*0 = none; + = slight; + + = moderate; + + + = high
†Cardiac effects are usually seen with high doses and may vary in severity.

and constipation are commonly seen. Tertiary amine tricyclics are more potent than secondary amine tricyclics in producing anticholinergic actions and hypotension. Trazodone, a second-generation antidepressant, has little anticholinergic effect.

In therapeutic doses, the tricyclics produce significant **cardiovascular effects** which, in cases of intoxication, can be life threatening. Postural hypotension (a consequence of peripheral α_1-adrenoceptor antagonism), mild tachycardia, and ventricular arrhythmia, particularly when bundle branch block is present, are common. Trazodone appears to have minimal effects on cardiac conduction.

With the exception of amoxapine, which blocks dopamine receptors, tricyclic antidepressants do not elicit significant extrapyramidal symptoms or tardive dyskinesias. Claims have been made that the newer second-generation antidepressants (amoxapine, maprotiline, trazodone) have faster onset of action, fewer anticholinergic effects, and less cardiotoxicity, but these claims are not yet firmly established.

Tolerance and Toxicity

Tolerance develops to the anticholinergic actions of these agents. Physical dependence, if any, is mild and is revealed as lethargy and muscle aches after abrupt discontinuation of long-term therapy. Intoxication may produce coma, respiratory depression, hyperpyrexia, seizures, cardiac arrhythmias, hypotension, bowel and bladder paralysis, and death. In some patients, tricyclics (and other antidepressants) can precipitate manic episodes. Cardiotoxicity is less with amoxapine intoxication, but the incidence of seizures and acute renal failure is increased. Tricyclic antidepressants are potentially lethal in overdose, and the patient should not be allowed to keep more than a 1-week supply of these drugs.

Drug Interactions

The tricyclic antidepressants interact with several classes of drugs. The anticholinergic activity of tricyclics should be considered when they must be used concurrently with antimuscarinic drugs. Tricyclics will reverse the antihypertensive action of guanethidine by blocking its uptake into noradrenergic nerve terminals; they also block the uptake of directly and indirectly acting (e.g., tyramine) sympathomimetic amines. Rarely, concurrent administration of a monoamine oxidase inhibitor and a tricyclic can produce hyperpyrexia, convulsions, and coma.

Monoamine Oxidase (MAO) Inhibitors

Three monoamine oxidase (MAO) inhibitors are marketed in the United States: phenelzine, isocarboxazid, and tranylcypromine (Fig. 5–4). They inhibit oxidative deamination of serotonin (5-hydroxytryptamine) and catecholamines, and increase their content in the brain. They produce, in normal subjects, a feeling of well-being, elevation of mood, and increase in motor activity. Tranylcypromine rapidly produces behavioral effects such as CNS stimulation and an increase in motor activity because of its amphetamine-like,

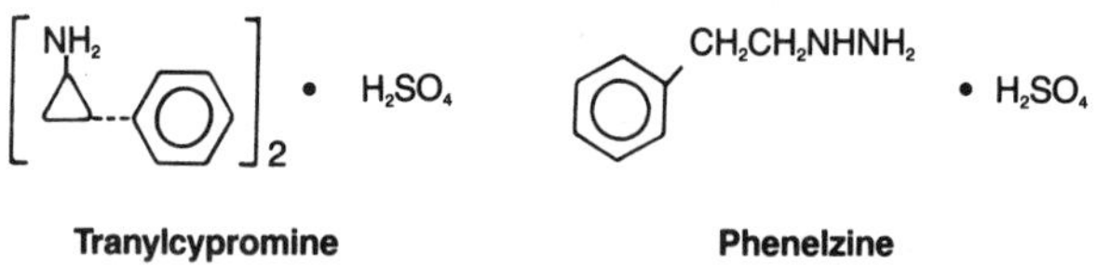

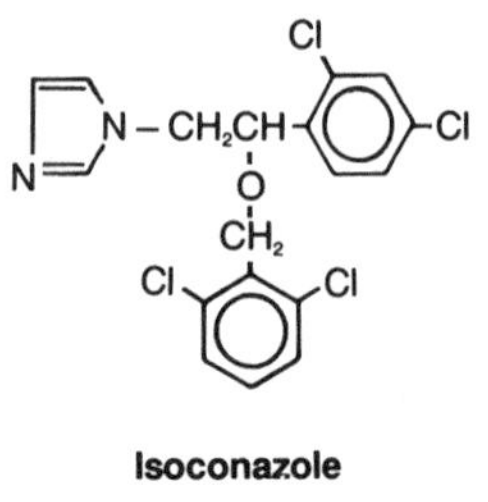

Tranylcypromine

Phenelzine

Isoconazole

Figure 5–4. Chemical structures of the MAO inhibitors currently in clinical use for the treatment of depression.

catecholamine-releasing action. However, the relationship between the anti-depressant effects of the MAO inhibitors and their ability to increase the brain amine content remains unproven. MAO inhibitors are readily absorbed following oral administration. Although maximal inhibition of enzymes occurs within 5 to 7 days, clinical antidepressant effects are not produced for 2 to 3 weeks. MAO inhibitors have a very limited role in the treatment of depression because of their **high toxicity** and **limited effectiveness**. In endogenous depression they may be no more effective than a placebo. They have been shown to be effective in the treatment of so-called atypical neurotic depression characterized by anxiety, phobias, and depression, which may include reactive depression.

Drug Interactions

These drugs inhibit not only the enzyme MAO but also other hepatic microsomal drug-metabolizing enzymes, thus decreasing the metabolism of several other classes of drugs. MAO inhibitors thus will prolong and intensify the effects of CNS depressant, tricyclic antidepressant, and anticholinergic drugs. Concomitant use of tricyclic antidepressant drugs or meperidine with MAO inhibitors may produce severe and catastrophic CNS toxicity.

Toxicity and Side Effects

The most serious adverse effects of intoxication involve the liver, brain, and cardiovascular system. Hepatoxicity is low with the drugs currently in use but is seen more with hydrazine derivatives (e.g., phenelzine). All MAO inhibitors produce postural hypotension and effectively suppress REM sleep. Central effects are manifest as various combinations of dizziness, agitation, insomnia, tremors, hallucinations, confusion, hyperreflexia, delirium, convulsions, manic episodes (in some patients), and atropine-like action (dry mouth, blurred vision, urinary hesitancy, and constipation).

Monoamine oxidase is involved in the regulation of the metabolism of biogenic amines, including tyramine. Tyramine is an excellent substrate for MAO, is endogenously formed, and is rapidly metabolized in the liver. Thus, the actions of indirectly acting sympathomimetic amines, such as tyramine and amphetamine, are potentiated by MAO inhibitors. Certain foods rich in tyramine (some cheeses, wines, and herring), when ingested during therapy with MAO inhibitors, may produce a **hypertensive crisis** and death. Hypertensive syndrome (hypertensive crisis with or without intracranial bleeding, headache, fever) may also occur when MAO inhibitors are used with other sympathomimetic amines such as methyldopa and dopamine, or when they are used concurrently with antihypertensive drugs such as guanethidine.

Lithium Salts

Lithium salts are highly effective and specific **antimanic** agents that normalize mood and cause cessation of racing thoughts without producing marked sedation. Lithium carbonate is the drug of choice for manic-depressive illness (bipolar affective disorder), especially during the manic phase. It is effective in 60 to 70 percent of patients within 2 weeks of initiating therapy. In addition, it is known to be useful prophylactically in preventing and will reduce the severity and the frequency of both mania and depression as well as prevent depressive episodes.

In mild mania, lithium alone is used. In agitated and hyperactive mania, therapy with less potent antipsychotic agents (e.g., chlorpromazine) is initiated simultaneously with lithium. The sedative properties of less potent antipsychotic agents allow better management of agitated manics. Lithium is less effective in the treatment of unipolar or major depressive illness, although it will suppress the severity and frequency of depressive episodes in manic-depressive illness.

Lithium can replace Na^+ in generating an action potential but cannot be substituted for Na^+ to maintain the membrane potential. Lithium **inhibits the Ca^{2+}-dependent release of norepinephrine and dopamine** but not of serotonin. Uptake and intraneuronal metabolism of catecholamines is enhanced by lithium, resulting in an overall decrease in the neuronal content of norepinephrine and dopamine. These observations support the hypothesis that mania may result from a hyperactivity of catecholaminergic systems.

Pharmacokinetics

Lithium salts are rapidly absorbed from the GI system. Lithium ion is not highly lipid soluble, does not bind to plasma proteins, and is not metabolized. Ninety-five percent of administered lithium is eliminated in urine unchanged; its elimination half-life is 20 to 24 hours.

Lithium has a **low therapeutic index** and therefore its plasma concentration must be regularly determined. The dose of lithium is optimized for maximal effect and minimal toxicity for each individual. Renal function is important in determining the clearance of lithium. Age and dehydration may decrease the clearance of lithium and thereby increase its toxicity.

Side Effects and Toxicity

Initially, sodium retention and edema are common but disappear after a few days. Polyuria and polydipsia, which are diabetes insipidus–like, are common and result, at least in part, from inhibition of the action of antidiuretic hormone on renal adenylate cyclase and an impairment of renal concentrating ability (nephrogenic diabetes insipidus). Patients reduce their water intake for fear of nocturia but should be discouraged from doing so because a reduction in water intake may reduce the clearance of lithium and increase its toxicity. Goiter with or without **hypothyroidism** may occur, probably due to inhibition of TSH (thyroid stimulating hormone)–mediated activation of thyroid adenylate cyclase. Acute intoxication may be manifest as an allergic reaction, leukocytosis, tremor, ataxia, diarrhea, vomiting, coma, and convulsions. More serious toxicity may be expressed as mental confusion, cardiac arrhythmias, seizures, hyperreflexia, hypotension, coma, and death. Structural renal damage associated with glomerular and tubular dysfunction may also occur.

CENTRAL NERVOUS SYSTEM STIMULANTS

Drugs classified as CNS stimulants comprise three distinctly different groups of compounds: analeptics (or convulsants), methylxanthines, and amphetamines and therapeutically related drugs.

Analeptics

Drugs categorized as **analeptics** (e.g., strychnine, picrotoxin, and pentylenetetrazole) produce CNS stimulation as their most prominent pharmacological action. These agents act generally by interfering with the action of endogenous inhibitory neurotransmitters (e.g., glycine and/or GABA) in the CNS, thereby blocking inhibitory neurotransmission. In the past, analeptic drugs were employed to reverse severe intoxication produced by general, nonselective CNS depressants (e.g., barbiturates), but this practice proved dangerous. Today these agents find little therapeutic application.

Methylxanthines

The **methylxanthines** (**caffeine,** theobromine, and theophylline) have a large number of pharmacological actions, only one of which is CNS stimulation. The methylxanthines are used widely, although usually in a nonmedical context inasmuch as they are contained in coffee, tea, and a variety of cola-flavored beverages. Among the methylxanthines, only theophylline and caffeine are potent CNS stimulants. Ingestion of caffeine helps overcome drowsiness and fatigue, increases the capacity for intellectual effort, and decreases reaction time. At increased doses, the methylxanthines will produce restlessness, agitation, insomnia, upset stomach, and tremors. The CNS stimulant effects are believed to arise primarily from inhibition of cyclic nucleotide phosphodiesterases or an antagonistic action at central adenosine receptors, or from both of these. Non-CNS actions of methylxanthines include cardiac stimulation, diuresis, and relaxation of smooth muscles. The use of theophylline in the treatment of bronchial asthma is discussed in Chapter 13.

Amphetamines

Unlike the analeptics, which today have virtually no therapeutic applications, and caffeine, which is consumed primarily in a nonmedical context, the amphetamines are employed therapeutically. Prior to 1970, amphetamines were indiscriminantly prescribed for a large number of conditions including depression, fatigue, and long-term weight reduction. In 1970, the Food and Drug Administration (FDA) restricted the legal use of amphetamines to narcolepsy, hyperkinetic syndromes (minimal brain dysfunction or attentional-deficit disorder), and short-term weight reduction. In addition to these therapeutic applications, the amphetamines also have a long history of abuse.

In addition to their effects in the CNS, amphetamines have widespread peripheral sympathomimetic effects (see Chapter 4). Effects of amphetamines are exerted primarily at noradrenergic and/or dopaminergic nerve terminals, both peripherally and centrally. In the CNS, amphetamines are indirect agonists (i.e., they are transported into vesicles in adrenergic nerve terminals and cause displacement and release of norepinephrine or dopamine or both). In addition, they block uptake of these neurotransmitters as well as inhibit monoamine oxidase. Further, amphetamines have some direct action at CNS adrenoceptors and may also be converted to false neurotransmitters. Thus, their pharmacology, while well understood, is complex. The indirect action of amphetamines (i.e., release of norepinephrine and/or dopamine) is considered most important. In addition to their action at noradrenergic and/or dopaminergic nerve terminals in the CNS, there is evidence that amphetamines may also release serotonin from serotonin-containing nerve terminals in the CNS. The consequences of these actions of amphetamines in the CNS include anorexia, insomnia, and CNS stimulation, including euphoria. Amphetamines also stimulate medullary respiratory centers and produce an analeptic effect. When abused in high doses, amphetamines can lead to compulsive and stereotyped behaviors and paranoia.

Amphetamine (Fig. 5–5) itself is a racemic mixture of *d* and *l* isomers. Other compounds in this class include the *d* isomer dextroamphetamine and methamphetamine. **Dextroamphetamine** is three to four times more potent as a CNS stimulant than is the racemic mixture. Methamphetamine is closely related structurally to amphetamine but has more pronounced central effects.

Clinical Applications

The principal therapeutic applications of these agents is in the short-term (i.e., 4 to 6 weeks) treatment of **obesity** and in the treatment of the sleep-

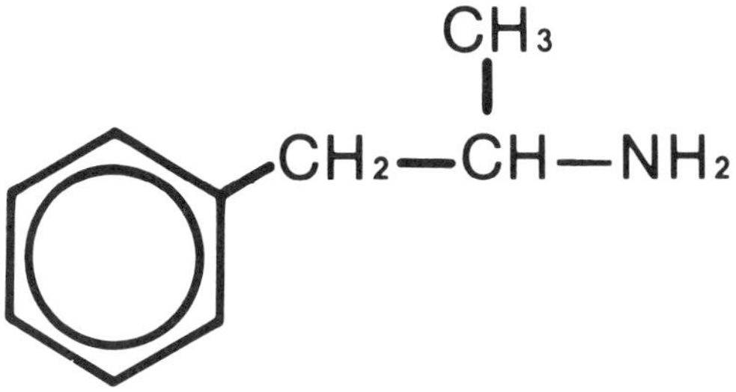

Figure 5–5. Chemical structure of amphetamine.

attack disorder **narcolepsy** and **hyperkinetic syndromes**. Tolerance develops to the anorexic, CNS stimulant, and euphoric effects of amphetamines. Thus, while a mild anorexic effect is produced by amphetamines and weight loss can be documented, tolerance develops over a period of 4 to 6 weeks (depending upon dose), and the use of amphetamines for weight reduction in place of other approaches (e.g., modification of eating behavior) is questionable.

Amphetamines are usually considered drugs of choice in the treatment of narcolepsy. Narcolepsy is characterized by sudden sleep attacks, loss of muscle tone, sleep paralysis, and often visual nightmares. The efficacy of amphetamine in the treatment of narcolepsy appears not to be diminished over time and, in the absence of tolerance, amphetamines have been used for long periods in the treatment of narcolepsy. However, prolonged treatment with amphetamines often leads to development of a paranoid psychosis (amphetamine psychosis), which must be carefully monitored.

The third FDA-approved use of amphetamines is in the treatment of hyperkinetic syndromes. In addition to the amphetamines (primarily dextroamphetamine), a piperidine derivative structurally related to amphetamine, **methylphenidate (Ritalin)** (Fig. 5–6), is also employed. Methylphenidate is also a CNS stimulant, and its pharmacologic properties are essentially the

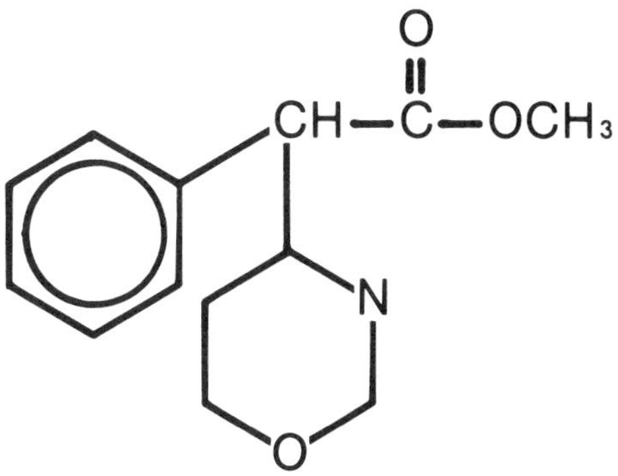

Figure 5–6. Chemical structure of methylphenidate.

same as those of the amphetamines. Similarly, methylphenidate is also subject to abuse. Controlled double-blind studies have clearly established that dextro-amphetamine or methylphenidate improve behavior, ability to concentrate, and learning in children with attention-deficit disorder. Both of these agents also have been reported to retard growth in these children, but they apparently "catch-up" following cessation of therapy. Other side effects of these agents include insomnia, anorexia, and irritability, which can often be controlled by reduction in dose. A significant problem in the use of amphetamines or methylphenidate in the treatment of hyperkinetic syndromes relates to diagnosis and indiscriminate application of these drugs to children who are disruptive in the classroom. Careful evaluation of the "problem" child is required.

Abuse and Toxicity

Another consideration associated with the use of amphetamines is their potential for abuse (see Chapter 6). Patterns of abuse include intermittent low-dose oral use, sustained low-dose oral use, and high-dose intravenous use. Dextroamphetamine and methamphetamine ("speed") have been abused most commonly. The euphoria produced following intravenous administration of methamphetamine is considered ineffable. Since the first experience with methamphetamine is almost uniformly reported as pleasurable, and the euphoria as ineffable, a rapid and significant psychological dependence develops with amphetamine abuse. In addition to the anorexia and insomnia associated with high-dose intravenous methamphetamine use, chronic use inevitably leads to compulsive and stereotyped behaviors, paranoia, and often violent behavior. Acute intoxication is associated with hyperpyrexia, anxiety, confusion, assaultiveness, chest pain, arrhythmias, and possible circulatory collapse.

Cocaine is discussed in Chapter 6.

OPIOID ANALGESICS AND ANTAGONISTS

Opioid agonists are employed primarily for symptomatic relief from pain but also possess therapeutically useful antitussive (cough suppressant) and constipative effects as well as undesirable respiratory depressant effects. Although opioids are undeniably the most efficacious agents available for relief from pain, their use is complicated by the development of tolerance as well as physical and sometimes psychological dependence.

Two widely employed opioids—codeine and morphine—are natural products contained in opium extracted from the poppy plant, *Papaver somniferum*. Other available opioids are either semisynthetic (i.e., modifications of morphine such as oxymorphone) or entirely synthetic (e.g., methadone, fentanyl, meperidine). None of the semisynthetic or synthetic opioids have been established as superior to morphine (Fig. 5–7) for relief from pain. Opioid analgesics differ primarily with respect to relative potency, duration of action, and effectiveness following oral administration; their effects as a group are qualitatively similar and differ little when compared at equipotent analgesic doses. Newer agents having mixed agonist **and** antagonist efficacy, however, are qualitatively different with respect to analgesic efficacy and respiratory depression. Thus, three therapeutically important groups of agents will be discussed: (1) opioid agonists, employed primarily for relief of pain; (2) mixed agonists/antagonists, also employed for relief of pain; and (3) opioid antagonists, employed only to antagonize or reverse the effects of opioids in the other two groups.

Opioid Receptors and Endogenous Opioids

Opioid receptors were discovered in the early 1970s. This discovery, coupled with the subsequent identification of endogenous substances that interacted at these receptors, has led to a clearer understanding of the pharmacology of the opioids. There are several subtypes of **opioid receptors,** each having different affinities for exogenously administered and endogenous opioids and each subserving overlapping as well as different physiological functions: **mu** (μ), **delta** (δ), **kappa** (κ), **epsilon** (ϵ), and **sigma** (σ). Opioid receptors are unevenly distributed throughout the CNS and also are found outside the CNS (e.g., smooth muscle). Each opioid receptor, in addition, has a unique distribution. The μ receptor, found throughout the CNS, is believed to mediate the major portion of opioid-produced analgesia, particularly at supraspinal sites. Morphine is the preferred ligand for the μ receptor, which also mediates, at least in part, opioid-produced respiratory depression, euphoria, and physical dependence. The δ receptor may mediate opioid effects on emotion, seizures, and perhaps respiratory depression; it is localized in structures related to those actions (e.g., amygdala, hippocampus, and cerebral cortex). The endogenous opioid peptide enkephalins are considered the preferred ligands

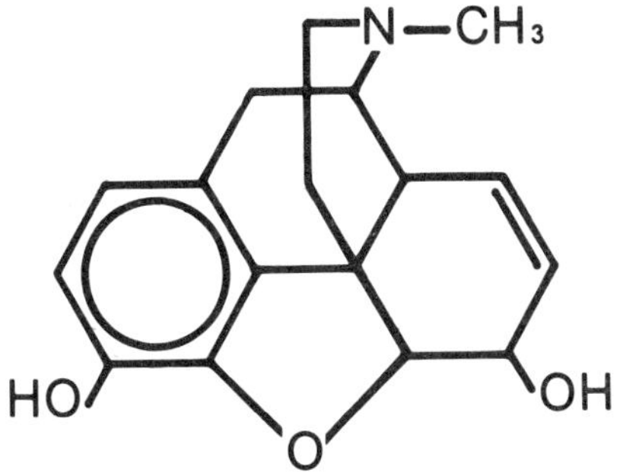

Figure 5–7. Chemical structure of morphine.

for the δ receptor. The central localization of κ receptors is similar to that of μ receptors, but κ receptors are believed to mediate spinal analgesia and to be the preferred receptors for the endogenous opioid peptide dynorphins. The ε receptor is less well understood than the μ, δ, or κ opioid receptors and is believed to mediate opioid-produced euphoria. The endogenous opioid peptide endorphins are considered the preferred ligand for the ε receptor. The fifth receptor designated as an opioid subtype, the σ receptor, may mediate opioid-produced dysphoria and hallucinations. Because the nonopioid phencyclidine (PCP) also appears to mediate effects at this receptor, it is not clear that the σ receptor should be classed as a subtype of opioid receptor.

Like the opioid receptors, the **endogenous opioid peptides** are also unevenly distributed in the CNS, and each family of endogenous opioids is uniquely distributed. There are three families of endogenous opioid peptides: **endorphins, enkephalins,** and **dynorphins**. The pentapeptide enkephalins (leucine- and methionine-enkephalin) were the first opioid peptides discovered and are now known to be derived from a large precursor, pro-enkephalin A. The dynorphins constitute the most recently discovered family of opioid peptides and are derived from a precursor referred to as pro-enkephalin B or prodynorphin. There are several dynorphins of differing lengths (8 to 17 amino acids) and other peptides derived from the same precursor (α neoendorphin and β neoendorphin). In addition to opioid peptides, the parent protein precursor for the endorphins (pro-opiomelanocortin) also gives rise to several important hormones, including ACTH. The opioid peptides derived from pro-opiomelanocortin arise from β lipotropin, a fragment of pro-opiomelanocortin that is 91 amino acids long. β endorphin constitutes the carboxy terminal 30-amino-acid sequence of β lipotropin and is considered the most important endorphin. In addition, α-, γ-, and δ-endorphin opioid peptides are derived from β endorphin, but their function(s) is unclear at present. β endorphin is present in the anterior and intermediate lobes of the pituitary from which it is released into the general circulation, and in neurons in the medial hypothalamus whose axons terminate in the amygdala, the midbrain periaqueductal gray, and the brain stem reticular formation. The enkephalin and dynorphin opioid peptides, on the other hand, are more widely distributed throughout the CNS where they may function as neurotransmitters or neuromodulators. Enkephalins, for example, are stored in nerve terminals of what are believed to be inhibitory interneurons. The physiologic roles of the opioid peptides, however, are not well understood. It might be expected that endogenous opioid peptides play a role in the response and reaction to pain. Indeed, endogenous opioid peptides and opioid receptors are ideally localized in the CNS to play important roles in pain perception (e.g., spinal cord, brainstem reticular formation, periaqueductal gray). However, neurons in which they are contained do not appear to be tonically active inasmuch as the administration of the opioid-receptor antagonist naloxone does not generally affect pain thresholds or responses to pain.

Sites and Mechanisms of Action

Mechanisms by which opioid effects are produced are still not well understood. Following the demonstration of opioid receptors, the periaqueductal gray in the midbrain was established as a focal point of opioid action and pain-suppressing systems. Electrical stimulation in this same area in humans produces an efficacious and long-lasting analgesia. Both morphine and electrical stimulation in the midbrain similarly inhibit the transmission of pain in the spinal cord, suggesting that an important aspect of opioid-produced analgesia is activation of descending inhibitory systems. However, both supraspinal and spinal sites of action of opioids have been demonstrated and, moreover, can act independently of each other. Thus, the interaction of opioid agonists at opioid receptors distributed throughout the CNS has been established as important for the analgesic, respiratory depressant, and other effects of opioids. It should be emphasized, however, that neither the opioid agonists nor the receptors involved exhibit total selectivity. For example, although morphine is the preferred agonist for μ opioid receptors, morphine interacts with and produces effects at other opioid receptors as well.

Regarding the biochemical events that occur following activation of opioid receptors, little is known. It is widely appreciated that cAMP functions as a second messenger for many extracellular stimuli. It is also well known that a wide variety of membrane ion channels can be modulated by cAMP-mediated phosphorylation events. One prevailing view is that opioid-receptor activation involves adenylate cyclase. Current evidence, however, suggests that opioid effects are not mediated by cAMP, except perhaps in cases of chronic administration of opioids. Electrophysiological studies suggest that the generally inhibitory action of opioids is a consequence of opioid receptor-mediated alterations in Ca^{2+} distribution or intraneuronal influx, or a change in neuronal K^+ conductance. In the first case, it is suggested that opioids may influence the Ca^{2+} channels necessary for stimulus-secretion coupling of neurotransmitter release; in the second case, it is suggested that an opioid-produced enhancement of K^+ conductance hyperpolarizes neurons.

Pharmacological Effects

Although primarily used for actions on the CNS, opioid effects on the smooth muscle of the GI tract were appreciated earlier and generally occur at lower doses than those required for effects on the CNS. Opioid effects on the CNS are a combination of stimulation and depression; these include analgesia, respiratory depression, depression of the cough reflex, miosis, sedation, initial stimulation of the medullary chemoreceptor trigger zone for emesis followed by its depression, euphoria/dysphoria, and suppression of the secretion of some gonadotropins.

The **analgesia** produced by morphine and other opioids occurs without loss of consciousness and is considered to be selective in that other sensory modalities such as vision, audition, and so on are not affected. It is generally considered that morphine and other opioids influence more significantly the reaction and response to pain (motivational-affective component) than they influence the threshold for pain perception (sensory-discriminative component), suggesting a prominent action at opioid receptors within the limbic system of the brain. Morphine and other opioids are more efficacious against continuous, dull pain than against intermittent, sharp pain. Elderly patients are generally more sensitive to opioids and experience greater pain relief at any given dose than do younger patients; however, successful management of pain with morphine or other opioids is achieved on an individual basis. The nature of the pain must be well understood, the response to morphine monitored, and the dose titrated to the needs of the patient. Despite adherence to these basic principles, pain in general—and in children in particular—is not well managed. Health professionals consistently underestimate the dose of opioid required for pain relief, overestimate the duration of action of the agent, and unreasonably fear "addicting" the patient in pain.

The second important CNS action of morphine and other opioids is **respiratory depression**. It is discernible even at therapeutic doses and is the primary undesirable side effect associated with opioid use. Opioids decrease the responsiveness of medullary centers to the concentration of CO_2 in blood and also directly depress brainstem centers that regulate respiratory frequency. Morphine and other opioids are also potent **antitussives,** although morphine itself is generally not employed for cough suppression. The antitussive action of the opioids generally occurs at doses lower than required to produce analgesia.

Morphine and most opioid agonists produce an easily observed **pupillary constriction** at therapeutic doses. Meperidine, which has atropine-like effects, does not. The miosis produced by morphine is a result of an action on the oculomotor nerve and not from a direct effect on musculature of the eye. At therapeutic doses, morphine and other opioids also produce a **drowsiness** from which patients can be easily aroused. It is important to emphasize, however, that opioids should not be used to promote sleep unless sleeplessness is due to pain. Morphine also directly stimulates the chemoreceptor trigger zone in the medulla, producing **nausea** and sometimes **vomiting.** Following the initial period of stimulation produced by morphine, the chemoreceptor trigger zone in the medulla is depressed and subsequent administration of other opioids or emesis-inducing agents is generally ineffective. This effect occurs at therapeutic doses and must be guarded against in postoperative patients. The nausea and vomiting produced also apparently includes a vestibular component, since nausea occurs more frequently in ambulatory than in recumbent patients. The dichotomous **euphoria/dysphoria** produced by morphine and many other opioid agonists is likely due to an action at opioid receptors in the limbic system.

Euphoria (a state of enhanced well-being and feeling of warmth) occurs primarily in the patient in pain; dysphoria (a state of anxiety and difficult mentation) more commonly occurs in pain-free patients. A final action of opioids in the CNS is depression of **gonadotropin secretion**. Morphine and other opioid agonists will decrease the secretion of luteinizing and follicle-stimulating hormones, which can lead to decreased libido and sexual activity; tolerance develops to this effect, however.

The effects of morphine and other opioids on the **gastrointestinal tract** are both significant and therapeutically important. Opium use for relief of diarrhea antedated by centuries its use for relief from pain. Morphine exerts a significant influence on smooth muscle all along the GI tract; the tone of smooth muscle is increased and the propulsive motility is decreased, resulting in **constipation**. While therapeutically useful, the effect of morphine on smooth muscle can also result in painful muscle spasms (e.g., biliary tract) and nonpropulsive muscle contractions. Morphine also increases muscle tone in smooth muscle of other organs (e.g., uterus, urinary bladder, ureters, and bronchioles). However, the effect of morphine on these muscles is generally unremarkable at therapeutic doses.

Morphine's effects on the **cardiovascular system** are also generally unremarkable at therapeutic doses. Blood pressure, heart rate, and cardiac work are generally unaffected and blood pressure is maintained near normal, even after intoxicating doses of morphine have been received. Indeed, morphine decreases cardiac work and, in addition to its analgesic and anxiolytic actions, is useful following myocardial infarction. Morphine does produce minor dilatation of the peripheral vasculature, due in part to a release of histamine, producing an overall sensation of warmth and occasionally itching of the face. Orthostatic hypotension occurs occasionally in some recumbent patients when the head-up position is suddenly assumed. This is believed to be due to a fall in peripheral vascular resistance in association with a central vestibular action produced by morphine. Morphine and other opioids also can produce a cerebral vasodilation secondary to depression of respiration and the resulting increase in arterial P_{CO_2}. Since cerebral vasodilation may lead to increase in intracranial pressure, opioids must be used cautiously in the presence of head injury.

Tolerance

The repeated use of morphine and other opioids is associated with the development of **tolerance** and **physical dependence**. Tolerance develops most rapidly to the depressant effects of opioids (analgesia, respiratory depression, depression of gonadotropin secretion, and drowsiness) and slower or not at all to their stimulant effects on the GI tract and pupil. The tolerance that develops to the respiratory depressant effect of opioids is not absolute, and although the lethal dose is increased significantly, there always exists a dose capable of producing death by respiratory depression. The rate at which tolerance develops is a function of dose and frequency of administration; the greater the dose and shorter the interval between administrations, the more rapid is the development of tolerance.

Development of tolerance to the analgesic effect of opioids is often therapeutically problematic. It is usually manifest as a shortened duration of action or patient-reported reduced analgesic effect, or both. Typically, doses of opioids are not appropriately titrated to the needs of the patient in pain and the first signs of tolerance are interpreted as complaining or, worse, "drug craving." It is important to emphasize that factors other than the drug *per se* (such as drug disposition affected by the disease, fear and anxiety associated with the disease, setting) also influence the patient's response to opioids. In addition to these nonpharmacological factors, the well-documented exaggerated concern by health professionals of addicting patients to opioids also plays an important role in pain management.

Physical Dependence

Like the development of tolerance, the development of physical dependence is also dose-related, and usually the two develop concurrently and at a similar rate. Physical dependence is defined by signs of withdrawal in the absence of the drug (e.g., salivation, lacrimation, perspiration, diarrhea) and is commonly confused with **addiction** by health professionals. Addiction is defined as the extreme of compulsive drug use, including drug-seeking behaviors, and typically encompasses both physical and psychological dependencies upon the drug. Thus, in the hospital setting, it is neither accurate nor appropriate to refer to the development of physical dependence as "addiction."

Intoxication

The combination of stupor, pinpoint pupils, and respiratory depression is virtually diagnostic of **acute opioid intoxication**. Initially, blood pressure is maintained near normal but falls as hypoxia associated with respiratory depression develops. If the course of the intoxication is not interrupted, pupillary dilation and shock caused by persistent hypoxia precede death. The intoxication, however, can be rapidly countered by administration of the opioid-receptor antagonist naloxone. In the absence of immediately effective opioid-receptor antagonism, establishing a patent airway for efficient pulmonary ventilation will prevent the hypoxia and cardiovascular sequelae of opioid intoxication.

Two notes of caution bear emphasizing regarding the use of naloxone. First, because its duration of action is shorter than that of most opioids (which also have most likely been given or taken in excess), careful monitoring and possible readminstration of additional naloxone is required in the acutely opioid-intoxicated individual. Second, administration of an opioid antagonist to an acutely intoxicated, opioid-dependent individual can precipitate a severe withdrawal syndrome, which may not be readily attenuated by an opioid agonist during the period of action of the antagonist (since opioid antagonists generally have greater affinity for opioid receptors). In this circumstance, the dose of opioid antagonist must be carefully titrated.

Absorption, Metabolism, and Excretion

Morphine and most opioids are generally well absorbed from the GI tract, but are not nearly as effective when given orally as when given parenterally in the same dose. Morphine, for example, is subject to significant first-pass metabolism in the liver, and its bioavailability may vary from 15 to 60 percent of the administered dose following oral administration. However, it is possible to adjust the dose of morphine to account for first-pass metabolism and to achieve adequate relief of pain by the oral route of administration. Flavored solutions of morphine for oral administration are now widely used for chronic pains. Given intravenously, morphine and other opioids act quickly; the more lipid-soluble analgesics penetrate the CNS quickly and have a rapid onset of action. When administered epidurally, morphine is retained for a significant period of time within the cerebrospinal fluid, providing significant pain relief and an extended duration of effect. However, cephalad flow of cerebrospinal fluid carries morphine to the brainstem, which often results in respiratory depression. Morphine is metabolized primarily by conjugation with glucuronic acid and is eliminated largely in the urine. A small percentage of morphine glucuronide also appears in the bile, and some free morphine may be found in the urine. The total excretion of an administered dose of morphine is approximately 90 percent complete after 24 hours.

Opioid Agonists (Analgesics)

There is both confusion and controversy regarding the use of heroin as an analgesic. Although more potent than morphine, heroin is not more efficacious. Several well-controlled, double-blind studies have established that heroin offers no advantage over morphine in the treatment of pain. Heroin is categorized in Schedule I and is unavailable for use as an analgesic. Indeed, given the widespread, often irrational concern among physicians relative to "addicting" patients whom they treat, it is not likely that the treatment of chronic pain would improve if heroin were made available.

Codeine is employed primarily as an orally administered analgesic and cough suppressant. It is metabolized primarily by the liver and is excreted in inactive forms chiefly in the urine. Approximately 10 percent of an administered dose of codeine is demethylated to form morphine *in vivo;* both free and conjugated morphine are found in the urine following administration of a therapeutic dose of codeine. Morphine has an analgesic potency approximately 10 to 12 times that of codeine, and many believe that codeine is a morphine prodrug. Like morphine, the analgesic and antitussive actions of codeine are central in origin, and codeine shares with morphine and other opioids the ability to depress respiration, constrict the pupils, and produce constipation, among other effects. It is a mistakenly held general impression that the analgesic efficacy of codeine is limited; this is supported by the manner in which it is employed—as a "mild analgesic" in doses providing analgesic relief equivalent to aspirin. At therapeutic doses, the side effects of codeine are relatively few and insignificant. At high doses, however, the frequency of nausea and vomiting and other side effects is increased.

Methadone (Dolophine) (Fig. 5–8) is a synthetic opioid analgesic qualitatively similar to other opioids in its basic pharmacology. Methadone, however, offers advantages over morphine in the treatment of conditions requiring long-term pain management. It retains a significant portion of its analgesic efficacy following oral administration, has a long duration of action, and provides stable, persistent blood levels for pain control with repeated administration. Like morphine, methadone exhibits depressant effects on respiration, cough, and the secretion of gonadotropins and increases smooth muscle tone while decreasing propulsive activity of the GI tract. In addition to its primary therapeutic application for relief from pain, methadone is also employed in the treatment of the opioid withdrawal syndrome and in maintenance programs for opioid-dependent individuals. In the latter regard, there still persists the mistaken notion that methadone "blocks" the effects of other opioids in opioid-dependent individuals, conferring upon methadone a pharmacological property it does not possess. Methadone is **not** an opioid-receptor antagonist. Methadone's use and "blocking" action in maintenance programs relates to cross-tolerance and cross-dependence among opioids. Cross-dependence allows the substitution of one opioid (e.g., methadone) for another (e.g, heroin) to prevent the development of withdrawal symptoms. Cross-tolerance implies

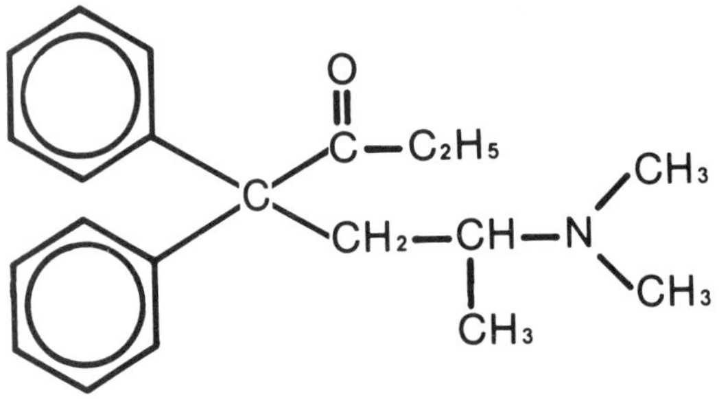

Figure 5–8. Chemical structure of methadone.

that tolerance also develops to the same effects (e.g., analgesia) of other drugs in the same class. Thus, the management of pain becomes difficult with the development of analgesic tolerance because the substitution of another opioid in an attempt to overcome the tolerance will be frustrated because of cross-tolerance. Cross-tolerance and cross-dependence among the opioids is not complete, however.

Propoxyphene (Darvon) is a synthetic opioid analgesic structurally related to methadone. Because propoxyphene was initially introduced and classified as a "non-narcotic," the belief persists that propoxyphene offers a significant advantage over other opioids, such as codeine, in that it is free of dependence liability. Propoxyphene is an opioid analgesic (and has now been appropriately placed in Schedule II), is subject to abuse, has been used in maintenance programs as a substitute for other opioids, binds to opioid receptors, and produces the full spectrum of central effects produced by other opioids (e.g., nausea, constipation, drowsiness, respiratory depression). There is, however, considerable disagreement regarding the analgesic efficacy of propoxyphene. Propoxyphene is considered to be approximately one-half as potent an analgesic as codeine when given orally, but in controlled trials it has often been difficult to demonstrate that propoxyphene is superior to placebo. Unlike morphine, codeine, and methadone, acute intoxication with propoxyphene has been associated with CNS stimulation (e.g., delusions, hallucinations, and occasionally convulsions), in addition to the more typical consequence of acute opioid intoxication (respiratory depression). It is believed that the CNS excitation is due to a metabolite, norpropoxyphene.

Meperidine (Demerol) was initially synthesized as an atropine-like drug, but was subsequently discovered to possess analgesic efficacy and was introduced as a powerful analgesic having an antispasmodic effect (rather than the spasmogenic effect that characterizes other opioids). It has since been demonstrated, however, that in addition to analgesia, sedation, respiratory depression, and other central actions common to the opioids as a class, meperidine is also spasmogenic to smooth muscles of the GI tract. When given in doses equi-analgesic to morphine, meperidine produces the same degree of respiratory depression and other undesirable effects. Meperidine is often abused by health professionals who erroneously believe that meperidine has a lower dependence liability and is easier to stop using than morphine or other opioids. Because the duration of action of meperidine is relatively short (2 to 4 hours), the administration of high doses at frequent intervals will lead to a rapid development of physical dependence, withdrawal from which includes CNS excitatory effects such as hallucinations and seizures. These excitatory effects are believed to be due to metabolism of meperidine to normeperidine, the accumulation of which also influences renal and hepatic functions. Because of its relatively short duration of action, meperidine is not generally useful in the long-term management of chronic pain, but is useful when a limited duration of analgesia is desired (e.g., obstetrical analgesia). An advantage meperidine may offer over other opioids is its reported lower incidence of respiratory depression in the fetus. Meperidine is not useful therapeutically in the treatment of diarrhea, but two chemically related compounds are employed therapeutically for their constipating effects. **Diphenoxylate,** in combination with atropine, is available as Lomotil, and **loperamide** is available as Imodium. Both agents slow GI motility, presumably by an action at opioid receptors in the GI tract, and are used in the treatment of diarrhea.

Fentanyl (Sublimaze) is a newer, wholly synthetic opioid estimated to be 80 to 100 times more potent than morphine. Used alone, fentanyl is employed primarily as an anesthetic supplement. In combination with the neuroleptic droperidol, fentanyl is used to produce a neuroleptanalgesia in place of general anesthesia; the combination is available as **Innovar.** Two congeners of fentanyl, sufentanil (Sufenta) and alfentanil (Alfenta), are similar to fentanyl in that they are potent opioids having rapid onset of action and relatively short duration of effect. These three agents are used in analgesic anesthesia as the principal component of balanced anesthesia (usually with N_2O and a neuromuscular blocking drug), particularly for cardiac surgery. They offer the advantage of providing cardiovascular stability during surgery, but they are **not** anesthetics. Disadvantages associated with their use include incomplete anesthesia, incomplete amnesia following surgery, and hypertension during sternotomy.

Other opioid agonist analgesics, as well as mixed opioid agonists/antagonists employed as analgesics, are listed in Table 5–9.

Mixed Opioid Agonists/Antagonists

A group of agents referred to as mixed agonists/antagonists or partial agonists have been recently introduced for use as analgesics in place of opioid agonists. These agents differ in their relative actions at the different opioid receptors; some act as agonists at some opioid receptors and as competitive antagonists at other opioid receptors. The objective in synthesizing and introducing into medicine this group of compounds relates to the longstanding desire to have available a potent analgesic free of abuse liability and reduced undesirable effects (e.g., respiratory depression). Indeed, many of these agents exhibit a **"ceiling effect"** on respiration, thus reducing the risk of respiratory depression by overdose. However, the analgesic efficacy of these agents is also somewhat limited and is less than other opioid agonists (e.g., morphine, methadone).

Pentazocine (Talwin) (Fig. 5–9) was the first of these compounds to be successfully introduced and was initially believed to be free of abuse liability. With frequent and repeated use, both tolerance and physical dependence develop, and it is not clear that pentazocine offers a significant advantage over codeine, which it was initially intended to replace. Pentazocine is an agonist

Table 5–9. COMPARISON OF OPIOID ANALGESICS

Nonproprietary Name	Proprietary Name	Usual Therapeutic Dose (mg)	Route of Administration*	Duration (Hours)	Dependence Liability
Agonists					
Alphaprodine	Nisentil	40–60	SC	1–2	High
Codeine	—	30–60	Oral	4–6	Low to moderate
Fentanyl	Sublimaze	0.05–0.1	IM	1.0–1.5	High
		0.05–0.1[†]	IV	0.5–1.0	
Heroin[‡]	—	3–5	IM	3–4.5	High
Hydrocodone	Dicodid	5–10	Oral	4–6	Moderate
Hydromorphone	Dilaudid	2	IM	4–5	High
		2–4	Oral	4–5	
Levorphanol	Levo-Dromoran	2–3	SC	4–7	High
		2–3	Oral	4–7	
Meperidine	Demerol	50–100	IM	2–4	High
		50–100	Oral	2–4	
Methadone	Dolophine	2.5–10	IM	4–5	Moderate
		5–15	Oral	4–6	
Morphine	—	10–15	IM	4–5	High
Oxycodone	In Percodan	5–10	Oral	4–5	High
Oxymorphone	Numorphan	1.0–1.5	IM	4–6	High
Propoxyphene[§]	Darvon	32–65	Oral	4–6	Low to moderate
Mixed Agonists/Antagonists					
Buprenorphine	Temgesic	0.3–0.6	IM	6–8	Low
Butorphanol	Stadol	1–4	IM	3–4	Low
		0.5–2	IV		
Nalbuphine	Nubain	10	IM	3–6	Low
Pentazocine	Talwin	30	IM	2–4	Low
	Talwin Nx	50	Oral	3–5	

Estimates of dependence liability are taken from the literature and do not pretend to be definitive.

*IM = intramuscular; SC = subcutaneous; IV = intravenous.

[†]Greater doses may be used for general anesthesia.

[‡]Heroin is a Schedule I drug and therefore is not available for routine clinical use.

[§]The analgesic efficacy of propoxyphene is a matter of controversy.

at κ and σ opioid receptors, and it is believed that its analgesic efficacy arises through action at the κ opioid receptor. At low to moderate doses, pentazocine produces effects similar to those of morphine-like opioids (e.g., analgesia, sedation, respiratory depression). At higher doses, however, the analgesic efficacy of pentazocine is limited by its weak antagonistic action at the μ opioid receptor. This antagonism requires caution when the drug is administered to individuals physically dependent on other opioids (such as morphine or meth-

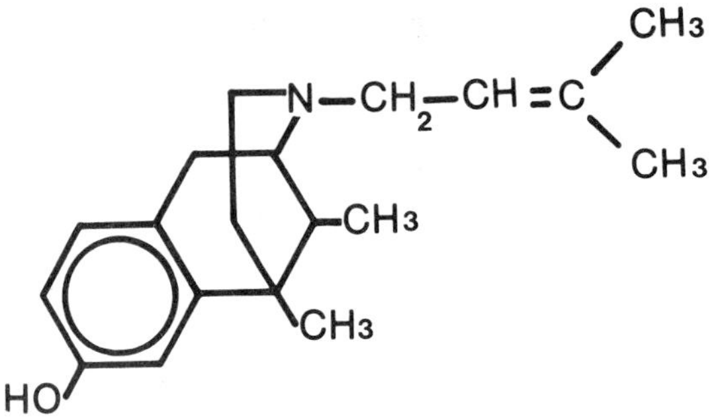

Figure 5–9. Chemical structure of pentazocine.

adone), in whom it can precipitate a mild withdrawal syndrome. Acute intoxication with pentazocine is associated with marked respiratory depression and, unlike morphine-like opioid agonists, with anxiety and psychotomimetic-like effects, increases in blood pressure and heart rate likely resulting from its action at the σ opioid receptor. Acute intoxication can be reversed by administration of the opioid-receptor antagonist naloxone.

The receptor antagonist action of naloxone is used to prevent the abuse of pentazocine. Typically, pentazocine tablets for oral use are crushed and self-administered intravenously, often in combination with the antihistamine tripelennamine. The tablets now are available only mixed with naloxone (50 mg pentazocine + 0.5 mg naloxone = **Talwin Nx**). When taken orally, the naloxone in the tablet exerts no antagonistic effect, and the pentazocine produces analgesia. When crushed and injected, however, the naloxone will prevent the desired effect of the pentazocine.

Butorphanol (Stadol) is a more potent analgesic than pentazocine but shares with pentazocine agonistic effects at κ and σ opioid receptors. **Nalbuphine (Nubaine)** is similar to pentazocine and butorphanol; it is believed that its analgesic efficacy arises from action at the κ opioid receptor. Nalbuphine is, however, a more potent μ opioid–receptor antagonist than pentazocine and may be used to reverse the respiratory depressant effects of opioid agonists (e.g., morphine). It has been reported that nalbuphine is capable of reversing opioid-induced respiratory depression without affecting opioid-induced analgesia. Nalbuphine is not very active at the σ opioid receptor, and therefore dysphoria or psychotomimetic-like effects are not likely at increased doses. **Buprenorphine (Temgesic)** is a semisynthetic mixed agonist/antagonist opioid analgesic having partial agonistic effects at the μ and κ opioid receptors. In this regard, buprenorphine is more morphine-like than pentazocine-like. Like nalbuphine, buprenorphine has little or no activity at σ opioid receptors.

Opioid Antagonists

Naloxone (Narcan) (Fig. 5–10) is the only "pure" opioid-receptor antagonist currently available. It is a competitive antagonist at all opioid receptors, but its affinity is greatest for the μ opioid receptor. Naloxone possesses no agonistic actions and thus, when given alone, will not produce analgesia, respiratory depression, or any of the other effects associated with agents previously discussed. The introduction of naloxone has made essentially obsolete a group of compounds having mixed agonist/antagonist efficacy but whose use was reserved for antagonism of opioid-induced intoxication (e.g., nalorphine and levallorphan). Naloxone is now the drug of choice for treatment of opioid intoxication. Because naloxone possesses no agonistic action at opioid receptors and thus will not produce any respiratory depression, its administration will not further embarrass respiration depressed by a nonopioid, centrally acting depressant (e.g., barbiturates). As indicated previously, the duration of action of naloxone is relatively short (1 to 4 hours) and in cases of acute opioid intoxication its administration will likely need to be repeated. When administered to opioid-dependent individuals, naloxone will precipitate a withdrawal syndrome of a severity and duration that will depend on both the dose of naloxone and the extent of physical dependence on the opioid agonists.

Naloxone is well absorbed after oral administration but is subject to significant first-pass metabolism by the liver such that it is approximately one-fiftieth as potent when given orally as when administered parenterally. As already explained, because of its poor activity when administered orally, naloxone has been incorporated into tablets containing pentazocine (**Talwin-Nx**) and methadone (**Methenex**) to prevent subversion of these oral preparations to illegal intravenous use.

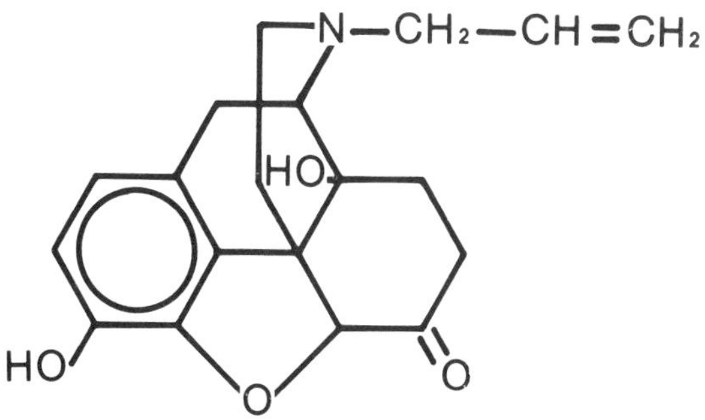

Figure 5–10. Chemical structure of naloxone.

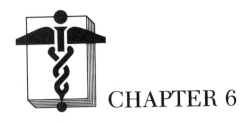

CHAPTER 6

Psychoactive Drugs

SEAN MURPHY, Ph.D.

TERMINOLOGY

Although the majority of psychoactive drugs (drugs that interact with the nervous system and affect "mood" or "state of mind") have been developed in the last 40 years, their "discovery" was based on explorations into traditional herbal medicines in a search for the active components. Thus, not only does the medical use of psychoactive substances have a long history, but so does their recreational use. Today, depending on the prevailing social and cultural attitudes, recreational use may be termed **abuse**.

Use of the term "addiction" for long-term abuse has, because of negative connotations, been replaced by **"drug dependency."** This term recognizes that there exists not only **psychological dependence,** a desire to administer a drug periodically or continually in order to produce pleasure (or to avoid discomfort), but also **physiological dependence,** an adaptive state manifested by intense physical disturbance when administration of the drug is suspended. Symptoms of such **withdrawal** vary with the drug and the individual, and their many manifestations illustrate how widespread are the effects of drugs that act on the nervous system. **Tolerance,** a diminishing response to a given dose of a drug (up to a lethal limit), is a common phenomenon. It can result from both metabolic changes, such as the induction of liver enzymes, and receptor desensitization.

A number of the stimulants and depressants to be discussed have been introduced earlier in Chapter 5; therefore, modes of action and routes of metabolism will not be repeated in detail here. In many instances, particularly the hallucinogens, the precise mechanisms by which psychoactive drugs achieve their effects remain unclear.

CNS STIMULANTS

In general, these drugs are fast acting, and their sympathomimetic effects (increased arousal, motor activity) are transient.

Amphetamines

Originally developed in the 1920s in the search for a synthetic source of ephedrine, amphetamine was widely used as a nonprescription bronchodilator (Benzedrine). During World War II, amphetamine was circulated officially by a number of governments to counteract battle fatigue, both in the military and civilian populations. In countries like Japan, unofficial use had reached epidemic proportions by the late 1940s.

Because of lipid solubility, amphetamines readily penetrate the blood-brain barrier. Their action is indirectly sympathomimetic, causing the release of dopamine and norepinephrine and also blocking the metabolism (through inhibition of monoamine oxidase [MAO]) and reuptake of catecholamines. Heart rate increases, and this, combined with vasoconstriction, elevates blood pressure. Behavioral effects include an increase in alertness and locomotion, as well as insomnia, anorexia, and hyperthermia. Overdose is fairly uncommon and daily intake can reach 4 g.

Barbiturates can counteract or potentiate the effects of amphetamine. Tricyclics and MAO inhibitors will potentiate their effects, and reserpine pretreatment will prevent the actions of amphetamine in the periphery. Khat, an alkaloid (cathinone) derived from the leaves of a North African plant, has properties similar to those of amphetamine.

Although once prescribed for the treatment of neurotic depression, today the medical use of amphetamines is restricted to the treatment of narcolepsy, to reverse "hyperkinesis" in children, and in the short-term treatment of obesity. Although such amphetamines are chemically transformed, their use still implies tolerance and dependency. Fenfluramine (Pondimin) selectively facilitates serotonin (not catecholamine) transmission, and its appetite-suppressing actions are not associated with euphoria or insomnia. Methamphetamine ("speed") is similar to the parent compound but with a substitution in the chain; there is little stimulation of autonomic activity associated with its use.

Associated with amphetamine abuse is a psychotic state very similar to paranoid schizophrenia that can be treated with a neuroleptic agent such as haloperidol. Ironically amphetamine, like ephedrine, was developed because it could be taken orally. Amphetamine abuse today almost invariably employs intravenous injection. Long-term intravenous use can induce necrotizing arteritis, a specific lesion that is often fatal owing to brain damage and kidney failure.

There is also a neonatal withdrawal syndrome manifesting as restlessness, hypoglycemia, tremor, and diaphoresis. Such infants may have limb deformities.

Cocaine

This drug has replaced amphetamine as the major stimulant of abuse. Derived from the leaves of the coca plant (*Erythroxylon* sp.), cocaine has a long history in South America, where it is still used by those performing hard manual labor as a source of energy and motivation, in the same way that alcohol was used in Europe before this century (Fig. 6–1). The use of cocaine was much favored medically in the late 19th century as a substitute for morphine, and it was a constituent of various cordials such as "Vin Mariani" and "Coca Cola," where, mixed with caffeine, it was sold as a remedy for headache.

The effects of cocaine and amphetamine are very similar. Cocaine inhibits

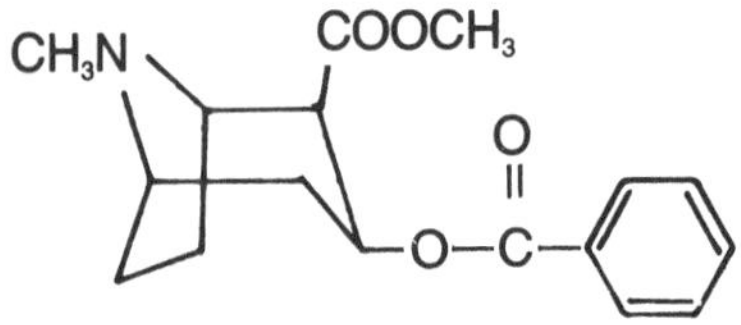

Cocaine

Figure 6–1. The chemical structure of cocaine.

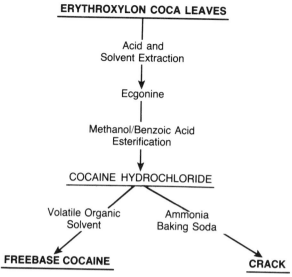

Figure 6–2. Derivation of cocaine from coca leaves.

MAO and the reuptake of endogenous monoamines. Blood pressure is increased, and there is mydriasis and increased locomotion.

While derivatives such as lidocaine and procaine find extensive use as local anesthetics, cocaine is employed today as an anesthetic only in eye surgery and in preparation for intubation.

Intravenous injection is uncommon, as it can be rapidly fatal as a result of decreased respiration, arrhythmias, cardiac arrest, and seizure. By inhalation, the stimulant effects peak within an hour and wear off slowly. The risk of overdose is especially pronounced with smoked pure cocaine ("crack," "freebase") (Fig. 6–2). Treatment with the dopamine receptor agonist bromocriptine will decrease the craving for cocaine. The usual treatment is to give a sedative (such as diazepam [Valium]) intravenously, together with propranolol and a tricyclic antidepressant such as desipramine.

Cocaine is lipid soluble and crosses the placental barrier. Although there is no neonatal withdrawal syndrome, infants exhibit symptoms of cocaine exposure and may have malformations, particularly of the muscles of the abdominal wall.

CNS DEPRESSANTS

Barbiturates and benzodiazepines share similar actions in that they potentiate GABA transmission and so depress neuronal activity.

Barbiturates

Developed and widely used clinically in the first part of this century as sedatives and hypnotics, the potential for barbiturates to create dependency was soon recognized. Their ability to cross the blood-brain barrier depends on lipid solubility. These drugs induce oxidative enzyme activity in the liver, resulting in metabolic tolerance, and there is cross-tolerance to alcohol and sedatives such as benzodiazepines.

Thiopental is rapidly taken up, has a short duration of action (minutes to hours), and so is used as an anesthesia-inducing agent; the uptake of barbital is so slow as to be inappropriate. Secobarbital (Seconal) is still a widely used sedative and hypnotic, and phenobarbital is employed as an anticonvulsant in the treatment of epilepsy; these two are the most widely abused barbiturates. Barbiturates with a long duration of action (4 to 8 hours) are used as hypnotics, though there is often a hangover effect.

Chronic barbiturate toxicity is associated with drowsiness, confusion, motor incoordination, and even psychosis. Physiological dependence follows doses of 500 mg per day; high doses can reach a lethal limit with depression of cardiovascular and respiratory centers. Withdrawal symptoms include anxiety, agitation, convulsions, nausea, rebound REM sleep, and orthostatic hypotension. Propranolol will relieve some of the symptoms of withdrawal. The abruptness of onset of withdrawal, and its severity, depends upon the half-life of the barbiturate. Those with shorter half-lives (8 to 24 hours) produce a rapidly evolving and severe withdrawal compared with barbiturates with half-lives of 2 to 4 days. Withdrawal symptoms from the latter are so slow to appear that the individual may be unaware of the very slight symptoms. Commonly, to combat severe withdrawal a barbiturate with a long half-life such as phenobarbitone is given to stabilize the condition. This can then be gradually withdrawn.

Benzodiazepines

Benzodiazepines readily cross the blood-brain barrier, and their duration of action depends upon the half-life, which varies widely. In addition to the ability of benzodiazepines to potentiate GABA transmission, it seems that, through an affinity for purinergic receptors, they may also potentiate the inhibitory actions of the transmitter adenosine, which itself has sedative and anxiolytic properties.

These drugs were developed in the 1950s as anxiolytic (diazepam), hypnotic (nitrazepam), and anticonvulsant (clonazepam) agents because of the problems with barbiturate dependency and overdose. Although overdosing with benzodiazepines is rare, it is now recognized that their long-term use invokes dependency.

Therapeutic doses of more than 60 mg per day can lead to withdrawal symptoms within a few days, and these include apprehension, tremor, anorexia, and sometime psychosis. Such symptoms can endure for 2 to 3 weeks. Doses of 500 mg can produce euphoria.

As benzodiazepines readily cross the placental barrier, there is danger of fetal growth irregularities such as cleft palate during the first trimester of pregnancy.

Opioids

These alkaloids, derived from opium poppy, have a long history in patent medicines (replacing codeine in cough cures) and in the production of analgesia. They can be naturally, synthetically, or semisynthetically produced. A major outbreak of morphine abuse followed the Civil War, when veterans who had been given morphine in field hospitals discovered their dependency on the drug (soldier's disease).

Opioids are well absorbed but cross the blood-brain barrier at different rates (heroin more quickly than morphine). Effects on the brainstem lead to cough-reflex suppression, decreased gastric secretion, nausea, miosis, and euphoria.

The medical uses of opioids, primarily in the symptomatic relief of pain, are discussed in Chapter 5.

There is evidence of both metabolic and cellular tolerance, and withdrawal leads to supersensitivity that is often the cause of death due to overdose. Most commonly abused opioids are heroin, morphine, oxycodone, and, among health professionals, meperidine. Abuse is mostly by intravenous injection, and 25 mg heroin can produce effects lasting 3 to 5 hours. Withdrawal begins about 5 hours later with symptoms akin to activating the sympathetic systems (i.e., lacrimation, rhinorrhea, sweating, hyperpnea), involuntary movements, and long-lasting hypertension. Clonidine is therefore useful in detoxification because it reduces sympathetic activity while not being addictive. Methadone is used for long-term detoxification as it can be taken orally, has long-lasting effects, and, because of cross-tolerance and cross-dependence with heroin, can be substituted for it. However, like other opioids, methadone induces dependency.

HALLUCINOGENS

There are a range of drugs within this category. The central effects of mescalin, psilocybin, and lysergic acid diethylamide (LSD) are very similar (Fig. 6–3). Phencyclidine is related to meperidine and, though used as a muscle relaxant, is most often abused because of its hallucinogenic properties.

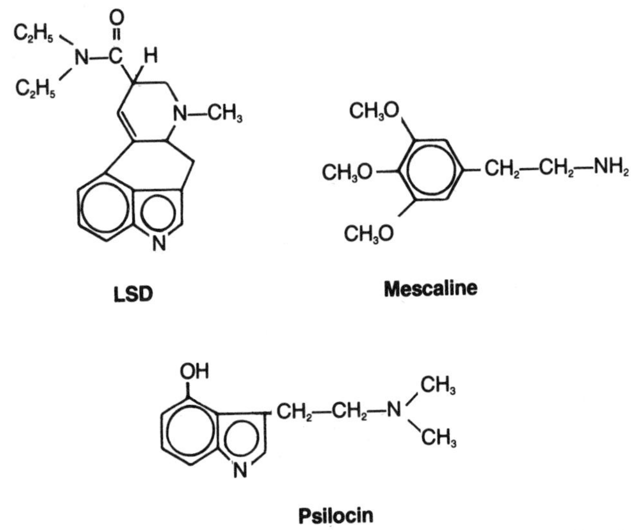

LSD

Mescaline

Psilocin

Figure 6–3. The chemical structure of LSD, mescaline, and psilocin.

Cannabis produces hallucinations only rarely, depending on the individual, the dosage form, and the dose.

LSD

Originally prepared in the 1940s as one of a series of semisynthetic ergot compounds, it is one of the most potent drugs available, with activity at doses of less than 100 μg. It has a half-life of 3 hours and concentrates in the hypothalamic and visual/auditory centers of the midbrain. Maximal effects are experienced after 4 hours and it is completely metabolized. The responses of the brain stem reticular formation to input from sensory collaterals are much enhanced. This is brought about by an agonist interaction of LSD with serotonin receptors on sensory perception neurons which project to the locus coeruleus.

The effects of LSD are sympathomimetic: tachycardia, pupil dilation, raised blood pressure, piloerection, hyperglycemia, hyperthermia, and often nausea, tremor, and numbness. Mood swings between panic and euphoria. Perception is heightened with recurring colorful visual illusions (micropsia) and distorted body illusions such as floating limbs. Time is suspended, thought is disjointed, and the user is highly introspective. Sensory modalities become mixed—for example, colors are "heard" (synesthesia).

LSD has limited clinical use as an "unblocker" in psychoanalysis and group therapy.

LSD can be antagonized by antipsychotic agents such as chlorpromazine. The paranoia that sometimes results from LSD can be treated with phenothiazine, and barbiturates/benzodiazepines are useful to ameliorate withdrawal. Morning glory seeds contain the monoethylamide of lysergic acid.

Mescalin and Psilocybin

Their effects are almost identical to those of LSD. Mescalin is a norepinephrine-like compound (3,4,5-trimethoxyphenylethylamine) found in the peyote cactus (*Lophophora* sp.). Compared with LSD, quite large doses of mescalin (5 to 15 mg) have to be taken and it has a long duration of action (9 to 12 hours). Mescalin is metabolized by alkaline phosphatase to psilocin, which is the potent compound. Synthetic derivatives of mescalin include DOM (2,5-dimethoxy-4-methylamphetamine), a much more potent agent with a long duration of action, often referred to as STP (Serenity, Tranquility, and Peace); and MDMA (3,4-methylenedioxy-N-methylamphetamine), which produces euphoria but without the psychotic effects—hence its name, "Ecstasy."

Psilocybin, a fungal compound, is a tryptamine derivative that is very similar to serotonin. It is less than 1 percent as active as LSD and requires much greater doses than mescalin. As with the metabolism of mescalin, psilocin is the active metabolite of psilocybin.

Phencyclidine

This is a stimulant that goes by the name of PCP or "angel dust" (Fig. 6–4). Its muscle relaxant/anticonvulsant effects are due to the binding of PCP to nicotinic receptors. However, it is now heavily abused because of its central hallucinogenic properties. Here it acts as an alpha-adrenergic receptor agonist, and also as a noncompetitive antagonist at glutamate pathways implicated in (among other processes) learning.

It produces marked sensory blockade and is therefore useful in anesthe-

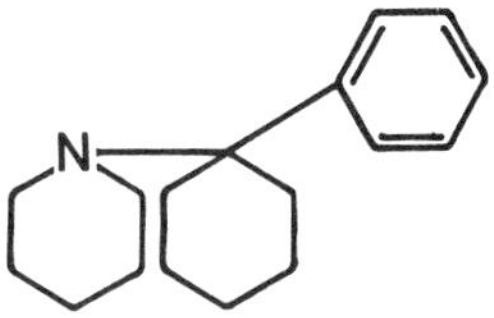

Phencyclidine

Figure 6–4. The chemical structure of phencyclidine ("angel dust").

sia, particularly in veterinary medicine where, marketed as Sernylan, it is used primarily for tranquilizing monkeys.

The user has feelings of detachment or disorientation, sweating, and hypertension. There are delusions of strength and attendant psychosis. Overdose can be fatal owing to respiratory arrest. As it is secreted from the circulation to the stomach and back again from the small intestine to the blood, symptoms wax and wane. Nasogastric suction is useful in removing PCP from the circulation, or its excretion can be promoted by acidification of the urine.

PCP crosses the placenta and can result in nystagmus, tremor, and even chromosome damage in infants.

Cannabis (Marijuana)

Probably the best-known drug of recreational use, its mechanism of action is not at all clear. Smoking the leaves of *C. sativa* produces effects within minutes, whereas ingestion has a slower onset. The active component is 1-Δ^9 tetrahydrocannabinol (THC), a lipid-soluble compound that has effects of cholinergic and monoaminergic pathways (Fig. 6–5). Synthesis, release, and degradation of acetylcholine are all decreased. THC is hydroxylated in the lungs and the liver and has a half-life of between 1 and 2 days. Isomerization of THC alters the potency dramatically, which suggests that a receptor exists, but the evidence is not conclusive.

Effects in individuals vary significantly. Pulse rate increases, blood pressure falls, and, while there is reddening of the eye, there is no change in pupil diameter.

Research into the risks of use has resulted in the production of a number of potential clinical applications for cannabis products. For example, there is a consistent drop in intraocular pressure associated with cannabis intake, leading to interest in its potential in the treatment of glaucoma. Levonantrodol, a homolog, has analgesic properties and can relieve muscle spasm and convulsion. Because of its antiemetic effects, cannabis has found use in relieving the

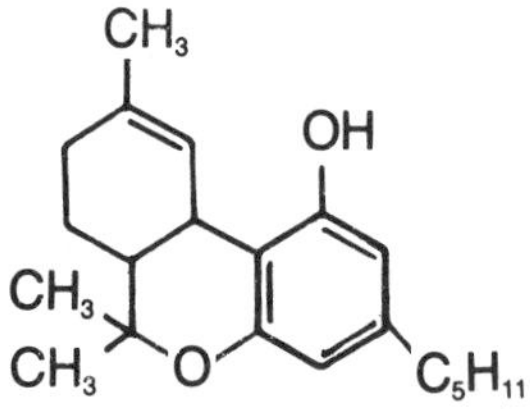

Delta-9-THC

Figure 6–5. The chemical structure of Δ-9-tetrahydrocannabinol (Δ^9-THC), the primary psychoactive constituent of marijuana.

Table 6–1. PSYCHOACTIVE DRUGS—SITES OF ACTION,
MAIN EFFECTS, AND TREATMENT

Drug	Site of Action	Main Effects	Treatment
Amphetamine	Catecholamine pathways	Sympathomimetic; increased heart rate, blood pressure, alertness, locomotion; insomnia, anorexia	Haloperidol for psychosis; sedative for anxiety
Cocaine	Same as for amphetamine	As for amphetamines; can be fatal, especially intravenously, owing to arrhythmias, cardiac arrest	Bromocriptine in withdrawal; sedative and propranolol for anxiety
Barbiturates	Potentiate GABA transmission	Sedative/hypnotic, hypotension, decreased respiration and cardiovascular center activity; psychosis, coma	Propranolol, substitution chemotherapy in withdrawal
Benzodiazepines	Same as for barbiturates. Facilitate adenosine transmission	As for barbiturates; drowsiness, ataxia; euphoria at high dosage	Substitution chemotherapy in withdrawal
Opioids	Activate specific receptors, e.g., in brainstem	Euphoria, cough-reflex suppression, nausea, miosis	Clonidine, substitution chemotherapy in withdrawal
LSD/Mescaline/ Psilocybin	Interaction with serotonin receptors; brain stem responses enhanced	Sympathomimetic; increased heart rate, blood pressure; euphoria, nausea, tremor, psychosis	Chlorpromazine for psychosis; phenothiazine for paranoia; sedatives for withdrawal
Phencyclidine	Alpha-adrenergic receptor agonist; glutamate receptor antagonist	Detachment, sweating, hypertension; psychosis, respiratory arrest	Nasogastric suction, acidify urine; sedative for anxiety, haloperidol for psychosis
Cannabis	Cholinergic, monoaminergic pathways	Hypotension, panic/ dysphoria; psychosis, antiemetic	Sedative for panic; haloperidol for psychosis

side effects of radiation therapy in cancer patients. This treatment is now sanctioned, and nabilone (Cesamet) and dronabinol (Marinol) have been approved for such use by the FDA.

Use can evoke panic, dysphoria, and even toxic psychosis. However, withdrawal effects are negligible, and for the most part tolerance is found only with long-term use. A number of wide-ranging studies have failed to find evidence of impairment or brain damage, though there are reports of lowering of serum testosterone and narrowing of the airways.

SUMMARY

Table 6–1 shows the principal targets for psychoactive drugs, their main effects, and established treatments for intoxication.

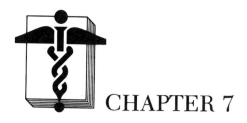

CHAPTER 7

Local Anesthetic Drugs

J. P. LONG, Ph.D.

M. D. SOKOLL, M.D.

Local anesthetic agents can be used either by topical application or by local infiltration, i.e., injection directly into tissue such as skin or subcutaneous tissue. The major clinical use is to block conduction of sensory nerve fibers and thus produce relief from pain. There are other specialized uses for these agents, but their ability to **stabilize membranes** is the basis for all use.

Cocaine was the first local anesthetic agent to be recognized. Use of coca leaves by natives in the Andes mountains precedes written history. Leaves of the plant were ingested to depress appetite and for actions on the central nervous system (CNS), but there is also evidence that the Indians recognized that the leaves produced regional anesthesia. Early Spanish explorers were fascinated by the plant and by the alkaloid cocaine, which is the active ingredient of the leaves and among the first substances to be isolated from plant origin. Köller first used cocaine in 1884 to produce **anesthesia of the cornea** following topical application. Its usefulness was soon recognized, and cocaine was the only agent of its kind available for about 25 years. Cocaine also possessed toxic actions (**e.g., convulsions and/or depressant actions involving the cardiovas-**

179

Table 7-1. LOCAL ANESTHETIC AGENTS

Compound	Structure	Dosage (% sol.)*	Duration (hours)	Use	Comments
Series A—esters					
Procaine	H_2N—⬡—$C(=O)$—$OCH_2CH_2N(C_2H_5)(C_2H_5)$	0.5, 1.0, 2.0, 4.0	0.3–0.7	Infiltration only, nerve block, spinal (max. 5%)	Ineffective topically, widely used for infiltration
Chloroprocaine	H_2N—⬡(Cl)—$C(=O)$—$OCH_2CH_2N(C_2H_5)(C_2H_5)$	1.0, 2.0, 3.0	0.2–0.5	Infiltration only, nerve block, epidural	Ineffective topically, short duration with epidural
Tetracaine	C_4H_9—N(H)—⬡—$C(=O)$—$OCH_2CH_2N(CH_3)(CH_3)$	0.25–2.0	6	Infiltration or topical (1–2%), nerve block, spinal (max. 0.5%)	Slow in onset and long duration, about 10 times more toxic than procaine following systemic inj.
Benzocaine	H_2N—⬡—$C(=O)$—OCH_2CH_3	10.0	>10	Topical only (10%)	Insoluble

180

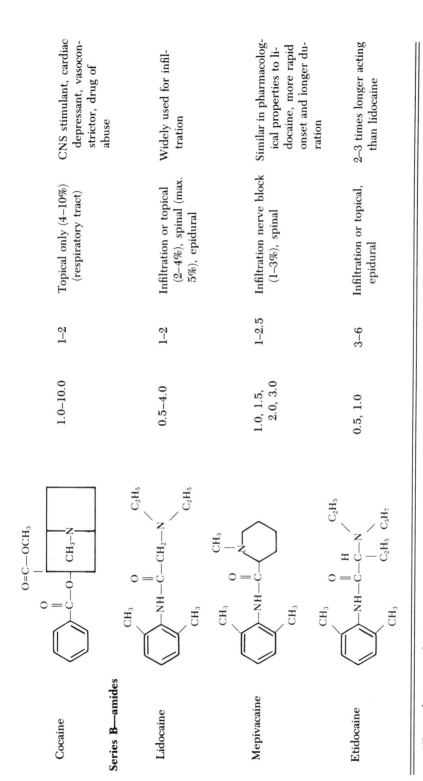

Cocaine		1.0–10.0	1–2	Topical only (4–10%) (respiratory tract)	CNS stimulant, cardiac depressant, vasoconstrictor, drug of abuse
Series B—amides					
Lidocaine		0.5–4.0	1–2	Infiltration or topical (2–4%), spinal (max. 5%), epidural	Widely used for infiltration
Mepivacaine		1.0, 1.5, 2.0, 3.0	1–2.5	Infiltration nerve block (1–3%), spinal	Similar in pharmacological properties to lidocaine, more rapid onset and longer duration
Etidocaine		0.5, 1.0	3–6	Infiltration or topical, epidural	2–3 times longer acting than lidocaine

*Epinephrine or other vasoconstrictor agents are often added to solutions of local anesthetic agents. Addition of a vasoconstrictor will prolong the duration of action, and it is often possible to reduce the amount of local anesthetic agent used.

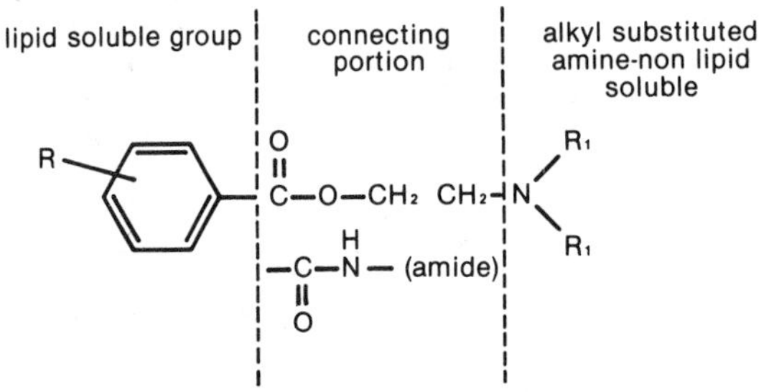

Figure 7–1. Chemical substituents required for local anesthetic agents. The connecting portion may contain an amide

$$(-\overset{\overset{\displaystyle O}{\|}}{C}-\overset{\overset{\displaystyle H}{|}}{N}-)$$

or an ester

$$(-\overset{\overset{\displaystyle O}{\|}}{C}-O-).$$

cular system), and ophthalmologists noted that it could "pit" the cornea following topical application.

The first synthetic local anesthetic, **procaine**, was prepared by Einhorn in 1905 and became the reference compound for the next 40 years. Lofgren's discovery of **lidocaine** in 1943 produced a potent agent that was effective either topically or by infiltration. Many structural analogs have been prepared and evaluated clinically, and several have now been introduced into therapy.

CHEMISTRY

Local anesthetic agents contain a lipid-soluble portion (an ester or amide moiety) and an alkyl-substituted amino group that tends to be non–lipid soluble. These relationships are illustrated in Figure 7–1.

Structures outlined in series A in Table 7–1 contain an **ester linkage,** and many of these agents are excellent **substrates for plasma cholinesterase.** Thus, they tend to have a shorter duration of action than agents having an amide linkage (series B), which are not substrates for plasma cholinesterase. In contrast to soluble local anesthetic agents, **benzocaine** is insoluble and is used only topically.

Local anesthetic agents are usually used as a hydrochloride salt. This salt form greatly increases the aqueous solubility of the compound, allowing concentrated solutions (10 to 50 mg per ml) to be formulated. Some agents (e.g., benzocaine) are very insoluble and their use therefore is restricted to topical application.

PHARMACOKINETICS

Mechanism of Action

All local anesthetic agents stabilize membranes by interfering with the large transient increase in membrane permeability to Na^+ that occurs during depolarization. These agents may also act as depressants of smooth, cardiac, and skeletal muscle. It is now believed that the agents penetrate to the interior side of the neuronal membrane in a noncharged form and, after crossing the membrane, become charged (gain a proton); it is this charged form that is believed to inhibit Na^+ flux and thus block neuronal conductance.

Sensitivity of Nerve Fibers to Local Anesthetics

Local anesthetic agents readily penetrate small-diameter nerves, which are more sensitive than large nerves. Nonmyelinated nerves are almost always of small diameter and more sensitive than nerves with a myelin sheath. Inhibition of neuronal conduction occurs with approximately the following order (most sensitive to least sensitive): **small-diameter unmyelinated and thinly myelinated pain fibers and postganglionic autonomic nerves, temperature sensory nerves, touch, proprioception,** and **somatic muscle tone.** The high sensitivity of the small and usually nonmyelinated pain fibers to these agents is fortunate and facilitates the use of the agents in pain control with minimal involvement of other modalities.

Absorption

Absorption from various sites is determined to a considerable extent by the chemical properties of an individual agent. **Benzocaine** is so insoluble that it is very poorly absorbed and is used topically. There are considerable differences in time required for onset of action, which is probably related to the rate at which an agent crosses the nerve membrane in the non-ionized form. As a rule, agents that are slower in onset of action also have a longer duration of action.

Absorption into the systemic circulation is of major concern following regional injections. None of the local anesthetic agents, except cocaine, induce vasoconstriction by mimicking the action of the sympathetic nervous system. Therefore, with the introduction of new synthetic local anesthetic agents, it was soon recognized that the addition of a **vasoconstrictor** agent (e.g., **epinephrine**) had definite therapeutic benefits. A vasoconstrictor will increase the duration of action of a local anesthetic agent by decreasing the rate of diffusion from the site of injection. This decreased rate of diffusion will decrease the systemic toxicity because degradative mechanisms will be able to keep up with rate of absorption into the systemic circulation. A number of vasoconstrictor agents are used, but epinephrine remains the most commonly used drug. Its dilutions are usually in the range of 1:50,000 to 1:200,000. However, one should use the lowest concentration possible to minimize toxicity. Epinephrine has its own potential side effects such as cardiac stimulation, vasopressor activity, and others. On occasion absorption of epinephrine into the systemic circulation will induce tachycardia in a sensitive individual. Inadvertent intravenous injection of a solution containing a combination of epinephrine and local anesthetic agent is dangerous and is discussed subsequently under the toxicology section of this chapter.

Metabolism

Ester-containing local anesthetic agents tend to be hydrolyzed by plasma cholinesterase. **Procaine** is an excellent example and is often used in clinical laboratories as a substrate to measure functional activity of this esterase. In general, ester-substituted agents are shorter acting than other types of linkages such as amides. **Amide-containing agents** are not hydrolyzed by plasma cholinesterase, but are metabolized mainly by mixed-function oxidases of the liver, which usually involve dealkylation of amino groups. The decreased rate of metabolism is the major reason these agents are of longer duration than ester-substituted compounds.

TYPES OF LOCAL ANESTHETICS

The following representative listing of available local anesthetic agents illustrates variations in potency, duration, and so on, that the clinician now can offer (structures are shown in Table 7–1).

Benzocaine. This agent has a long duration of action (>10 hours) and is very insoluble. It is used only for **topical application** and only in very high concentrations.

Some soluble agents with ester substitution are outlined below:

Procaine. The duration of action is less than 1 hour and, because the compound is not effective following topical application, it must be administered by injection.

Chloroprocaine. This compound has a shorter duration of action than procaine but is more potent. It is quite widely used in obstetrics.

Tetracaine. This compound has a long duration of action and is a very potent agent. It may also be used **topically**. Topical use of hydrogen iodide salt may have a duration of action >24 hours. It is sometimes used for **spinal anesthesia** and is much more active and toxic than procaine.

Cocaine. This agent is used only by topical application, and 1.0 to 10 percent solutions are available. Cocaine is the only local anesthetic agent that is a vasoconstrictor resulting from inhibition of amine I transport in adrenergic nerve terminals. It is the only local anesthetic agent controlled by Federal drug-abuse regulations.

Some of the agents with amide substitution are outlined below:

Lidocaine. This is a widely used local anesthetic agent. It is used for infiltration and regional nerve block, for spinal and topical anesthesia, as well as to treat arrhythmias. Unfortunately absorption following oral administration is erratic.

Mepivacaine. The duration of action of mepivacaine is about 30 percent longer than that of lidocaine. It is not effective following topical application. Note its close structural similarity to lidocaine.

Etidocaine and Bupivacaine. These compounds have a longer duration of action than lidocaine. Their major use is for regional blocks, including epidural anesthesia. Bupivacaine may have significant cardiac toxicity.

Many other agents are now available, and the clinician has a wide selection depending upon desired use. The available agents do vary in potency, duration of action, tissue irritation, selectivity for nerves, metabolism, and toxicity.

CLINICAL USES

These agents are widely used in many areas of clinical practice. They are unique agents in that one can block neuronal conduction at the site desired without altering neuronal modalities in other areas. Some uses of these agents are outlined below:

1. **Surface anesthesia.** Local anesthetic agents may be applied to abrasions, burns, and so on. These agents penetrate denuded skin slowly and can be used safely, e.g., benzocaine.
2. **Infiltration anesthesia including intradermal, subcutaneous, or deeper injections.** A 0.5 percent solution of lidocaine combined with epinephrine (1:100,000) is a commonly used combination.
3. **Induction of a nerve block.** For example in dental work or pudendal block in obstetrics, lidocaine combined with epinephrine is commonly used.
4. **Spinal anesthesia (subarachnoid or intrathecal).** Injection is often made into the subarachnoid space at level L2 to L5. The level of anesthesia may be controlled by the specific gravity of the injected solution or by the position of the patient. This route of administration inhibits conduction of nerves, ganglia, and perhaps the spinal cord itself. The dose may vary depending on the drug and with the administration technique employed. A definite advantage is that the patient is awake and muscle relaxation is complete. The clinician must remember that sympathetic neuronal outflow to the lower extremities will be inhibited and that there will be pooling of venous blood and lowering of arterial pressure. Therefore, severe hypotension may occur and on occasion a vasopressor agent will need to be administered to combat this untoward effect.
5. **Epidural anesthesia.** The injection is made into the space between

the periosteal lining of the spinal canal (ligamentum flavum) and the dura mater. Usually the injection is made below level L2, as the dura sack ends at L2. The major advantage is that the subarachnoid space is not entered. One potential disadvantage is that often a higher concentration of the local anesthetic agent must be administered to obtain the desired level of anesthesia.

6. **Caudal anesthesia.** This is sometimes regarded as a form of epidural block. The injection is made into the sacral hiatus. This technique is used in obstetrics. One advantage of caudal anesthesia is that, unlike in the use of epidural anesthesia, good results can be achieved without placing the patient in a sitting position. However, an even larger dose of local anesthetic may be needed, and the procedure is technically difficult.

TOXICOLOGY OF LOCAL ANESTHETICS

The major cause of toxic reactions is related to overdose and is due to **rapid absorption** from the site of injection. Great care must be exercised, to be sure that inadvertent intravenous administration of the drug does not occur. Likewise, one must remember that there can be rapid absorption of topically applied agents from areas where the skin has been denuded. Less severe signs of systemic toxicity include perioral paresthesias, salivation, tinnitus, anxiety, tremors, shivering, hypotension, tachycardia, and cardiac conduction defects. Severe symptoms of toxicity of most agents involve **convulsions or cardiovascular and respiratory collapse.** Convulsions may be treated by intravenous administration of a barbiturate such as **pentothal sodium.** If the respiration is impaired, it must be assisted and the cardiovascular system monitored; with evidence of impending collapse, intravenous fluids (lactated Ringer's solution) must be administered. In more severe cases, vasopressor drugs should be administered. In extreme toxic responses, external cardiac massage may be required. Other toxicities involving these agents are more related to **allergic phenomenon such as skin rashes**. It has been estimated that 10 percent of the population is sensitive to procaine; consequently a patient must always be questioned about potential allergic phenomena. If there is evidence of potential allergic responses, quite often an agent with a different chemical structure can be used successfully. For example, if an individual is sensitive to procaine (an ester) the individual may not be sensitive to lidocaine (an amide).

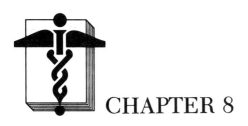

CHAPTER 8

General Anesthesia and General Anesthetic Drugs

M. D. SOKOLL, M.D.

J. P. LONG, Ph.D.

The aim of this chapter is to present various aspects of the **pharmacology, uptake, metabolism,** and **excretion of general anesthetic agents.** The principal pharmacological aspects of these drugs will be presented primarily as they

187

apply to the **cardiovascular and respiratory systems.** The concept of **minimum alveolar concentration** (MAC) will also be introduced.

HISTORY

The discovery of general anesthesia is one of the most important contributions of the United States to the practice of medicine. There has been considerable disagreement about who should receive credit for the first use of general anesthesia. Although Crawford W. Long of Georgia anesthetized James Venable on March 30, 1842, for excision of a tumor, he failed to document the occurrence in the medical literature. As a result, the first reported use of general surgical anesthesia was the use of ether by W. T. G. Morton on October 16, 1846, at the Massachusetts General Hospital.

In truth, the development of the entire field of surgery awaited the discovery of anesthesia. Prior to the advent of anesthesia patients were held still by strong attendants for operations. As a result, operations were few. In 1846 only 37 operations were performed at the Massachusetts General Hospital. A number of these were performed with anesthesia, following the first use of ether.

STAGES OF INHALATION ANESTHESIA

In the early 1920s **Guedel** published his well-known signs of ether anesthesia. The system rigidly divided ether anesthesia into four stages:

a. Stage 1, providing **amnesia and analgesia**
b. Stage 2, characterized by **excitement**
c. Stage 3, or the stage of **surgical anesthesia,** which consists of four planes (Table 8–1)
d. Stage 4, characterized by **respiratory and cardiovascular failure** and finally death

UPTAKE AND DISTRIBUTION OF VOLATILE OR GASEOUS ANESTHETICS

Delivered (Inspired) Concentrations

In the administration of general anesthesia it is preferable for the anesthesiologist to have an accurate knowledge of the **concentration** of anesthetic being delivered from the anesthesia machine. If one has available a well-

Table 8–1. SIGNS OF SURGICAL ANESTHESIA (Stage 3)
Seen with Commonly Used Halogenated Agents*

	Respiration		Eyes				
	Inter-costal Muscles	Diaph.	Pupil Size	Pupil Light Reflex	Tearing	Response to Incision Resp. or BP	Carinal Reflex‡
Plane 1			◎	+	+	+	
Plane 2			◎	+	–	–	
Plane 3†			◎	–	–	–	
Plane 4			◎	–	–	–	

*The signs of anesthesia presented here apply particularly to the halogenated agents (halothane, enflurane, and isoflurane). They have no application to intravenously administered agents.

†Although respiration is maintained to deep levels of anesthesia, the minute volume becomes inadequate in plane 3 as determined by elevated Pa_{CO_2}.

‡Note that the carinal reflex remains intact until very deep levels of anesthesia.

Diaph. = diaphragm contributions to ventilation.

functioning (temperature and flow compensated) vaporizer, the concentration of the anesthetic delivered from the machine can be read directly from the dial with considerable accuracy. If one has available a vaporizer such as the Copper Kettle, it is necessary to calculate the concentration of the delivered anesthetic. This can be accomplished if one knows the partial pressure of the volatile anesthetic at the temperature delivered, the gas flow through the vaporizer, and the flow rate of the background gas into which the anesthetic is being diluted.

Alveolar Tension of Inhalation Anesthetics

The rate at which alveolar and, as a consequence, arterial tension of an anesthetic rises is dependent on a number of factors. Among these are:

1. the minute volume of ventilation
2. blood-gas coefficient of the particular anesthetic

3. rate of redistribution of anesthetic from blood to tissue
4. the concentration of the anesthetic in the inspired mixture
5. the flow rate at which the anesthetic is being delivered into the inspired gas mixture.

The plot of the relationship between the alveolar or arterial concentration of anesthetic gas (often expressed as a percentage of the inspired concentration of anesthetic gas) versus time depicts the **uptake curve**. All other factors remaining constant, the rate of rise of the initial part of the uptake curve depends primarily on the magnitude of alveolar minute ventilation. The steepness of the slope will be affected, to some extent, by the rate of administration of the agent. As can be seen in Figure 8–1, decreasing flow rate from non-rebreathing to 10 liters per minute into the circle decreases the rate of rise of alveolar concentration.

The **blood-gas partition coefficient** (the ratio of the concentrations in each of two phases of a substance in equilibrium between the phases: e.g., halothane has a blood-gas partition coefficient of 2.36; therefore, at equilibrium

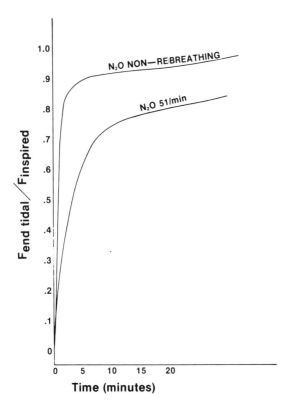

Figure 8–1. Effect of changing anesthetic gas flow rate on uptake of inhalation agents. For any one agent, the F_E/F_I ratio will rise more rapidly with higher flow rates. The F_E/F_I ratio is decreased by the mixing of the incoming gas with that exhaled by the patient, which has had some of the anesthetic agent removed in the patient's lungs. The higher the inflow rate, the less it will be diluted by the exhaled gas mixture. F = fraction; E = end tidal; I = inspired.

the blood will contain 2.36 times the number of molecules of halothane as will be in the gas phase) is primarily responsible for the height of the "knee" of the uptake curve (Fig. 8–2). As a general rule, the lower the blood-gas partition coefficient, the higher the knee of the uptake curve. This is based on the simple fact that the lower the blood "partition" of a given anesthetic agent, the more slowly it will diffuse from the alveolus into the blood and, therefore, the more rapidly will the alveolar concentration rise.

During the induction phase of an inhalation anesthetic, the alveolar concentration rapidly approaches that of the inspired concentration of the anesthetic gas. At the same time, anesthetic is being removed from the alveolus by blood perfusing the alveolar capillaries. This slows the rate of rise of the alveolar concentration of anesthetic drug and creates the knee of the uptake curve.

The final phase of the uptake curve is primarily determined by the tissue blood coefficient. Again, as with the blood-gas partition coefficient, the lower the tissue blood coefficient, the steeper the final slope of the uptake curve.

A number of other factors have effects of lesser magnitude on the uptake curve. The **concentration effect** is based on the fact that, if the lung is filled with a 100 percent concentration of an anesthetic, the concentration will remain 100 percent despite the volume removed by the blood. However, if the lung is filled with 80 percent anesthetic and 20 percent insoluble gas, the an-

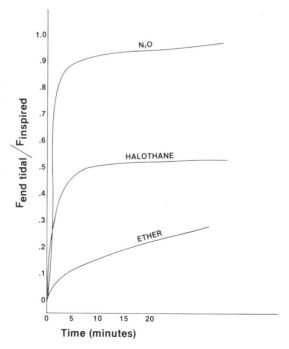

Figure 8–2. All else remaining constant, an anesthetic uptake curve is composed of three parts. The initial rapid rise is controlled primarily by alveolar ventilation. The final, almost horizontal, slope is determined by the tissue/blood solubility coefficient. The area in between, the "knee" of the curve, is determined by the uptake of anesthetic from the alveolae by the blood. This is controlled by the blood-gas partition coefficient; the lower the partition coefficient, the higher will be the knee of the curve.

esthetic concentration will decrease as the anesthetic is absorbed by the blood while the insoluble gas is not. The diluent gas now represents a higher percentage of the alveolar gas and the anesthetic a lower concentration (Fig. 8–3). A second aspect of the concentration effect is that when anesthetic is absorbed from the lung, the organ does not collapse, instead the volume inspired with the next breath increases, bringing in more anesthetic. A third aspect of the concentration effect is seen in the following. If an agent is used in low concentration, uptake by the blood can significantly decrease the concentration in the alveolus. The same agent, or one of similar solubility given in higher concentration, will leave the alveolar concentration less affected by uptake. Clinically, the concentration effect applies principally to nitrous oxide because it is the only anesthetic used in high (60 percent or greater) inspired concentrations. **The second gas effect** is produced by the concomitant administration of two anesthetics; the uptake of one of the anesthetic gases will result in an increased concentration of the other anesthetic (Fig. 8–4). Though this concept applies to all mixtures of anesthetics, from a practical aspect it is of significance only with nitrous oxide since only this drug is used in sufficiently high concentration to have adequate volumetric uptake.

From a clinical point of view, changes in cardiac output can cause signifi-

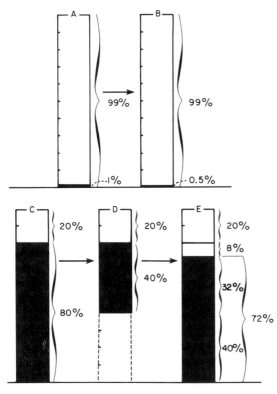

Figure 8–3. The columns represent gas concentrations in the lung. With low concentrations, uptake of half of the anesthetic decreases the concentration to one half of the original. (*A* and *B*). With high concentrations, considering that uptake of anesthetic causes additional gas mixture to be drawn into the lung, the resultant decrease is only 10 percent. (From Eger, EI, II: Anesthetic Uptake and Action. Williams & Wilkins, Baltimore, 1974, p. 114, with permission.)

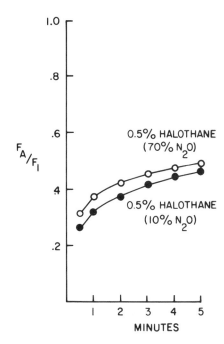

Figure 8–4. Effect of the second gas effect on the uptake of halothane. The uptake of greater amounts of nitrous oxide at the higher concentration results in a more rapid rise of the alveolar halothane concentration. (From Eger, EI, II: Anesthetic Uptake and Action. Williams & Wilkins, Baltimore, 1974, p. 117, with permission.)

cant alterations of uptake of inhaled anesthetics. Although a hyperactive circulatory system appears to have little effect on induction of anesthesia, a decreased cardiac output, particularly when caused by blood loss, can result in significant effects by the following two mechanisms.

First, with a hypovolemia-mediated decrease in cardiac output there is decreased blood flow through the lung, resulting in a lessened rate of removal of anesthetic from the alveolus. This results in an increased rate of rise of the alveolar concentration of anesthetic and, therefore, an elevated concentration of anesthetic in the arterial blood. It should be remembered that alveolar and arterial tensions of inhalation gases, for all practical purposes, equilibrate within 3 to 5 minutes when the inspired concentration is held constant. Second, during hypovolemia **there is shunting of cardiac output away from skin, muscle, and most viscera** because of adrenergically mediated vasoconstriction; **blood flow to the brain and myocardium,** whose vasculatures are less responsive to catecholamines, is **preserved.** Because of the maintained tissue perfusion to the brain and heart and the more rapid rise of alveolar drug concentrations, induction of anesthesia can be quite rapid in hypovolemic patients with the possibility of rapid and profound decreases in blood pressure.

It must be remembered that these uptake curves represent only changes in the alveolar concentration of inhalational anesthetics. The potency of the individual anesthetic is an entirely separate consideration. As an example, **cyclopropane** and **nitrous oxide** both have low blood-gas solubility coefficients, and as a result, the alveolar tension of these gases rises rapidly. The potency of these anesthetics, however, is markedly different; cyclopropane is an extremely potent anesthetic, whereas nitrous oxide has a relatively low potency.

Minimum Alveolar Concentration

Minimum alveolar concentration (MAC) is a concept that permits the pharmacological comparison of inhalational anesthetics in terms of potency. Strictly speaking, MAC is the ED_{50} for the specific anesthetic agent. It is the point on the dose-response curve at which 50 percent of subjects will not respond to a noxious stimulus. The concept of MAC has been applied to both humans and experimental animals. One of the shortcomings of the concept is that MAC measures only a single point on the dose-response curve. To its credit, however, MAC is of surprisingly small variability within a given species and the correlation of the values between humans and animals is high.

MAC is affected by a number of factors. With the exception of a slight increase in MAC at puberty, the value tends to decrease progressively with age. In general terms it appears to mimic the curve for basal metabolic rate. MAC is diminished by decreasing body temperature and agents that depress the CNS.

Elimination of Inhalation Anesthetic Agents

The same factors that govern the uptake of inhalation anesthetics into blood are also responsible for their elimination. These are pulmonary ventilation, blood flow, partition of the anesthetic in blood and tissue, and rate of administration of the anesthetic gases. With termination of the administration of the anesthetic, the inspired concentration decreases. This is rapidly followed by a decrease in alveolar, and then finally blood and tissue concentrations of anesthetic. Because of its relatively high blood flow, the brain is one of the earliest organs cleared of anesthetic agent, thus accounting for the rapid awakening from anesthesia noted with relatively insoluble agents such as nitrous oxide. The curves representing elimination of inhaled anesthetics are mirror images of the uptake curves. Nitrous oxide and cyclopropane, drugs having relatively low blood-gas partition coefficients and a rapid rise of alveolar concentration on induction, will also have rapid elimination once administration of the anesthetic has been terminated (Fig. 8–5).

Diffusion Hypoxia

Diffusion hypoxia is the reverse of the concentration effect and can occur during rapid elimination of inhalational anesthetics. As administration of the anesthetic agent is discontinued, the drug moves from the blood into the alveolae. As this occurs the anesthetic displaces the gases in the alveolus in

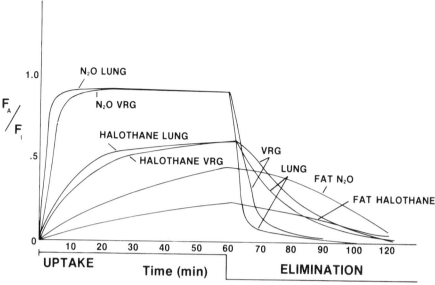

Figure 8–5. Uptake and elimination curves for nitrous oxide and halothane. The flow rate is 10 lpm. Anesthetic concentrations are N_2O, 70 percent; halothane, 1 percent. VRG = vessel rich group of tissue including brain, heart, liver, and kidney. Note the continued slow rise of the alveolar-blood concentration of halothane compared to nitrous oxide due to the high tissue/blood coefficient for halothane. (Modified from Smith, TC, et al: History and principles of anesthesiology. In: Gilman, AG, Goodman, LS, and Gilman, A: The Pharmacologic Basis of Therapeutics, ed 6. Macmillan, New York, 1980, p. 264.)

terms of volume and partial pressure. One of the gases so affected is oxygen, the result being a decrease in alveolar oxygen tension. Diffusion hypoxia is sometimes seen in the early minutes following the discontinuation of the administration of nitrous oxide when room air is breathed. The hypoxia is usually quite mild. Diffusion hypoxia occurs only with nitrous oxide because this is the only anesthetic gas used in sufficiently high inspired concentration. Diffusion hypoxia requires the combination of a rapid shift from a high nitrous oxide containing atmosphere to a high nitrogen containing atmosphere with concomitant alveolar hypoventilation. If either of these is not present, then diffusion hypoxia is not likely to occur.

MECHANISMS OF ACTION OF ANESTHETICS

The actual mechanism by which general anesthetics act, whether administered by inhalation or intravenous injection, is unknown. A number of theories have evolved, and there has been considerable effort to formulate a unified theory of anesthesia that would combine, under one theory, the modes of action of local, intravenously administered, and inhalational anesthetics.

Lipid solubility of anesthetics appears to be of some importance, and some theories would suggest that lipid solubility and potency are closely interrelated. Also of considerable interest, particularly in those theories relating potency to solubility in lipid membranes, is the observation that increases in ambient pressure can reverse the state of general anesthesia, a phenomenon referred to as "**pressure reversal**" of anesthesia.

INHALATIONAL ANESTHETIC AGENTS

The chemistry, physiology, and pharmacology of some inhalational anesthetics, primarily **nitrous oxide** and the **halogenated hydrocarbons,** will be discussed here. Physical characteristics of selected inhalational anesthetics are shown in Table 8–2.

Some pharmacological properties of the more important anesthetics are summarized in Table 8–3. A few pertinent clinical properties are listed under "advantages" and "disadvantages."

Table 8–2. PHYSICAL AND CHEMICAL SYSTEMS OF SELECTED INHALATIONAL AGENTS

Agent	Flamma-bility	Vapor Pressure at 20°C	Partition Coefficients		MAC in 100% O_2
			Oil-Gas	Blood-Gas	
Nitrous oxide	No	800 psi (5515 kPa)	1.4	0.47	105.00
Cyclopro-pane	Yes	90 psi (620 kPa)	11.2	0.42	9.20
Diethyl ether	Yes	400 mmHg (59 kPa)	65.0	12.10	1.92
Enflurane	No	184 mmHg (24 kPa)	98.5	1.80	1.68
Isoflurane	No	250 mmHg (33 kPa)	99.0	1.40	1.20
Halothane	No	243 mmHg (32 kPa)	224.0	2.30	0.75
Methoxy-flurane	No	22.5 mmHg (3 kPa)	825.0	13.00	0.16

Table 8–3. SOME PROPERTIES OF GENERAL ANESTHETIC

Drug	Min Ventilation	Cardiovascular* Blood Pressure*	Myocardial Contractility	Peripheral Resistance	Skeletal Muscle Relaxation	Advantages	Disadvantages
Diethyl ether	Decreased	Little change	Decreased	Decreased	Marked	Cardiovascular stability	Explosive; objectionable odor
Cyclopropane	Decreased	Little change	Decreased	Increased	Moderate	Very rapid induction	Explosive; arrhythmias, especially with catecholamines
Halothane	Decreased	Decreased	Decreased	Little change	Moderate	Pleasant odor; rapid induction and recovery	Arrhythmias, especially with catecholamines; possible hepatotoxicity
Enflurane	Decreased	Decreased	Decreased	Decreased	Moderate	Pleasant odor	Marked depression of blood pressure, seizures, hepatotoxicity
Isoflurane	Decreased	Decreased	Little change	Decreased	Moderate	Stable cardiac rhythm	Somewhat objectionable odor
Nitrous oxide	Unchanged	Unchanged	Decreased	Increased	None	No odor; rapid effect	Must be combined with other agents
Thiopental	Decreased	Decreased	Little change†	Arterial resistance and venous capacity increased	None	Rapid IV induction (30 sec); short duration with proper dosage	Must be combined with other agents; decreases ICP
Methohexital	Decreased	Decreased	Little change†	Arterial resistance and venous capacity increased	None	Rapid IV induction (30 sec); very short duration with proper dosage	Must be combined with other agents; decreases ICP
Ketamine	Little effect	Increased	Increased	Little change	None	Can be used IV or IM for induction	May produce hallucinations
Etomidate	Decreased	Little change	Little change	Little change	None	IV induction	Purposeless movements, adrenal suppression

*Ether and cyclopropane cause little change in blood pressure in the intact animal, because of elevated endogenous catecholamine.

†Blood pressure decrease with barbiturates is related primarily to venodilation and decreased venous return.

Nitrous Oxide

Nitrous oxide is a colorless, odorless, tasteless gas that is commercially prepared by heating ammonium nitrate. The gas is then passed through a series of scrubbers to remove residual nitric acid, ammonia, and higher oxides of nitrogen. In the cylinder, nitrous oxide is pressurized to about 700 lb per square inch and exists in both liquid and gas phases. The tank will register 700 lb until all of the liquid has evaporated, at which time only about one tenth of the original amount of nitrous oxide remains as a gas within the cylinder. **Nitrous oxide does not burn but will support combustion.**

The blood-gas solubility coefficient of nitrous oxide is 0.47, a relatively low value. The MAC of nitrous oxide is 105 percent, indicating that true anesthesia with nitrous oxide can be produced only under hyperbaric conditions.

Under clinical circumstances nitrous oxide is always combined with other anesthetic or analgesic agents. It is important that the amount of nitrous oxide administered be limited to 60 to 70 percent of inspired air at sea level and even lesser percentage at higher altitudes, so that an adequate tension of oxygen can be supplied. Though nitrous oxide has long been considered to be devoid of any cardiovascular side effects, recent studies have demonstrated that the drug produces slight myocardial depression. This, combined with a concomitant increase in peripheral vascular resistance, results in no change in blood pressure. Nitrous oxide is compatible with the use of exogenously administered catecholamines.

With relatively few exceptions, such as the **gut, middle ear,** and **paranasal sinuses,** there are no air-containing cavities that are not in direct communication with the ambient air pressure. In these noncommunicating areas, as well as in pneumothoraxes, the administration of an inhalational anesthetic requiring use of a high inspired concentration of the anesthetic may result in an increased pressure within the air-containing space. This results from the diffusion of the anesthetic from the capillaries into the air-containing space because of the high partial pressure of the anesthetic between the blood and the air-containing space. The resultant diffusion of gas into this space causes an increase in pressure within the space. The use of a mixture containing 75 percent nitrous oxide to 25 percent oxygen can cause the pressure in the cerebroventricular system to double if the patient has pneumocephalus, as might occur with a basilar skull fracture. Thus, it would appear to be **potentially dangerous to use nitrous oxide and oxygen mixtures in patients with pneumothoraxes or in the presence of pneumocephalus.** It can also result in intestinal distension, which may make intra-abdominal procedures more difficult.

Nitrous oxide has been demonstrated to have significant hematologic effects. When administered >24 hr for sedation in the respiratory management of tetanus patients, a megaloblastic bone marrow depression resulted. The mechanism by which this alteration of hematopoiesis occurs is most likely related to the interaction of nitrous oxide with folate and cobalamine metabolism. **Neurological defects** have been reported in patients exposed to high environmental concentrations or when nitrous oxide has been an agent of chemical abuse. Motor and sensory coordination and neurological reflex defects have been reported. These usually regress with discontinuation of inhalation of nitrous oxide. The drug has been reported to cause some **gestational defects,** among which are an increase in (1) spontaneous abortion rate, (2) fetal death rate, and (3) visceral abnormalities. These associations are still controversial.

Nitrous oxide has been reported to cause a slight increase in intracranial pressure. The increase is less than that caused by the **halogenated agents**.

Halothane

Halothane (Fig. 8–6) was first prepared by Raventos in 1956. It is a volatile liquid that is heavier than water and has a sweet smell. Halothane does not react with soda-lime, in contrast to **trichloroethylene** which can react with it to form phosgene. (Soda-lime [a mixture of 20 percent NaOH and 80 percent $Ca(OH)_2$] absorbs exhaled CO_2, permitting the use of partial or total rebreathing systems. The monetary savings achieved with soda-lime, versus CO_2 elimination with a nonrebreathing system, are appreciable.) When used for anesthesia it contains thymol as a preservative.

When combined with oxygen, **MAC for halothane is about 0.75 percent;**

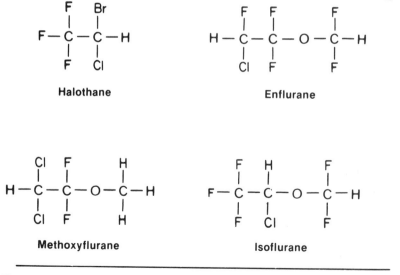

Figure 8–6. Structures of commonly used halogenated inhalational anesthetics.

MAC is only 0.3 percent when combined with 70 percent nitrous oxide. The blood-gas coefficient is 2.3 and is in the range of medium solubility. The tissue-blood solubility coefficient of halothane is, for most tissue, in excess of 2.0. This is quite high compared with that of other anesthetic agents, and leads to a prolonged uptake of halothane by the body.

Halothane is both a **respiratory and a cardiovascular depressant,** as are most anesthetic agents. The degree of depression of both systems is **concentration-dependent.** The mechanism underlying the myocardial depression is, to some extent, related to enzyme inhibition in cardiac muscle. Halothane has many effects on the sympathetic nervous system. It appears to decrease central adrenergic output and, concomitantly, blocks the vasoconstrictor action of norepinephrine in some peripheral vessel beds. The drug causes a decrease in both renal and hepatic blood flow.

Halothane causes a **direct relaxation of uterine muscle** that is dose related. **Increased blood loss** has been documented during therapeutic abortions when halothane was used compared with a barbiturate-narcotic anesthetic technique. Halothane causes a **dilatation of the cerebral vascular system** and results in an **increase in intracranial pressure.** This increase in intracranial pressure can be ameliorated if the patient is hyperventilated before the addition of halothane and the delivered concentration is limited to ≤ 1 percent.

Seventy-five to 95 percent of absorbed halothane is excreted either through the lung or by other routes. **Some inhaled halothane is metabolized,** usually by an oxidative pathway (cytochrome P-450), to trifluoroacetic acid. This metabolite, along with the fluoride and chloride ions simultaneously released, is relatively innocuous. In addition, an anaerobic "reductive biotransformation" of halothane has been postulated. It is felt that this type of metabolism can result in the formation of active metabolites, which have the potential for cellular toxicity. This mechanism, along with hypoxia, has been postulated as a possible source of "halothane hepatitis." The exact origin of this hepatic cellular injury, the existence of which has been the subject of considerable debate and some research, is unknown. A number of possible etiologies have been considered for the generation of "halothane hepatitis." These include (1) **direct cellular hepatotoxicity, such as that caused by chloroform,** (2) **hypersensitivity,** and (3) **biotransformation.** It is the last of these, with the formation of reactive metabolites, mentioned earlier, that is currently considered to be the prime candidate for the genesis of jaundice sometimes noted to appear following the administration of halothane. The incidence of "halothane hepatitis" is about 1 in 10,000 anesthesias, an occurrence rate not significantly different from that of other anesthetic agents. Once jaundice has occurred, the mortality is about 50 percent. Worldwide, halothane is still a very commonly used anesthetic, although its use in the United States has decreased because of the unique medicolegal climate. It should be noted that jaundice has also been noted to occur following the administration of both **enflurane** and **isoflurane,** halogenated anesthetics that are not known to undergo metabolism to a significant extent.

Enflurane

Enflurane (see Fig. 8–6) is a methyl-ethyl ether first synthesized in 1963. It is a colorless, nonflammable liquid that is heavier than water. The drug, as it is available clinically, is chemically stable and compatible with soda-lime.

MAC for enflurane is about 1.68 percent in 100 percent oxygen and approximately 0.6 percent when combined with 70 percent nitrous oxide. Its blood-gas solubility coefficient is 1.8, which places it between nitrous oxide and halothane. The tissue-blood solubility coefficient for most tissues is considerably lower than that for halothane.

Enflurane is a potent **respiratory depressant.** At 1 MAC enflurane is a stronger respiratory depressant than either halothane or isoflurane, whereas at 1.5 MAC the three drugs are respiratory depressants of equal potency.

As with other **volatile anesthetics,** enflurane is a direct **myocardial depressant.** There is also some decrease in peripheral vascular resistance. At 2 MAC, enflurane-induced hypotension was of sufficient magnitude that the studies being performed had to be terminated. Enflurane has little effect on the sympathoadrenal system and appears not to sensitize the myocardium significantly to the administration of exogenous catecholamines.

In experimental animals and in humans, **electroencephalographic patterns suggesting seizure activity** have been noted when deep levels of enflurane anesthesia have been combined with hypocarbia. Although a few instances of twitching have been noted, no seizure activity has been reported during clinical anesthesia.

Enflurane has effects on both smooth and skeletal muscle. In addition to the cardiovascular effects, enflurane depresses contraction and tone of both gravid and nongravid myometrium. Skeletal muscle is relaxed by enflurane and other inhalational anesthetics. There is a direct interference of action potential generation in skeletal muscle produced by inhalational anesthetics resulting in an enhancement of the activity of nondepolarizing neuromuscular blocking agents.

Enflurane is relatively nontoxic compared with other anesthetic agents. Although postoperative jaundice has been reported, its incidence has not been determined. Most of the drug is excreted unchanged *via* the lung or through the skin, with a relatively small percentage (about 2.5 percent) found in the urine as fluorinated metabolites. Some fluoride ion is released in the metabolism of enflurane, but peak blood levels are only about one half of the level usually accepted as being nephrotoxic.

Isoflurane

Isoflurane is an isomer of enflurane and is therefore also a methyl-ethyl ether. It is a colorless, nonflammable, chemically stable liquid. It has a slightly irritating odor that, to some extent, limits the rate of induction of anesthesia. On the other hand, isoflurane has a relatively low blood-gas solubility coefficient, leading to a fairly rapid induction of anesthesia. Compared with other anesthetics it is only very slightly metabolized and yields low blood bromide levels. In young adults, **MAC for isoflurane is about 1.3 percent** in oxygen and about 0.6 percent with 70 percent nitrous oxide.

The drug is a reasonably potent **respiratory depressant** and, in the absence of surgical stimulation, results in a $PaCO_2$ of approximately 50 mmHg at 1.5 MAC. Surgical stimulation decreases this elevation in $PaCO_2$ considerably. The ventilatory response to hypoxia is also markedly decreased by isoflurane.

Although animal studies suggest significant myocardial depression by isoflurane, similar studies in humans indicate relatively little cardiac depressant effect at 1 to 2 MAC. Total peripheral vascular resistance is reduced in a dose-related fashion resulting, in the absence of an increased cardiac output, in a decrease in arterial blood pressure.

Isoflurane produces a significant increase in blood flow to both muscle and skin. It sensitizes the myocardium to exogenously administered catecholamines to a lesser degree than **halothane** does, so that the administration of epinephrine with isoflurane is much better tolerated. Isoflurane has little effect on intracardiac conduction mechanisms.

Isoflurane produces cerebral vasodilation and an increase in both cerebral blood flow and intracranial pressure. These effects may be ameliorated to some extent by a dose-dependent decrease in cerebral oxygen demand produced by the drug.

As with the other halogenated anesthetic agents, isoflurane produces uterine relaxation, which may make the drug useful for operative obstetrical maneuvers such as version and extraction. The drug is not advised for use with termination of pregnancy or similar procedures.

Other Inhalational Agents

Diethyl ether is a colorless liquid having a vapor pressure of approximately 425 mmHg at room temperature. The liquid is **highly flammable** in air and **explosive** when combined with oxygen. The blood-gas solubility coefficient of ether is 12:1, leading to a relatively slow induction of anesthesia. In contrast to other anesthetic agents, ventilation is not depressed at surgical levels of anesthesia. The drug has a **wide margin of safety** with respect to the cardiovascular system. In the heart-lung preparation ether is a myocardial depressant, but in the intact animal, as a result of increased catecholamine secretion, the drug produces little change in blood pressure or pulse rate. Ether causes **no sensitization of the myocardium to exogenously administered cate-cholamines.** The drug depresses renal blood flow and reduces the tone of the gravid uterus in low concentrations. As are the other drugs considered here, ether is compatible with soda-lime.

Methoxyflurane is a volatile liquid with a characteristic pleasant odor. The vapor pressure at room temperature is only 23 mmHg. The only current use of this drug is self-administration of low concentrations to provide analgesia for labor. In higher concentrations, particularly if administered over a long period of time, the drug causes progressive degrees of renal impairment that can culminate in oliguric renal failure. The renal injury is caused by high blood levels of fluoride ion produced by metabolism of methoxyflurane.

INTRAVENOUSLY ADMINISTERED ANESTHETICS

This section will be devoted to a consideration of the rapidly acting thiobarbiturates, ketamine, and etomidate (Fig. 8–7).

The uptake and distribution of the intravenously administered agents are markedly different from those of the inhalationally administered drugs. With the intravenous agents, the drug is administered directly into the vascular system and is removed from the vascular system by distribution, metabolism, or excretion. **Thiopental** is the prototype intravenously administered general anesthetic.

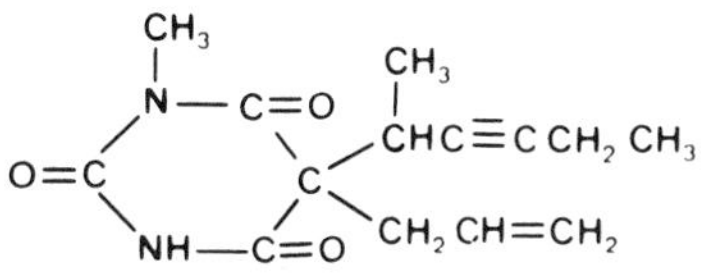

Methohexital (Brietal, Brevital)

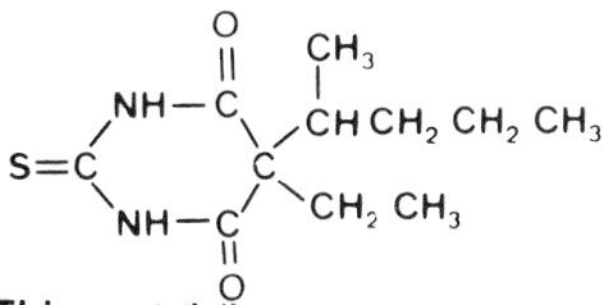

Thiopental (Intraval, Pentothal)

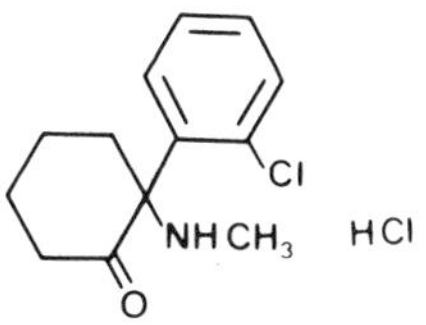

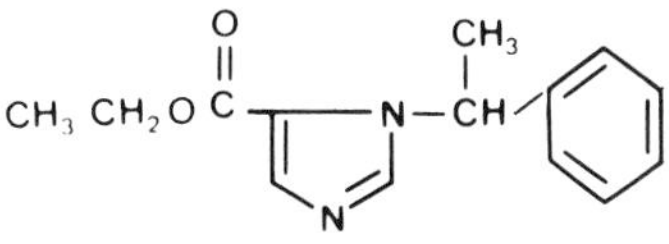

Ketamine Hydrochloride (Ketalar)

Etomidate

Figure 8–7. Structures of some commonly used intravenous anesthetics.

The **distribution of thiopental** following bolus intravenous administration is shown in Figure 8–8. The **thiobarbiturates** are remarkable in that they have a **high fat solubility**. It was initially believed that redistribution to fat was the reason for rapid recovery following the bolus administration of a modest dose of drug. Further studies, including those of Price,[39] suggested that the prime reason for the rapid recovery was distribution from the vessel-rich tissue, which includes the brain, to lean muscle. This is followed later by further redistribution to the fat and vessel-poor tissue. As the distribution sites in muscle are saturated, the rate of decline of thiopental concentration in the plasma and vessel-rich tissue will be markedly modified, leading to a much longer effect of a relatively small dose of drug.

Thiopental

Thiopental, the thio analog of pentobarbital, is a weak acid. The clinically available drug contains sodium carbonate, and the freshly mixed solution has a pH of 10 to 11. Because of its high lipid solubility, thiopental rapidly crosses cell membranes and, with the administration of a "sleepdose" (3 to 4 mg/kg) onset of sleep occurs in about 30 seconds. In the fit adult this dose has little cardiovascular effect. The patient awakens in 4 to 6 minutes. Thiopental is a **profound respiratory depressant** and the administration of a bolus dose suffi-

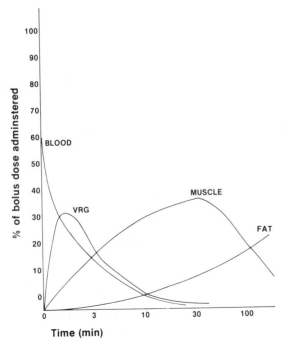

Figure 8–8. Set of curves representing the distribution of thiopental from the CNS to other compartments. VRG = vessel rich group (heart, brain, and so forth). Note log time scale.

cient to cause sleep will also cause a transient apnea. The drug is not a profound depressant of pharyngeal or tracheobronchial reflexes and, as a result, its use is not advocated in patients having asthma.

The effects of thiopental on the cardiovascular system are diverse. Small doses of thiopental cause dilatation of skin and muscle vascular beds and a compensatory constriction in the gut and viscera. As a result, total peripheral resistance, cardiac output, and blood pressure are not altered. In larger doses, blood pressure and cardiac output decrease, probably resulting from peripheral vasodilation primarily in the venous circulation and possibly also from direct myocardial-depressant actions of high blood levels of the drug.

Thiopental has little effect on neuromuscular transmission. It crosses the placental barrier freely and can depress neonatal respiration. The administration of a sleep-inducing dose of thiopental to the mother should not cause significant respiratory depression in the infant.

Following intravenous administration, 70 to 80 percent of the administered dose of thiopental is initially bound to plasma protein. The percent of binding of a given dose depends on the dose administered and the presence of other drugs that compete with thiopental for binding sites on plasma protein. **Thiopental is metabolized in the liver.**

Thiopental decreases cerebral oxygen consumption and cerebral blood flow concomitantly. Drug-induced cerebral vasoconstriction decreases intracranial pressure.

Because of the tissue toxicity reported with higher concentrations, thiopental should not be administered in solutions exceeding 2.5 percent. Accidental intra-arterial injection of a 2.5 percent solution usually causes little problem, but a 5 percent solution produces a profound chemical vasculitis distal to the site of injection with resultant arterial thrombosis. Surgical amputation of the distal extremity has sometimes been necessary. Should the drug be injected intra-arterially the following steps are suggested. First, leave the needle or catheter in the artery if at all possible. Second, 10 to 20 ml of either 0.5 percent **procaine** or 1 percent **lidocaine** should be injected through the needle into the artery. **Papaverine, heparin,** or **a small dose of sodium nitroprusside may also be used**. One must be aware of the profound hypotension-inducing properties of nitroprusside.

Methohexital

Methohexital is an oxybarbiturate that is approximately twice as potent a CNS depressant as is **thiopental**. The clinically available preparation is a white powder having a pKa of 7.9 to 8.3 in solution and is combined with sodium carbonate. The pH of the usual solution is 10 to 11.

The pharmacological actions of **methohexital** are very similar to those of **thiopental**. Consciousness is lost rapidly and there is a significant **incidence of hiccups and skeletal muscle twitching** following the intravenous administration of methohexital. These phenomena occur with thiopental at a lesser frequency. The cardiovascular and respiratory effects of methohexital are similar to those of thiopental. The drug is metabolized in the liver by oxidation, demethylation, and cleavage of the ring.

Sleeping time from a dose of 1 mg per kg body weight is only 2 to 3 minutes. The drug is therefore frequently **used for outpatient surgery.** It should be remembered, however, that **driving skill is impaired** for up to 8 hours following the administration of a dose of 2 mg per kg to young healthy adults.

Ketamine

Ketamine, a cyclohexanone derivative, is a white crystalline powder that is soluble in water. In adequate dosage it will produce a state characterized by sedation, amnesia, and marked analgesia referred to as "dissociative anesthesia."

The drug may be used either intramuscularly or intravenously for induction of anesthesia. Intravenous administration of 1 to 2 mg per kg results in **analgesia lasting about 15 minutes.** Some degree of analgesia may persist for another 30 to 40 minutes.

With moderate doses of ketamine, respiration is usually well maintained, although some respiratory depression may be seen immediately following intravenous administration of the drug. This may be particularly so in very young infants. The upper airway tends to remain patent, probably because the drug produces little or no muscular relaxation. Hypercarbic or hypoxic stimulation of respiration appears to be little depressed following usual dosages of the drug. Laryngeal and pharyngeal reflexes are also well maintained.

Blood pressure and heart rate are usually somewhat increased. This may result from increased sympathetic activity as the concentrations of both epinephrine and norepinephrine in the circulation are increased. Both cerebral blood flow and intracranial pressure, as well as intraocular pressure, are increased by ketamine.

Ketamine produces some interesting mental changes. Following the administration of the drug most adults will have a period of vivid, **anxiety-producing dreams or even hallucinations.** Hallucinations occur with considerable frequency. These psychiatric disturbances can be decreased in frequency by the administration of diazepam or thiopental near the end of the anesthesia. The "flashback" phenomenon has been reported.

Etomidate

Etomidate, an imidazole carboxylate derivative, is a nonbarbiturate hypnotic. Following rapid intravenous injection, **etomidate produces hypnosis in**

about 1 minute. The duration of the hypnosis is dose-dependent, but recovery is usually rapid. Pain at the site of injection is common.

Although etomidate was initially thought not to cause hypotension, more recent observations have documented the rather frequent occurrence of this side effect. As with other anesthetics, etomidate possesses some respiratory-depressant activity, and short periods of apnea are commonly seen following intravenous administration of large doses. Intravenous administration of etomidate frequently causes some purposeless movement.

There is increasing evidence of adrenal cortical suppression following long-term administration of etomidate as a sedative in intensive care settings. Modest adrenal suppression has been noted with shorter-term administration of the drug.

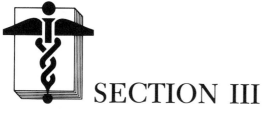

SECTION III

Pharmacology Related to Other Major Organ Systems

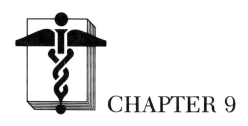

CHAPTER 9

Cardiovascular Drugs

MICHAEL J. BRODY, Ph.D.

ROSS D. FELDMAN, M.D.

R. KENT HERMSMEYER, Ph.D.

From the early use of digitalis as a folk remedy to the most recently approved drugs such as TPA, the pharmacological treatment of disease of the heart and blood vessels has been central to clinical management. This chapter explores the extensive variety of drugs used in the treatment of hypertension, angina pectoris, cardiac arrhythmias, and congestive heart failure, as well as thrombolytic and anticoagulant agents and the lipid-lowering drugs used in the prevention and treatment of atherosclerosis.

ANTIHYPERTENSIVE AGENTS

Pharmacological management of **hypertension** represents a major medical accomplishment. In only 30 years, the field has advanced from the introduction of ganglionic blocking agents to the now diverse spectrum of drugs that offer the promise of blood pressure control relatively free of side effects and tailored to the individual patient. Knowledge about arterial pressure regulation, pathogenesis of hypertension, and the mechanisms of antihypertensive agents provides a framework around which rational and effective treatment of hypertension can be accomplished.

Epidemiology of Hypertension

The incidence of hypertension is high in industrialized societies and involves approximately 25 percent of the total American population, a figure that translates into approximately 55 million adults and 2.7 million children.

The specific etiology of **essential hypertension** has not been identified, although there is increasing awareness of subpopulations of this large group (which comprises 90 percent of all patients with hypertension). One subgroup includes **borderline hypertension,** in which the elevated pressure is not fixed and in which pressure may vary proportionately with the level of stress and anxiety. Other groups are patients with relatively high or low plasma renin activity and those with relatively low or high circulating plasma catecholamines or urinary catecholamine secretion. Although these classifications are potentially useful in the application of specific antihypertensive therapies, no widespread consensus has developed about their reliability or predictability. The remaining 10 percent of subjects with hypertension have potentially curable forms of the disease. Most common among these are **renal hypertension,** including renal artery stenosis, which can be alleviated by nephrectomy, renal artery replacement, or balloon angioplasty; **mineralocorticoid-dependent hypertension** produced by adrenal adenomas; and **intermittent hypertension** produced by tumors of chromaffin tissue (**pheochromacytoma**) that produce high circulating levels of catecholamines. Other secondary causes include hyperthyroidism, Cushing's disease, hypercalcemia, and oral contraceptives.

The epidemiological data relating to the consequences of hypertension and its prevention by antihypertensive agents are striking. Diastolic arterial pressures in excess of 90 mm Hg are regarded as hypertensive because of increased risk of cardiovascular fatality. For example, there is at least a doubling of cardiovascular mortality in patients with arterial pressures in excess of 160/95, with proportionately lower but nonetheless graded risks for subjects between this level and 140/90. These risks exist in the absence of symptoms. By comparison with the normotensive subject, the patient with hypertension is three times as likely to develop coronary artery disease, is four times as likely to develop congestive heart failure, and is seven times as likely to develop stroke.

Control of arterial pressure confers substantial protection from the secondary consequences of the disease. Furthermore, the closer the control is monitored and the more strict the compliance, the better is the protection from cardiovascular disease. A disturbing feature, which tempers an otherwise outstanding record of success with antihypertensive drug therapy, is that morbidity and mortality from myocardial infarction is reduced to a much lesser extent than that from heart failure or stroke. It appears from these considerations that the progression of coronary atherosclerotic disease may not be greatly altered by antihypertensive therapy.

Relatively little is known about which specific antihypertensive agents confer the greatest protection on patients with elevated blood pressure. Most trials that have established the beneficial effects of treating hypertension have employed multiple therapies. Several recent trials employing monotherapy have led to the suspicion that simply lowering arterial pressure by itself may not protect against secondary cardiovascular disease. In the Multiple Risk Factor Intervention Trial (MRFIT), increased incidence of sudden death was observed with diuretics, whereas protection without increased risk was observed in several trials employing β-adrenoceptor antagonists such as propranolol.

Mechanisms of Hypertension

Investigations into the pathogenesis of hypertension have contributed importantly to our understanding of the normal processes that regulate arterial pressure. A complex interplay among neural, humoral, and local vascular systems maintains arterial pressure within normal limits and also provides the adaptations necessary for adjustments in arterial pressure required during physical exertion, changes in posture, and so forth. Hypertension is a disease of abnormal regulation in which vasoconstrictor mechanisms prevail over these adaptive systems. Antihypertensive agents, in turn, although not capable of reestablishing normal homeostasis, can return arterial pressure to normal or nearly normal levels.

Neural Mechanisms

A schematic representation of peripheral and central structures involved in arterial pressure control is seen in Figure 9–1. Sympathetic discharge appears to originate primarily from a group of cells in rostral ventrolateral medulla, some of which are adrenergic in nature (i.e., employ **epinephrine** as an excitatory neurotransmitter at the intermediolateral column of the spinal cord). Many other putative excitatory transmitters that influence the pregan-

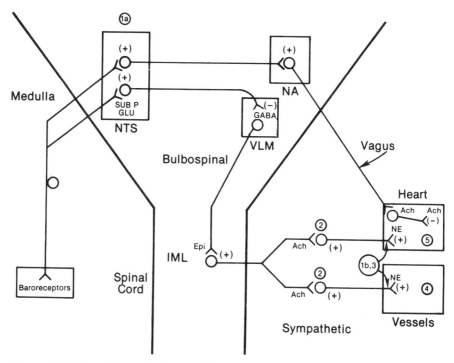

Figure 9–1. Central control of sympathetic nervous system discharge. Afferent fibers from baroreceptors in the aortic arch and carotid sinus project to the nucleus of the solitary tract (NTS) where they synapse with excitatory and inhibitory interneurons. Excitatory interneurons project to the nucleus ambiguous and increase vagal tone to the heart. Interneurons to the rostral ventrolateral medulla (VLM) inhibit the high tonic discharge of bulbospinal neurones that project to the intermediolateral column (IML) of the spinal cord where an excitatory synapse with the preganglionic sympathetic neuron is made. Sites of action of antihypertensive agents are labeled numerically. *1a* and *1b*, postsynaptic α_2-adrenoceptors on interneurons and presynaptic α_2-adrenoceptors (clonidine). *2*, Ganglionic synapse (ganglionic blocking agents). *3*, nerve terminal (reserpine and guanethidine). *4*, Vascular smooth muscle (vasodilators, α-adrenoceptor antagonists). *5*, Cardiac muscle (β-adrenoceptor antagonists). Putative or known neurotransmitters are shown: SUB P = substance P, GLU = glutamate, GABA = γ-aminobutyric acid, Epi = epinephrine, Ach = acetylcholine, NE = norepinephrine. Excitatory (+) and inhibitory (−) actions of these transmitters are designated.

glionic sympathetic nerve originate at brainstem or higher central levels. These include **norepinephrine, vasopressin** and **oxytocin, substance P,** and **5-hydroxytryptamine (serotonin)**. The excitatory sympathetic activity originating in the rostral ventrolateral medulla is modulated by inhibitory input from the nucleus of the solitary tract (NTS), the site of termination of both high and low pressure baroreceptor afferents. Control of heart rate is achieved through modulation of sympathetic outflow and outflow from vagal motor neurons connected by excitatory interneurons from the NTS. The hypothalamic paraventricular and median preoptic nuclei (not shown) are connected reciprocally with the NTS and rostral ventrolateral medulla, and not only modulate vasomotor outflow over the sympathetic nervous system but also integrate other key visceral functions including thirst, blood volume, sodium excretion, and the release of vasopressin.

A hallmark of hypertension is elevated or inappropriately high **sympathetic nervous system activity** that contributes significantly to an increase in total peripheral resistance while cardiac output is maintained in the normal range. Several abnormalities contribute to increased sympathetic activity in hypertensive states. **Baro-receptor reflex mechanisms** on both the arterial and low pressure sides of the circulation are impaired, with deficits in function found at the level of the pressure receptor as well as in the central nervous system (CNS). Impaired reflex inhibition contributes to increased central sympathetic discharge. Enhanced central responsiveness to a variety of stimuli that increase sympathetic activity has also been implicated. These stimuli include environmental stress and circulating humoral factors (sodium chloride and **angiotensin**) that act on the CNS. Enhanced vascular smooth muscle sensitivity to norpinephrine is often observed and contributes to increased vasomotor tone of neurogenic origin.

Humoral Mechanisms

Several **humoral systems** involved in arterial pressure homeostasis have been implicated in the pathogenesis of hypertension. In hypertension originating from abnormalities in renal function, excessive secretion of **renin** leads to high circulating levels of angiotensin. This form of hypertension can be reversed with inhibitors of the renin-angiotensin system and is potentially curable with nephrectomy or repair of a partially occluded renal artery. Several mechanisms contribute to the hypertensive properties of angiotensin. Angiotensin directly causes vasoconstriction, directly stimulates the secretion of **aldosterone,** and increases sympathetic nervous system activity by actions at both central and peripheral sites.

Hypersecretion of mineralocorticoid from adrenal adenomas increases arterial pressure. Sodium retention alone does not explain this form of hypertension, as there is a rapid escape from the sodium-retaining properties of mineralocorticoids. This escape has been attributed to the release of **natriuretic factors,** one of which has digitalis-like properties, that is, inhibits sodium potassium ATPase (atrial natriuretic factor does not have ATPase inhibitory action). This effect leads to vasoconstriction as well as natriuresis, and this natriuretic factor has been implicated in mineralocorticoid-induced hypertension. Interestingly, sympathetic activity is also elevated in this form of hypertension, perhaps by central actions of mineralocorticoids.

Blood levels of the antidiuretic hormone, vasopressin, are increased in mineralocorticoid hypertension and in some subjects with essential hypertension. Using competitive antagonists of vasopressin, it has been found that direct vasoconstrictor actions of the peptide are not responsible for the increase in arterial pressure. However, interactions of vasopressin with the sympathetic nervous system and with fluid-electrolyte balance may be involved in long-term adjustments that sustain increased pressure.

Local Vascular System Abnormalities

Intrinsic abnormalities in local control of **vascular smooth muscle** probably provide a background against which neural and humoral factors contribute to the pathogenesis of hypertension. In general, enhanced sensitivity to vasoconstrictor agents is a characteristic of hypertensive states. Several mechanisms contribute to this exaggerated responsiveness.

In chronic hypertension most vascular beds show **vascular smooth muscle hypertrophy** in response to the chronic pressure load. This adaptation of increased vascular wall mass provides a structural basis for increased sensitivity to vasoconstrictor stimuli. With an increased ratio of wall thickness to lumen diameter, increases in vascular resistance are greater for a given stimulus than are those found in vessels with normal dimensions. Vascular hypertrophy appears to depend in part on a trophic (or growth-promoting) action of the sympathetic nerves.

Abnormalities in **membrane properties** of vascular muscle also contribute to increased vasoconstrictor responsiveness. Increases in α-adrenoceptor density and enhanced membrane depolarization have been documented.

Finally, changes in local formation of **vasodilator and vasoconstrictor substances** related to activation of endothelium have been demonstrated to contribute to enhanced vasoconstrictor sensitivity. Both reduction in the formation of a vasodilator (**endothelial-derived relaxation factor,** or **EDRF**) and enhanced production of a vasoconstrictor have been observed in vascular muscle with damaged or abnormal endothelium. The ability of free radical scavengers to attenuate the contribution of endothelial factors suggests that the formation of free radical intermediates may be essential (see also discussion on nitrates under antianginal agents). Recently, an extremely potent peptidergic vasoconstrictor, **endothelin,** has been isolated from endothelium and characterized structurally.

Pharmacology of Antihypertensive Agents

Agents used for the control of hypertension are derived from a number of drug classes. They share the common property of arterial pressure reduction but accomplish this through several unrelated mechanisms of action. The agents are conveniently classified into four major groups: (1) diuretics, (2) direct-acting vasodilators, (3) inhibitors of the sympathetic nervous system, and (4) inhibitors of the renin-angiotensin system. Table 9–1 lists the most commonly used representative drugs of these classes.

Diuretics

The rationale for the use of diuretics in the treatment of hypertension derives from the efficacy of **sodium restriction** as an independent arterial pressure–lowering intervention. In certain individuals, classified as sodium-sensitive, sodium restriction alone produces a marked hypotensive effect. The natriuretic action of the commonly used diuretics is widely employed as the first step in the treatment of hypertension. The agents are used alone, as well as in conjunction with other antihypertensive drugs. For a detailed discussion of the overall pharmacology of the diuretics, refer to Chapter 10.

Diuretics produce a fall in arterial pressure that is relatively slow in onset. The maximum hypotensive effect obtained in essential hypertension is mild. The agents are usually well tolerated and are used chronically as monotherapy for the management of mild hypertension. Initially, the fall in arterial pressure is accompanied by a reduction in cardiac output resulting from a fall in blood volume and cardiac filling pressure. This effect does not persist, however, and within weeks cardiac output and blood volume return toward normal while peripheral resistance and arterial pressure remain reduced.

The mechanism by which diuretics lower arterial pressure is unknown. Their ability to decrease arterial pressure due to a fall in cardiac output does not explain the persistent antihypertensive action. Local vascular effects of the diuretics, perhaps because of depletion of sodium from vascular smooth muscle, reduce the sensitivity of the vasculature in a rather uniform manner to vasoconstrictor stimuli. This vasodilator effect is more profound than is apparent from the modest fall in arterial pressure produced by the agents. Diuretics (and salt restriction) lower arterial pressure despite the recruitment of three major adaptations that tend to sustain pressure when sodium is depleted from the body. Diuretics increase sympathetic nervous system activity and circulating blood levels of angiotensin and vasopressin. In fact, the antihypertensive efficacy of diuretics is enhanced if any of these pressor systems is blocked pharmacologically.

There are no known differences in mechanism of action among such agents as **thiazides, loop diuretics,** and **potassium-sparing diuretics.** The more potent diuretics with higher ceiling effects may be employed in patients with more severe hypertension, whereas thiazides are ordinarily used in those with mild or moderate elevations in arterial pressure.

As a class, diuretics are well tolerated and relatively free of side effects. Hypokalemia can be anticipated with chronic use of any of these agents, with the exception of potassium-sparing diuretics. This effect is thought to contribute to increased incidence of arrhythmias seen in subjects taking these drugs.

Table 9–1. ANTIHYPERTENSIVE AGENTS

| Class | Site of Action (See Figs. 9–1 and 9–3) | | Mechanism |
	Number	Location	
Diuretics			
Thiazides ⎫	Major	Vessel	Depress vascular muscle responsiveness to vasoconstrictor stimuli.
Furosemide ⎬	4		
Ethacrynic acid ⎭			
	Minor	Nerve terminal	Impair release of norepinephrine.
	3		
Spironolactone ⎫			
Amiloride ⎬		Unknown	Unknown
Vasodilators			
Hydralazine	4	Vessel	Hyperpolarization of cell membrane- intracellular Ca^{2+} action?
Minoxidil	4	Vessel	Unknown.
Diazoxide	4	Vessel	Unknown.
Nitroprusside	4	Vessel	Increase intracellular cGMP-suppress Ca^{2+} action.
Verapamil ⎫			
Diltiazem ⎬			Reduce entry of calcium through calcium channels.
Nifedipine ⎭	4	Vessel	
Inhibitors of Sympathetic Nervous System			
α-Adrenoceptor antagonists			
Phentolamine	4	Vessel	Competitive inhibition of vascular α_1 and α_2 receptors.
Phenoxybenzamine	4	Vessel	Irreversible binding with vascular α_1 and α_2 receptors.
Prazosin	4	Vessel	Competitive inhibition of α_1 vascular receptors.
β-Adrenoceptor antagonists			
Propranolol ⎫	Minor	Heart	Competitive inhibition of cardiac β_1 receptors.
Metoprolol ⎪	5		
Atenolol ⎬	Minor	Nerve terminal	Inhibition of presynaptic β_2 receptors that facilitate release of norepinephrine (except for β_1 selective agents).
Pindolol ⎪	3		
Nadolol ⎭			

219

Table 9–1. (*Continued*)

| Class | Site of Action (See Figs. 9–1 and 9–3) | | Mechanism |
	Number	Location	
	Minor 1a	Brainstem	Reduce central sympathetic activity.
	Minor 7	Kidney	Inhibition of renal β_1 receptors that stimulate release of renin.
	Minor 4	Vessel	Unknown
α_2-Adrenoceptor agonists			
Clonidine	Major 1a	Brainstem	Activation of postsynaptic α_2 receptors in CNS that excite inhibitory interneurons.
α-Methyldopa Guanabenz	Minor 1b	Nerve terminal	Activation of presynaptic α_2 receptors in CNS that inhibit release of norepinephrine.
Neuronal Blockers			
Reserpine	3	Nerve terminal	Deplete norepinephrine from nerve terminals by blocking uptake into storage granules.
Guanethidine	3	Nerve terminal	Deplete norepinephrine from nerve terminal by displacement.
Ganglionic Blockers	2	Autonomic ganglia	Competitive inhibition of ganglionic nicotinic receptors.
Renin-Angiotensin Inhibitors			
Captopril ⎱ Enalapril ⎰	6		Competitive inhibition of angiotensin converting enzyme—block of angiotensin II synthesis.
Saralasin	Major 4	Vessel	Competitive inhibition of vasoconstrictor angiotensin II receptors.
	Minor 8	Adrenal cortex	Competitive inhibition of angiotensin III receptors activating aldosterone secretion.

The increased risk of sudden death observed in the Multiple Risk Factor Intervention Trial (MRFIT) of the National Heart, Lung, and Blood Institute has increased awareness about the need to monitor carefully the electrolyte status of subjects taking diuretics chronically.

The major interaction of consequence is with the cardiac glycosides. **Hypokalemia** is a major contributor to the high incidence of myocardial toxicity observed with the glycosides. Another area of concern with the use of diuretics is their ability to increase serum lipids. The issue of whether diuretics as a class represent a risk factor for the progression of atherosclerotic disease remains to be resolved.

Vasodilators

Arterial pressure is controlled successfully with agents that produce vasodilation by direct actions on vascular smooth muscle. These agents exhibit excellent efficacy; however, because they act beyond the level at which sympathetic nervous system function can be altered, they exhibit several side effects that are the direct consequence of sympathoexcitation. For this reason they are almost always used in conjunction with β-adrenoceptor antagonists.

Mechanisms of Action. Vascular muscle contraction is triggered by increased **intracellular calcium,** and vascular muscle cells are among the smallest that exist in mammals. However, what would otherwise seem to be a simple situation, in which calcium from the extracellular fluid could diffuse through **calcium channels** to activate contraction, is much more complex, with several steps and modulatory mechanisms involved. Figure 9–2 shows a simplified model of excitation-contraction coupling in the vascular muscle cell. In addition to calcium channels, important regulatory sites include the sarcoplasmic reticulum (which is the major storage and release site for calcium) in at least two subcategories, and the surface membrane. Intracellular calcium release, although only poorly understood at present, appears to provide the most important source of calcium for control of the contractile state.

In addition to agents acting on calcium entry or calcium release *per se,* vasodilators act on membrane potential to affect the trigger mechanism for increases in intracellular calcium. Agents that depolarize vascular muscle cells (e.g., norepinephrine and angiotensin) cause contraction because calcium levels increase within the cell, and possibly because intracellular second messengers increase contractile state at a given intracellular free calcium concentration. Recent evidence indicates that several of the vasodilators cause muscle cell hyperpolarization by stimulation of an **electrogenic ion pump** (probably the sodium-potassium membrane ATPase transport system), which would remove the normal trigger step for contraction.

Vascular muscle can also be relaxed by interference with entry of calcium by direct blockade of surface membrane calcium channels. A large new class of vasodilators, called **calcium antagonists** (or calcium entry blockers), directly

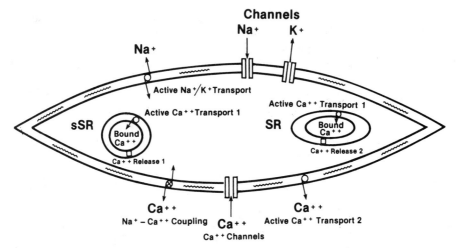

Figure 9–2. Vascular muscle cells contain several important points where contraction can be modified. The E–C coupling model shown here includes composite mechanisms that may be more or less important in different blood vessels, making selectivity of vasodilators possible. Receptors (not shown) may be present for a number of vasoactive agents. Membrane potential is controlled by ion conductances and electrogenic ion transport, and strongly influences contractile state. Calcium entry through calcium channels is essential for long-term and short-term contraction. Calcium release and re-uptake from sarcoplasmic reticulum (SR) in both the center or near the cell surface (sSR) is important. Several second messengers and modulation factors are thought to importantly influence contraction in vascular muscle cells of certain blood vessels (see text).

interfere with calcium channels believed to be the principal route by which calcium enters these cells. Even though the calcium may have entered during previous activation, blockade of calcium entry effectively blocks contraction in many blood vessels because the calcium has an **intracellular trigger** role (directly releasing intracellular calcium stores) as well as directly activating contractile proteins. Drugs acting at this locus include **verapamil, gallopamil** (D600), **nifedipine,** and **diltiazem.**

The calcium removal pathway is extremely important in vascular muscle, as a significant portion of intracellular calcium is recycled during contraction by **calcium pumps** that activate as soon as calcium concentration rises. Stimulation of calcium pumps in sarcoplasmic reticulum would reduce contraction by shifting the balance more toward uptake than release. Stimulation of surface membrane calcium pumps would not only remove calcium from the cell, but also (if electrogenic) would hyperpolarize the cell, removing the condition for calcium entry and release.

The activation of the actomyosin system within vascular muscle depends on calcium interaction with **myosin light chain kinase** (MLCK), which is modulated by the calcium-binding protein, **calmodulin**. Vasodilators would be effective at decreasing contraction, even in high calcium, if calmodulin were inhibited from interaction with MLCK.

The calcium release mechanism has been postulated to involve **inositol triphosphate (IP$_3$)** formation at the inner surface of the cell membrane. If this hypothesis is correct, interference with formation of IP$_3$ would provide another important vasodilator mechanism.

The notably small vascular muscle cells in various regions of the vascular tree appear to be significantly different, allowing for selectivity of vasodilator agents. Certain vessels are very dependent on calcium entry on a continuous basis, while others have calcium stores that support contraction even when calcium entry is prevented. Other variables are the ratio of different ion channels, the resting membrane potential, the activity of the sodium pump, activity of the calcium pump, level of production of intracellular second messengers, number and type of surface membrane receptors, and interactions of these variables. The diversity of vascular muscle types found in the cardiovascular system is understandable considering all of these factors importantly influencing contraction.

Hydralazine. Through its direct action on vascular smooth muscle, **hydralazine** (Apresoline) lowers arterial pressure exclusively by peripheral arterial vasodilation. This reduction in pressure, by engaging the baroreceptor reflex, increases sympathetic nervous system activity. The two major side effects of hydralazine, **tachycardia** and **sodium retention,** are the direct result of this reflex mechanism. The increase in sympathetic tone to the heart is responsible for the increase in heart rate; increased renin secretion results from the increase in sympathetic activity to the juxtaglomerular cells. This leads to increased aldosterone secretion with consequent sodium and water retention. In susceptible individuals hypervolemia, increased body weight, and frank edema can be observed. Because of these undesirable side effects, hydralazine is ordinarily combined with a β-adrenoceptor antagonist or diuretic, or both. The β-blocker prevents the reflex tachycardia and limits the increase in renin secretion mediated by adrenergic mechanisms. Diuretics relieve or prevent the retention of sodium and water. When employed chronically at high doses, hydralazine can induce in a few patients a **lupus-like syndrome** that is reversed when administration of the drug is terminated.

Minoxidil. The cardiovascular profile observed with **minoxidil** (Loniten), another arterial vasodilator, is qualitatively identical to that seen with hydralazine. Although there are chemical similarities between minoxidil and hydralazine, minoxidil is more potent on a molar basis. Reflex tachycardia and sodium and water retention are observed with minoxidil and can be prevented with the use of β-adrenoceptor antagonists and diuretics. The antihypertensive action of minoxidil is probably attributable to enzymatic conversion by a sulphotransferase to minoxidil sulfate. The sulphated form is more lipophilic and probably penetrates vascular smooth muscle membranes to a greater extent than does the parent compound. Because minoxidil sulfate is a more potent vasodilator than minoxidil, the metabolite probably makes a major contribution to the overall vasodilator efficacy of the agent. Although the side effects related to sympathoexcitation are similar for minoxidil and hydralazine, minoxidil has another therapeutic application owing to its ability to **enhance hair growth (hypertrichosis)**. Topical application to the scalp stimulates hair growth in approximately 30 percent of subjects with male-pattern baldness.

Agents Used for Management of Hypertensive Crises. Diazoxide and **sodium nitroprusside** are used exclusively for acute management of uncontrolled arterial pressure (i.e., **hypertensive crises** or emergencies). The agents lower arterial pressure in situations when other antihypertensive drugs have lost their efficacy. They are extremely potent, exhibit steep dose-response curves, and must be used with caution in a controlled setting in which arterial pressure is monitored continuously, preferably with an intra-arterial catheter. Diazoxide (Hyperstat) is an unusual vasodilator that is relatively selective for the arterioles. It is closely related chemically to the thiazide class of diuretics, which have no direct vasodilator effects. After administration of a single dose, the hypotensive effects of diazoxide are unusually long lasting and may persist for over 10 hours. The mechanism of this persistent vasodilator action is not fully understood but may be assumed to be related to a poorly reversible intracellular or membrane effect on either the release or entry of calcium. The toxicity of diazoxide is not of great consequence, because it is used for relatively short periods of time. Excessive hypotension is potentially the most serious danger of the agent, especially in view of its poorly reversible effects. **Hyperglycemia** resulting from inhibition of insulin release and sodium and fluid retention are other effects of this agent.

Sodium nitroprusside (Nipride) is a cyanonitroso-complex of iron used intravenously for its direct and potent vasodilator effect. It is a less specific arteriolar vasodilator than diazoxide, having additional effects on the capacitance side of the circulation, and its actions are relatively short acting; sustained hypotension is produced only with continuous intravenous infusion. Acute toxicity with sodium nitroprusside is cardiovascular in nature with excessive hypotension representing the primary adverse effect. It should be noted, however, that the short duration of action allows for relatively precise adjustment of the hypotensive action, and excessive hypotension would tend to be of short duration. Because the agent produces **venodilation** and reduction in cardiac filling pressure, impairment in cardiac output is potentially more significant than with diazoxide. Extended use of nitroprusside leads to the danger of toxicity produced by **thiocyanate,** the major metabolite of nitroprusside. This includes acute psychosis and thyroid dysfunction.

Diazoxide and sodium nitroprusside also may be efficacious for the acute management of severe congestive heart failure. Both agents reduce afterload, and nitroprusside also reduces preload. Improved ventricular performance may be observed in subjects with heart failure refractory to inotropic interventions or other hypotensive interventions.

Calcium Antagonists (Calcium Channel Blockers). The calcium antagonists nifedipine, diltiazem, and verapamil have been documented in clinical trials to be efficacious in normalizing the blood pressure of hypertensive individuals. At present, only verapamil is approved in the United States for treatment of hypertension. The hemodynamic mechanism of reducing arterial pressure is a fall in total peripheral vascular resistance by reduction of calcium influx into arterial muscle cells. The antihypertensive action of calcium antagonists occurs without the marked reflex increase in heart rate found with vasodilators like hydralazine, making calcium antagonists usable as monotherapy. Other advantages include the absence of plasma renin level increase or sodium retention.

Inhibitors of the Sympathetic Nervous System

Arterial pressure is maintained by tonic vasoconstrictor and cardiac stimulant activities of the sympathetic nervous system. Regardless of site of action, interference with this tonic sympathetic outflow will lower arterial pressure by any combination of vasodilation and reduced cardiac output. From a historical standpoint, the first effective antihypertensive agents were the ganglionic blockers. Although highly efficacious, these agents produced numerous autonomic side effects, the major of which was **orthostatic hypotension**. Orthostasis is a potential limitation of any agent that interferes with sympathetic control of arterial pressure, but it is now clear that certain specific sites of action are associated to a much smaller degree with this disturbing limitation to the use of antisympathetic agents.

Figure 9–1 illustrates the major sites of action of the agents of this class. Peripheral vasodilation is produced by α-adrenoceptor antagonists that interfere with the action of neurotransmitters at the level of vascular smooth muscle. Reduced secretion of neurotransmitter is produced by agents that interfere with the release and/or storage of norepinephrine from sympathetic nerve terminals. Blockade of the postganglionic excitatory effects of **acetylcholine** in the ganglionic synapse also reduces the level of sympathetic activity. Finally, peripheral sympathetic activity may be reduced by several classes of agents that inhibit sympathetic outflow through direct or indirect actions on the CNS.

α-Adrenoceptor Antagonists. The **α-adrenoceptor antagonists phentolamine** and **phenoxybenzamine** are used primarily for diagnostic purposes and to a lesser extent in treatment of pheochromacytoma. **Prazosin** (Minipress) is a widely employed α_1-adrenoceptor antagonist in the treatment of hypertension. Prazosin is unusual in that it produces less reflex tachycardia than nonselective α-adrenoceptor antagonists (e.g., phentolamine or phenoxybenzamine). Central inhibition of sympathetic activity could explain why reflex tachycardia is relatively mild with this agent. Because prazosin is quite selective for α_1-adrenoceptors, it does not impair feedback inhibition of the release of norepinephrine, as occurs with nonselective antagonists such as phentolamine, which block **presynaptic α_2-adrenoceptors**. The inhibition of negative feedback probably contributes to reflex tachycardia observed with the nonselective agents. Orthostatic or postural hypotension is ordinarily encountered with α-adrenoceptor antagonists but appears to be less significant with prazosin. The mechanism that underlies the relative absence of orthostasis is unclear. It can be speculated, however, that the agent may impair more selectively those peripheral or central adrenergic mechanisms involved in maintenance of tonic vasomotor activity than those systems that are activated through the baroreceptor reflex when arterial pressure is lowered. It is appreciated that one of the major reasons for poor compliance with inhibitors of sympathetic nervous system function is **impairment of sexual function**. Prazosin and other agents of this general class can produce impotence and delayed or reflux ejaculation.

β-Adrenoceptor Antagonists. **β-Adrenoceptor antagonists** are used very widely for the control of high arterial pressure. Their mechanism(s) of action has not yet been clearly identified but could include reduction of cardiac output, reduction of central sympathetic discharge, peripheral nerve terminal actions, and suppression of renal secretion of renin. Blockade of cardiac β-adrenoceptors causes a reduction of heart rate and force of contraction, reducing cardiac output and reducing arterial pressure. However, with persistent treatment, cardiac output returns toward normal levels and lowered arterial pressure is sustained by a reduction in total peripheral resistance. As the agents have little or no direct vasodilator effects, their prolonged hypotensive action is probably caused through indirect mechanisms that reduce vasoconstrictor tone. Several of these indirect actions may reside at the level of the nerve terminal.

Propranolol (Inderal) is taken up into peripheral nerve terminals by amine uptake mechanisms and partially displaces norepinephrine. This effect is moderate, probably contributes in only a minor way to any impairment in peripheral neurotransmission, and is not found with all agents of the class. Neurotransmission could also be impaired by blockade of presynaptic β adrenoceptors, which facilitate the release of norepinephrine. Whether β-adrenoceptor antagonists exert influences on central sympathetic discharge is controversial. Propranolol, which easily penetrates into the CNS, has been documented to reduce central sympathetic discharge and to reduce plasma levels and excretion of catecholamines. The major argument used against this potential mechanism is that other β-adrenoceptor antagonists, which share the excellent hypotensive properties of propranolol, do not enter the CNS. However, this argument may have limited validity because key parts of the CNS involved in autonomic control are accessible to penetration *via* the leaky portions of the **blood-brain barrier** found in the **circumventricular organs**. It can be anticipated, therefore, that all β-adrenoceptor antagonists would reach the CNS in these key sites and therefore would have the potential to reduce central sympathetic discharge.

The hypotensive action of β-adrenoceptor antagonists can also involve inhibition of renin secretion stimulated by catecholamines. This β_1 adrenoceptor–mediated phenomenon is especially prominent in high renin states. Combined β_1- and β_2-adrenoceptor antagonists such as propranolol are efficacious in such high renin states in part through this renal action; however, they are also efficacious in normal or low renin states, and selective β_1-adrenoceptor antagonists are also efficacious.

The pharmacology and toxicity of β-adrenergic receptor antagonists such as propranolol, **metoprolol (Lopressor)**, **nadolol (Corgard)**, **atenolol (Tenormin)**, and **pindolol (Visken)** are covered in detail in Chapter 4. Labetalol (**Normodyne**), which antagonizes both α and β adrenergic receptors, is employed as an antihypertensive agent and has the potential to antagonize both cardiac and vascular adrenergic receptors.

α_2-**Adrenoceptor Agonists.** α_2-Adrenoceptor agonists are believed to lower arterial pressure through CNS actions that result in inhibition of sympathetic nervous system activity. They also have the capacity to lower arterial pressure through their peripheral presynaptic actions on α_2 adrenoceptors that inhibit the release of norepinephrine. The net effect of the putative central and peripheral actions is the same (i.e., vasodilation resulting from a reduction in the amount of norepinephrine available for interaction with vascular and cardiac adrenoceptors whose activation sustains arterial pressure). Agents commonly employed in the treatment of hypertension are **clonidine, α-methyldopa**, and **guanabenz**. Although their ultimate mechanism of action involves activation of α_2 adrenoceptors, the pharmacology of these agents differs in several key aspects. As shown in Figure 9–1, the central site of actions of these agents is probably in the brainstem. Inhibitory interneurons in the NTS, when activated postsynaptically by α_2-adrenoceptor agonists, inhibit discharge of bulbospinal neurons in the ventrolateral medulla. Recent evidence suggests that this ventrolateral neuronal pool may also be inhibited directly by α_2-adrenoceptor agonists. In fact, an endogenous α_2-adrenoceptor ligand whose structure is not yet determined has been identified in receptor-binding assays after extraction from ventrolateral medulla.

Clonidine (Catapres), originally intended as a nasal decongestant, exerts both α_1- and α_2-adrenoceptor agonist activity; however, α_2-adrenoceptor activation is much more prominent. The pressor activity characteristic of α_1-adrenoceptor activation on blood vessels is observed only upon rapid intravenous administration. Clonidine reduces central sympathetic outflow and lowers plasma concentration and urinary excretion of norepinephrine. Heart rate and cardiac output are reduced, with a relatively small overall change in peripheral vascular resistance; however, regional vascular resistance, especially in the kidney, is lowered. An interesting aspect of this class of agents is that they produce relatively little postural hypotension despite interrupting central sympathetic outflow. It remains to be determined whether separate central neuronal pools involved in vasomotor regulation differentially control tonic sympathetic outflow and the reflexly induced increments in sympathetic outflow required for vasomotor adjustments to changes in posture. The major side effects associated with clonidine are **dry mouth** and **sedation**. Drowsiness can be severe enough to drastically limit the drug's usefulness. A prominent feature of clonidine in selected individuals is a **withdrawal syndrome,** characterized by severe hypertension that can be malignant in nature. The syndrome is best counteracted by readministration of clonidine or by giving labetalol, an α- and β-adrenoceptor antagonist.

α-Methyldopa (Aldomet) must be converted to specific metabolites in order to exert antihypertensive effects. It is taken up into both peripheral and central catecholaminergic nerve terminals and enters the biosynthetic cascade for catecholamines. α-**Methylnorepinephrine,** the major active metabolite, α-**methylepinephrine,** and α-**methyldopamine** have all been documented to be end products of α-methyldopa administration, and all three of these metabolites are capable of activating α_2 adrenoceptors with greater efficacy than norepinephrine. Thus, all are candidates for mediation of the antihypertensive actions. The sites of action in the brain of α-methyldopa are similar to those of clonidine. However, intact catecholaminergic synthetic mechanisms are required for α-methyldopa to produce its effects. Side effects seen with α-methyldopa are similar to those of clonidine; sedation, drowsiness, and related signs of CNS depression are most prominent. **A positive Coomb's test** result is observed in approximately 20 percent of patients; however, less than 5 percent of these exhibit autoimmune hemolytic anemia.

Guanabenz (Wytensin) is an agent with pharmacological properties very similar to those of clonidine. It interacts directly with CNS postsynaptic α_2 adrenoceptors and exerts similar central actions. Several reports suggest that the agent may produce less sodium and water retention as a result of a more prominent renovasodilator action; however, it remains unclear whether this represents an important therapeutic advantage.

Adrenergic Neuronal Blockers. The adrenergic neuronal blockers reserpine and guanethidine (and related guanethidine-like drugs, bethanidine and guanadrel) are potent antihypertensive agents. However, their utility is limited owing to serious side effects, and as a class these drugs are not widely used in contemporary treatment of hypertension. **Guanethidine** (Ismelin) initially **inhibits the release** of norepinephrine from sympathetic nerve terminals and then subsequently **depletes stores** of norepinephrine. The stabilizing effect on the nerve terminal occurs immediately after administration, whereas the depleting effect requires chronic administration. Guanethidine is taken up into the nerve terminal and ultimately displaces norepinephrine from its binding sites. Antagonists of uptake such as cocaine and tricyclic antidepressants prevent the action of guanethidine. **Reserpine** depletes norepinephrine, dopamine, and serotonin from their central and peripheral storage sites but without any guanethidine-like effect on the release of norepinephrine. The action of reserpine involves interference with a neurotransmitter **uptake mechanism** within storage granules dependent upon magnesium and ATP. Repletion of catecholamines and serotonin occurs slowly after administration of reserpine is terminated.

The ability of adrenergic neuronal blocking agents to lower arterial pressure is dependent on interference with the function of both cardiac and vascular innervation. Heart rate and cardiac output as well as peripheral vascular resistance are reduced. The side effects and toxicity of adrenergic neuronal blocking agents are frequent and prominent. Orthostasis, GI side effects, impotence, and retrograde ejaculation are major consequences of treatment with guanethidine, especially at larger doses. Reserpine produces postural hypotension less frequently than does guanethidine, but the remaining side effects are similar. In addition, reserpine, which, unlike guanethidine, depletes central catecholamines, produces a wide variety of CNS disturbances, including sedation, **depression,** and **extrapyramidal signs** (presumably resulting from depletion of dopamine).

The **ganglionic blocking** agent **trimethaphan** (Arfonad) has a very short duration of action and is used intravenously for controlled hypotension, for example during surgery and hypertensive emergencies.

Renin-Angiotensin Inhibitors (ACE Inhibitors)

Inhibitors of the renin-angiotensin system block **angiotensin-converting enzyme** (ACE) and prevent the synthesis of the key endogenous peptide, angiotensin II. The biosynthetic pathway for the production of angiotensin and its relationship to the synthesis and degradation of **bradykinin** are illustrated in Figure 9–3. ACE is identical to the **kininase** responsible for degradation of bradykinin, and is a dipeptidyl carboxypeptidase. The major conversion of angiotensin I to angiotensin II occurs in the lungs; the enzyme is located in crypts of pulmonary and other endothelial blood vessels. The dipeptide sulfhydril containing **captopril** (Capoten) and the de-esterified product of the tripeptide nonsulfhydryl derivative **enalapril** (Vasotec) are competitive ACE inhibitors with higher affinity for the enzyme than that of the normal decapeptide substrate angiotensin I. Although early analogs of these ACE inhibitors were larger peptides with poor oral absorption, these two agents are relatively well absorbed and highly effective by the oral route of administration. Enalapril has a somewhat longer half-life and may be administered less frequently than captopril.

Angiotensin II is fundamentally important in elevating arterial pressure in renin-dependent hypertension through its capacity to stimulate secretion of aldosterone and by its direct and indirect vasoconstrictor actions, the latter mediated through activation of the sympathetic nervous system at both central

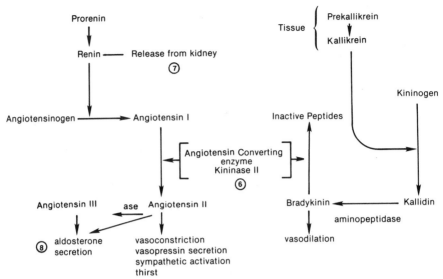

Figure 9–3. Relationship between the renin-angiotensin and kinin systems. Angiotensin-converting enzyme and kininase II are identical. Sites of action for antihypertensive agents are designated numerically. 6 = Captopril and enalapril, 7 = β_1-adrenoceptors on juxtaglomerular cells, 8 = angiotensin receptors on adrenal glomerulosa cells.

and peripheral sites. An interesting aspect of converting enzyme inhibitors is that they are also efficacious in lowering arterial pressure in **non**renin-dependent states. Clearly these agents produce their greatest antihypertensive effects in subjects with hypertension of renal origin or with normal renal function and elevated plasma renin activity. In such states the antihypertensive action is directly attributable to removal of the vasoconstrictor effects of angiotensin and to its ability to interfere with sodium retention mediated by aldosterone.

The mechanism by which captopril lowers arterial pressure in nonrenin-dependent states remains unclear. Inhibition of kininase with subsequent accumulation of vasodilator concentrations of bradykinin could contribute in part to the hypotensive action. Potential central actions have been suggested that involve inhibition of a separate brain renin-angiotensin system. Although the agents are thought not to penetrate the CNS to any appreciable extent, localized effects in and around circumventricular organs probably occur. Peripherally, interference with a renin-angiotensin system localized within the blood vessel wall has been hypothesized, and evidence has also been provided for a mild effect on the release of norepinephrine from peripheral sympathetic nerve terminals.

ACE inhibitors lower arterial pressure primarily by lowering peripheral vascular resistance. The fact that heart rate is not increased in the face of reduced arterial pressure makes ACE inhibitors unusual vasodilators. The absence of reflex tachycardia implies that effects on CNS integration sites contribute to the antihypertensive action. An important renal vasodilator action, mediated through relaxation of efferent arterioles, decreases glomerular capillary pressure and makes the agents beneficial in chronic renal failure. A variety of side effects have been encountered with converting enzyme inhibitors. These include **cough, rash, proteinuria,** abnormalities in **taste,** and infrequent allergic and rare neutropenia reactions. Severe hypotension can be encountered when sodium restriction or diuretic therapy results in primary maintenance of blood pressure by the renin-angiotensin system.

ANTIANGINAL AGENTS

Coronary artery disease is now appreciated to produce symptomatology related to a variety of abnormalities in regulation of the coronary circulation. **Angina pectoris,** the referred pain of myocardial ischemia, has a complex etiology. Mechanical obstruction of the coronary arteries associated with **atherosclerotic lesions** is the primary cause of angina. However, a variety of other physiological and pathophysiological factors involved in regulation of the coronary circulation can contribute to the production of cardiac pain. The treatment of coronary artery disease and its symptomatology has become complex. Surgical interventions, including **coronary artery bypass** and **balloon angioplasty,** remove or alleviate mechanical obstruction to coronary blood flow. These treatments are well documented to relieve the symptoms of coronary artery disease; however, their long-term efficacy in altering the course of coronary atherosclerosis remains uncertain. Pharmacological management of angina pectoris employs traditional vasodilators such as **nitroglycerin,** calcium antagonists, and β-adrenoceptor antagonists. These treatments involve a number of pharmacological mechanisms, but all appear to be efficacious because they produce a more favorable balance between myocardial blood flow and cardiac oxygen requirement.

Regulation of Coronary Blood Flow

The mechanisms by which antianginal agents exert their effects are best appreciated with a full understanding of the inter-related factors that determine the magnitude of coronary blood flow and its relationship to myocardial work. In the coronary circulation there is moment-to-moment interplay between four major regulatory factors: mechanical, metabolic, neural, and humoral.

Mechanical Factors

Coronary vessels are subjected to **cyclic compression,** which reduces flow. During systole, compressive forces associated with shortening of myocardial fibers are sufficiently great to reduce coronary blood flow to zero. Flow proceeds during diastole, and changes in left ventricular coronary blood flow are almost exclusively diastolic in origin. The distribution of coronary blood flow across the ventricular wall is also dependent upon physical factors. **Left ventricular pressure** is highest at the **endocardial surface** with the diminishing gradient transmitted to epicardial vessels. Although the transmural flow at rest usually favors endocardium over epicardium, increases in myocardial oxygen requirement produce relatively greater deficits in endocardial than epicardial flow in patients with coronary artery disease.

Metabolic Factors

The coronary circulation is also exquisitely sensitive to changes in **metabolic demand.** Increases and decreases in coronary blood flow in response to alterations in myocardial oxygen requirement have been demonstrated to occur within a single beat. For example, increased coronary blood flow occurs immediately upon initiation of increased heart rate. Coronary blood flow is sensitive to changes in cardiac filling pressure (preload), arterial pressure (after load), heart rate, and contractile force. Increases in any of these hemodynamic parameters increase oxygen requirement of the myocardium and lead to an increase in coronary blood flow directly proportional to the increased metabolic need. This close linking of metabolism and flow is mediated by local vasoactive factors. A prime candidate for metabolic regulation of coronary blood flow is **adenosine,** a product of adenine nucleotide metabolism. The hypothesis that adenosine is the mediator of metabolically induced coronary vasodilation is supported by its rapid action, short duration of effect, ease of diffusion, and direct linkage to the metabolism of high-energy phosphates which provide energy for myocardial work. The hypothesis, however, has not been strongly supported by studies on interference of adenosine action using adenosine receptor antagonists and blockers of adenosine uptake and metabolism.

Neural Factors

The third major factor regulating coronary blood flow is **neurogenic control.** Coronary vessels are innervated by both the parasympathetic and the sympathetic branches of the autonomic nervous system. Sympathetic nervous system activation, mediated by α adrenoceptors, produces direct coronary vasoconstriction of larger arteries. This constrictor effect is ordinarily masked by simultaneous myocardial stimulation, which produces net increases in coronary blood flow through metabolically induced vasodilation. The direct constrictor effect may be unmasked using β-adrenoceptor antagonism to prevent myocardial stimulation of catecholaminergic origin. Direct vasodilation is produced by activation of the parasympathetic innervation to the coronary circulation. Because parasympathetic stimulation reduces both heart rate and force of contraction, myocardial oxygen requirement is diminished and the loss of metabolic vasodilation produces a net reduction in coronary blood flow. The direct vasodilator effect of the parasympathetic innervation can be unmasked by maintaining heart rate constant through pacing.

Humoral Factors

Humoral factors constitute the fourth major regulator of coronary blood flow. Circulating catecholamines stimulate the myocardium and lead to net vasodilation. Norepinephrine is a coronary vasoconstrictor whose effects can be observed following β-adrenoceptor blockade. Epinephrine has the capacity to interact with β adrenoceptors to produce coronary vasodilation. The antidiuretic hormone vasopressin is also a coronary vasoconstrictor; however, rather large concentrations of this peptide are required to unmask coronary vasomotor effects. Local generation of prostaglandin metabolites in the coronary circulation can produce significant vasomotor effects. **Prostacyclin** is a potent coronary vasodilator, whereas **thromboxane** is a coronary vasoconstrictor.

Mechanisms of Myocardial Ischemia

Abnormalities in regulation of the coronary circulation are associated with coronary artery disease. As illustrated in Figure 9–4, partial coronary artery obstruction does not change resting coronary blood flow despite the existence of a significant pressure gradient. Until almost 90 percent obstruction occurs, marked vasodilation of vessels on the downstream side of the obstruction produces a reduction in vascular resistance sufficient to offset the increase in resistance in the tributary vessel. These downstream vessels are dilated maximally. Increases in metabolic requirement in myocardium perfused by a partially obstructed coronary artery will not therefore be associated with an appropriate increase in coronary blood flow, because the downstream vessels are incapable of metabolically induced vasodilation. The increase in oxygen requirement without attendant increased delivery of oxygen produces ischemia and presumably activation of pain receptors. The failure of coronary vasodilation in vessels perfused from an obstructed coronary artery has been well documented by the almost complete **absence of reactive hyperemia**.

It is now appreciated that obstructive lesions of the coronary circulation are not necessarily fixed. **Active vasomotion** of obstructed arteries has been documented. These abnormal segments of coronary vessels are hyper-respon-

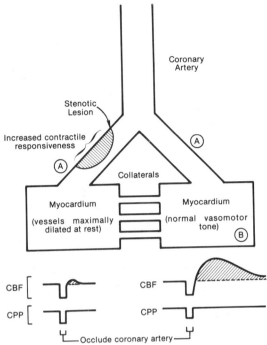

Figure 9–4. Schematic representation of coronary blood supply through normal and stenosed branches of the coronary arterial tree. Obstruction to blood flow produced by the stenotic lesion results in maximal dilation of vessels beyond the obstruction. A brief occlusion of a normal coronary artery produces a marked increase in flow (reactive hyperemia). The absence of reactive hyperemia in vessels beyond the stenosis provides evidence that these vessels are maximally dilated. Putative coronary vascular sites of action of vasodilator agents are shown alphabetically: *A,* Large arteries susceptible to the relaxant effects of nitroglycerin and calcium entry blockers. These vessels are involved in vasospastic forms of angina. *B,* Small vessels dilated by dipyridamole, an agent that "steals" coronary blood flow from vessels downstream from a stenosis through collateral vessels. CBF = coronary blood flow; CPP = coronary perfusion pressure.

sive to vasoconstrictor stimuli, perhaps as a result of altered properties of endothelium. Such enhanced contractile activity in the coronary vessels results from the absence of normally released vasodilator factors or from excessive production of vasoconstrictors. **Adhesion of platelets** to altered endothelium can lead to **vasospasm** induced by serotonin released from platelets. The constrictor activity of serotonin is enhanced when endothelium is damaged because its contractile effect is normally opposed by the release of endothelial-derived relaxing factor (EDRF).

Neurogenically mediated coronary vasoconstriction is enhanced in vessels downstream from a coronary stenosis. Since metabolically induced vasodilation is already maximal in such vessels, the direct constrictor effects of sympathetic stimulation are both prolonged and intensified. Patients with coronary artery disease have been documented to be more sensitive to the coronary constrictor effects of emotionally induced activation of the sympathetic nervous system.

A subset of patients with angina pectoris have symptomatology despite the absence of coronary artery obstruction. This syndrome is referred to as **variant angina** and appears to result from vasospasm of selected coronary arteries. The precise mechanism of this phenomenon is not known, but such subjects have been documented to be more sensitive to provocative tests for vasoconstrictor sensitivity such as the administration of **ergonovine,** an agent with serotonin-agonistic properties.

Pharmacology of Antianginal Agents

Nitrates

The prototypical drug of the nitrate/nitrite class of antianginal agents, nitroglycerin, is physically a volatile liquid that is ordinarily administered in highly soluble sublingual tablets. More recently it has been employed in longer-acting drug delivery forms such as ointments and transdermal patches. Agents of this class provide relief from the symptoms of angina pectoris by effects related to their vasodilator activity. Nitroglycerin and related analogs are general relaxants of vascular and other types of smooth muscle. Although they are capable of producing relaxation of coronary arterial vascular muscle, their antianginal action is probably more closely related to peripheral vasodilation. In a classic study, subjects with angina were administered nitroglycerin by direct intra-arterial injection at the time of coronary angiography. This did not suppress pacing-induced angina, whereas the sublingual route of administration was efficacious. It is now believed that relief of anginal pain in obstructive coronary artery disease by nitroglycerin and other antianginal agents results from reduction in **myocardial oxygen requirement** as opposed to direct improvement of coronary blood flow. Nitroglycerin dilates both arterial and venous smooth muscle, which reduces afterload and preload. Reduction in myocardial oxygen requirement is produced by a fall in ventricular volume and force of contraction and can be the result of a selective fall in preload.

The mechanism of action of the nitrate/nitrite class of agents probably involves activation of **guanylate cyclase** and increased synthesis of **cyclic guanosine monophosphate (GMP)**. This stimulation is believed to result from the intracellular formation of free radical nitric oxide (NO). Nitroglycerin, **pentaerythritol tetranitrate** (Peritrate), and **isosorbide dinitrate** (Isordil) all share this common mechanism of action. The vasodilator actions of these agents are not dependent upon endothelially mediated relaxation mechanisms; in fact, NO has been suggested as a candidate for the EDRF. The hemodynamic effects of nitrate vasodilators are predictable. Total peripheral resistance is reduced; however, heart rate and cardiac output may be increased because of reflex activation of the sympathetic nervous system. These reflex effects tend to offset the antianginal effects of the agents because they increase oxygen requirement of the myocardium. Although agents of this class are clearly effective in the treatment of angina, their efficacy increases when they are used in combination with β-adrenoceptor antagonists. The agents differ with respect to their pharmacological properties. Nitroglycerin and isosorbide dinitrate are very short acting (30 to 60 minutes), whereas pentaerythritol tetranitrate has a duration of action exceeding 4 to 6 hours. Longer-acting forms of this class are used for prophylaxis of angina, especially for so-called **nocturnal angina** in which coronary blood flow is reduced in parallel with hypotension associated with sleep.

The side effects of these agents—**headaches,** hypotension and orthostasis, nausea, and flushing and warmth—can be observed with excessive doses. **Tolerance** to headache is developed with repeated use. The question of whether tolerance to the antianginal effects of these agents develops with chronic administration remains controversial. Severity of coronary artery disease is often progressive and it has been difficult to separate tolerance to nitrates and nitrites from a true increase in drug requirement associated with increased severity of the disease.

β-Adrenoceptor Antagonists

β-Adrenoceptor antagonists have proven to be exceptionally effective in the treatment of angina pectoris. Controlled clinical trials have documented that β-adrenoceptor antagonists **increase survival** and **reduce the incidence of sudden death** in patients with documented **myocardial infarction.** It has not yet been determined whether such protection is afforded to patients with coronary disease prior to infarction. The mechanism by which β-adrenoceptor antagonists produce their antianginal effect is directly related to reduction of myocardial oxygen requirement. Reduction in heart rate, wall tension, contractility, and stroke volume produce a strong improvement of the ratio of myocardial oxygen delivery to oxygen requirement. It is interesting to note that the antianginal effect is produced despite the tendency for β-adrenoceptor blockade to lower coronary blood flow as a result of reduced metabolically related vasodilation. It is very common for antianginal therapy to include combined use of nitrates and β-adrenoceptor antagonists. Nitroglycerin, for example, may be employed to manage acute episodes of angina, whereas long-term prophylaxis is achieved with a β-adrenoceptor antagonist. Controlled trials have documented that the need for nitroglycerin is sharply decreased in the presence of β-adrenoceptor blockade. The combined use has the additional benefit of enhancing the antianginal effect of nitrates because reflexly medi-ated sympathoexcitation of the heart, an effect that increases myocardial oxy-gen requirement, is prevented by β-adrenoceptor antagonism.

Calcium Antagonists

The **calcium antagonists** verapamil (Calan, Isoptin), diltiazem (Cardizem), and nifedipine (Procardia, Adalat) are highly effective antianginal agents. Their efficacy is primarily attributable to reduction of **myocardial oxygen re-quirement**. The agents appear to reduce both preload and afterload and, through their ability to interfere with calcium entry into myocardial cells, di-rectly to depress myocardial contractility. In addition to the capacity of this class of agents to diminish myocardial oxygen requirement, they are perhaps the most efficacious drugs for the treatment of angina originating from coro-nary vasospasm.

Although this class of agent shares a common mechanism of action, there are significant differences in pharmacological properties among the three drugs. Nifedipine appears to have the most significant hypotensive action and has the greatest intrinsic capacity to reduce work demand on myocardium. Verapamil is more efficacious in depressing atrioventricular (AV) conduction than the other two agents but has the greatest negative inotropic effect on the myocardium. The agents as a class produce a number of common side effects including gastrointestinal disturbances, headache, and edema.

ANTIARRHYTHMIC AGENTS

Mechanisms of Arrhythmias

Abnormal rhythms of the heart can result from at least three different functional alterations. The first is **automaticity**. In the normal function of the heart, the action potential spontaneously originates in the sinoatrial (SA) node without any stimulation by nerve cells and is thus called "automatic" or "pace-making." Normally automaticity in the SA node has the highest intrinsic fre-quency, followed by the AV node, with Purkinje cells a distant third. Increased sympathetic activity releases norepinephrine and speeds the firing of the SA node, while increased parasympathetic activity (vagus nerve) re-leases additional acetylcholine and slows the spontaneous firing of the SA node. Norepinephrine and acetylcholine cause increases or decreases, respec-tively, in the spontaneous automatic activity of the SA node by alterations of inward current carried by two ions (sodium and calcium as depolarizing agents) and of outward current carried by one ion (potassium as a repolarizing agent). Action potentials are normally initiated by the SA node and conducted to atrial muscle, the AV node, conductile cells, and ventricular muscle, in that order (Fig. 9–5). Atrial or ventricular muscle only shows automaticity abnormally, as action potentials should first originate in the SA node. However, the AV node would initiate action potentials to drive the ventricle should the SA node fail.

The second property leading to arrhythmias is the **effective refractory period** (the time during which excitation cannot occur because of inactivation), which normally protects against repeat action potentials in a given cell but which can be shortened under certain conditions to give rapid repeat excitation. The refractory period is approximately equal to the duration of the action potential, which makes it roughly one half of the total time between beats (the interbeat interval includes both the diastolic time and the contraction time). When the action potential is shortened, the time during which re-excitation cannot occur is shortened. The most important example of this arrhythmia is **fibrillation** (the firing of myocardial cells at 350 to 600 per minute).

The third alteration leading to arrhythmias is **decreased conduction velocity,** in which the excitation of cells in the depressed conduction area may

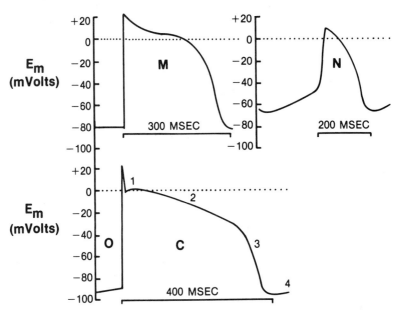

Figure 9–5. Cardiac action potentials of muscle (M), nodal (N), and conductile (C) cells have characteristically different shapes due to different proportions of underlying ion conductances. The phases of the cardiac action potential are labeled on the conductile cell action potential. Notice that spontaneous, pacemaker depolarization is absent in the muscle cells (M); that the cells of the conduction system (C), specialized for high-velocity conduction, have very rapid upstroke and long duration; and that the nodal pacemaker cells (N) have a very slow upstroke, and therefore low conduction velocity. E_m = membrane potential.

occur when the normal cells have repolarized and ended their effective refractory period. **Cell-to-cell conduction** in the heart appears to be a modulated process that depends on special junctions, and it is likely that there are preferential pathways created by regions of relatively lower resistance that are crucial for normal conduction to occur. An identified type of arrhythmia based on conduction is re-entry, in which slowed conduction can include unidirectional conduction block. Action potential propagation fails in the forward (normal) direction but not in the reverse (abnormal) direction, leading to re-excitation of part of the heart.

These three properties of the heart can vary independently: automaticity depends on a pacemaker mechanism; the effective refractory period depends on the duration of the action potential; and the conduction velocity depends on the maximum rate of rise of the action potential and cell-to-cell junctions.

Pharmacology of Antiarrhythmic Agents

Antiarrhythmic agents can be grouped into five major categories: Na^+ channel depressors, β-adrenoceptor antagonists, Na^+ channel restorers, Ca^{2+} channel blockers (Ca^{2+} antagonists), and membrane-stabilizing agents. **Ion channels** that open (activate) and close (inactivate) in response to voltage and time provide not only the basis for cardiac action potentials, but also abnormal electrical activity and the drugs used to control it. Na^+ and Ca^{2+} channels are two of the targets.

Sodium Channel Depressors

Na^+ channel depressors are the classic antiarrhythmic agents and include **quinidine, procainamide, disopyramide,** and the local anesthetic drugs **lidocaine** and **tocainide.** All of these agents depress fast Na^+ channels, decrease conduction velocity, and depress the tendency toward automaticity. The **local anesthetics** are perhaps the superior therapy for arrhythmias owing to increased automaticity. Quinidine and similar agents are used against ectopic focus arrhythmias. An important, indirect (atropine-like) effect of quinidine and related drugs can lead to blockade of the vagal influence on the heart. Quinidine—and to a lesser extent procainamide but to a greater extent disopyramide—blocks the action of the vagus normally to slow heart rate and decrease conduction through the AV node. The most important role of the tonic vagal influence is decreased conduction through the AV node, in terms of both conduction velocity and frequency of action potentials that can pass through the AV node. The decrease in frequency of action potentials passing through the AV node (which, in electrical terms, is the gateway to the ventricles) normally protects the ventricles from being excited at frequencies higher than they can follow without difficulty. Thus, in atrial fibrillation, it is important to increase vagal tone to counteract the atropine-like action of quinidine. For this purpose, the digitalis-like drugs are most often used as pretreatment for quinidine or disopyramide. Quinidine, procainamide, and disopyramide can all be used as oral preparations with efficacy against common types of arrhythmias, and are often presribed for long periods of time. The short duration of action of procainamide (2 to 3 hours) makes it less popular, although sustained release forms are now available. Disopyramide, with longer duration of action (6 to 8 hours), is a newer option for the many patients who show adverse reactions to quinidine.

Local anesthetic antiarrhythmic agents are perhaps the most potent agents available to treat ventricular arrhythmias. Lidocaine, which can be used only intravenously, is very effective in emergency situations against serious **ventricular tachycardias** and fibrillation and has the advantage of a very rapid and short duration of action. The agent is also useful for suppression of ventricular arrhythmias immediately and for days following myocardial infarction. Tocainide and mexiletine are new, long-duration (10- to 15-hour) local anesthetics very effective against ventricular arrhythmias.

β-*Adrenoceptor Antagonists*

β-Adrenoceptor antagonists compose the second category of antiarrhythmic drugs and have indirect effects *via* the sympathetic nervous system, as well as direct effects on myocardial cells. The indirect effect (β-adrenoceptor antagonism and decrease of sympathetic drive to the heart) allows the vagus to predominate, but also decreases the contractility of the heart (which is dependent on tonic adrenergic stimulation). Much of the beneficial effect of propranolol may be through a **membrane-stabilizing effect,** which would cause myocardial cell hyperpolarization and tend to improve conduction velocity. β-adrenoceptor blockade also may be quite important because of the decrease in heart work and the subsequent improvement in the ratio of blood flow delivered to the myocardial cells to that required. **Propranolol** is the prototype agent used for this purpose, although propranolol is a nonselective β_1- and β_2-adrenoceptor antagonist which also causes bronchoconstriction. **Metoprolol** is a β_1-selective adrenoceptor antagonist that avoids at least part of the bronchoconstriction problem. Blockade of β_1 adrenoceptors in the myocardium appears to have a beneficial effect without as pronounced an action on bronchial smooth muscle. **Nadolol** is a long-acting β-adrenoceptor antagonist that, like propranolol, is nonselective.

Sodium Channel Restorers

The third type of antiarrhythmic agent is the Na^+ channel restorer, for which there is only one example, phenytoin. **Phenytoin** (Dilantin) seems to have direct membrane actions only, causing the conductile cells to repolarize more completely in certain situations, especially when digitalis toxicity has occurred. The restored conduction through the depressed area appears to allow normal function where an overdose of digitalis had caused partial depolarization and slowed conduction. Phenytoin is used only as an intravenous agent and, therefore, only in certain cases in the hospital setting.

Calcium Channel Blockers

The fourth class of antiarrhythmic agents, Ca^{2+} antagonists, act at least partly by blocking Ca^{2+} channels: (1) inhibiting slow action potentials that occur in muscle or conductile cells as abnormal phenomena (transient inward currents); and (2) blocking contraction of the coronary vessels, dilating coronary arteries, and thus improving coronary blood flow. Because of decreasing Ca^{2+} entry through the surface membrane, coronary vasodilators, especially the first ones introduced, are potentially cardiodepressant, and there is concern over the decreased cardiac performance (Table 9-2). The first to be approved was verapamil, which is effective against supraventricular tachycardia,

TAble 9-2. COMPARATIVE CLINICAL EFFECTS OF CALCIUM CHANNEL BLOCKERS

	Verapamil	Diltiazem	Nifedipine
Coronary vaso-dilatation	+ +	+ + +	+ + +
Peripheral vaso-dilatation	+ +	+	+ + +
Myocardial con-tractility	↓	− −	↓, reflex ↑
Heart rate	↓ ↑	↓	reflex ↑
AV nodal con-duction	↓ ↓	↓	− −
Dosage (mg/day)	Oral: 240–480 IV: 5–10	120–240	30–120
Indications	Oral: Angina IV: Supraventricular tachyarrhythmia	Angina	Variant angina
Side effects	Oral: headache, dizziness, conduction disturbances IV: bradycardia, hypotension, exacerbation of heart failure	Conduction disturbances, edema, rash, headache	Peripheral edema, dizziness, aggravation of myocardial ischemia

Adapted from McCauley, KM and Brest, AN: McGoon's Cardiac Surgery: An Interprofessional Approach to Patient Care. FA Davis, Philadelphia, 1985, p 265.

atrial fibrillation, and atrial flutter, but which can be depressant to the myocardium and to the AV node. Diltiazem, a newer agent, is a stronger coronary vasodilator and also blocks Ca^{2+} entry into myocardial cells. Both verapamil and diltiazem have been found to eliminate certain **refractory arrhythmias,** although they often also trigger a drop in blood pressure and, therefore, a reflex-increased sympathetic outflow to the heart, which may aggravate the arrhythmia. These agents are often used in combination with other antiarrhythmic agents or as a last resort when other drugs of this class have failed.

Membrane Stabilizers

The fifth category of antiarrhythmics includes newer agents that have in common membrane stabilization. The prototypes for this group are lidocaine, which is also a Na^+ channel depressant, and bretylium, which interferes with norepinephrine release. Lidocaine and associated local anesthetic–type antiarrhythmic agents stabilize the myocardial cell membrane by **increasing K^+ conductance,** leading to **hyperpolarization.** The more negative resting membrane potential decreases or eliminates pacemaker activity. Bretylium interferes with norepinephrine release from adrenergic nerve endings and stabilizes myocardial cell membranes. These actions also decrease the tendency for pacemaker activity and high-frequency conduction.

DRUGS USED TO TREAT CONGESTIVE HEART FAILURE

Treatment for **congestive heart failure** is currently only partially effective because of a lack of understanding of the mechanisms that lead to heart failure. Cardiac output has four major determinants: (1) contractility, which is the point at which the myocardial contraction process fails; (2) heart rate; (3) diastolic volume, or preload; and (4) blood pressure against which the heart must pump, or afterload.

In order to understand the changes that occur on administration of agents given to alleviate heart failure, it is necessary to recall the **length-tension relationship,** otherwise known as the Starling mechanism, by which cardiac output is regulated by the central venous pressure (Fig. 9–6). In the normal heart, an increase in end-diastolic pressure results in an increase in the strength of the successive contraction, thereby increasing stroke volume and cardiac output (at a given heart rate). The alignment of thick and thin filaments in cardiac muscle results in striations of the cells. These represent the overlap of thick and thin filaments, for which there is an optimum length for development of force. As end-diastolic volume increases, the amount of overlap of thick and thin filaments is believed to approach the optimum, resulting in increased cardiac output. The entire relationship, which is plotted as a curve relating cardiac output to end-diastolic volume, is a **Starling curve** and represents one state of contractility (see Fig. 9–6).

Thus, contractility is not represented by a particular force, but by an entire curve relating the force at a given end-diastolic volume. A further important regulator of contractile force in the heart is **adrenergic innervation,** which is capable of shifting the heart to a higher Starling curve. Thus, under the influence of either neural or humoral adrenergic stimulation, at a given end-diastolic volume, the contractile force—and thus the cardiac output— will be greater. The combination of the two mechanisms (adrenergic stimulation and the Starling mechanism) can result in a five-fold increase in cardiac output when the metabolic demand of the organism requires increased blood flow.

Failure of the heart often occurs because of decreases in contractility and is most frequently associated with atherosclerosis, infarction, and embolism. All of these limit or reduce coronary blood flow and thus the blood supply to the myocardium. Other causes of heart failure include pericarditis, arrhythmias, and cardiomyopathies. These seriously impair the ability of the heart to develop sufficient contractile force and therefore to pump enough blood (cardiac output). Although the cellular pathophysiology of heart failure is not known, it appears to be related to the **lack of sufficient Ca^{2+} for contraction.** It is possible that the sarcoplasmic reticulum and other membranes within the cardiac muscle cell that store and release Ca^{2+} for contraction become impaired.

Treatment of congestive heart failure is rationally based on two strategies. The first is to increase with cardiac glycosides the development of contractile force in cardiac muscle cells; this is achieved at the expense of poisoning of the Na^+ pump that regulates the intracellular Na^+ and K^+ concentrations in the myocardial cell. The second is reduction of myocardial oxygen require-

Figure 9–6. Contractility curves for four different states would define four levels of cardiac performance. Each contractility state (e.g., normal) consists of a family of points representing different cardiac filling (end-diastolic pressure). Increases in stroke volume at a given end-diastolic pressure mean an increase in contractility (by definition) and would occur with increased sympathetic drive and β-adrenoceptor stimulation. Depressed contractility would be increased by positive inotropic agents (e.g., digitoxin) because contraction is improved in each myocardial cell by increased stores of intracellular Ca^{2+}.

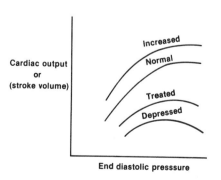

ment by treatment with a vasodilator, which decreases preload, afterload, or both.

Digitalis

Treatment of heart failure with **digitalis** (Table 9–3) is based upon the observation that partial poisoning of the Na^+/K^+ pump, which is the most notable action of digitalis on the myocardium, is accompanied by significant increases in the development of contractile force. The explanation is believed to be a **countertransport** mechanism that normally uses the inwardly directed Na^+ gradient to constantly pump Ca^{2+} out of the myocardial cell, which would become less active when the Na^+ pump was poisoned, thereby allowing accumulation of intracellular Na^+ and a buildup of intracellular Ca^{2+} in stores that are released to cause contraction.

With treatment by digitalis, there is an improvement of contractile force similar to that found with norepinephrine, but with a very important difference. The increase in contractile force produced by digitalis requires less oxygen supply to the myocardium in exchange for the increased force than is produced by adrenergic stimulation. While increased cardiac output with a smaller requirement of additional oxygen would at first seem paradoxical, the increase in contraction produced does come with a considerable, although indirect, penalty. As digitalis poisons the Na^+ pump, there is an increased intracellular supply of Ca^{2+}. If the problem in the myocardial cells that led to heart failure was the inability of intracellular organelles to take up and release Ca^{2+}, the improvement in contractile force comes with the danger that a small, further increase in Ca^{2+} could lead to overload and contractile failure in the cell.

Digitalis has the **lowest therapeutic index** of any drug now in use. The low therapeutic index (<2) results from (1) the delicate balance to allow just enough additional Ca^{2+} to be released for improved contraction, without overloading the cell and causing its failure to relax and therefore to function; and (2) poisoning of the Na^+ pump, which dissipates a portion of the K^+ gradient, causing depolarization of the cell and predisposing toward arrhythmias. The relatively low concentrations of digitalis used for beneficial therapeutic effect should cause only a minor depolarization of the cells which normally are only latent pacemakers, especially those of the Purkinje-His bundle branch system. With slightly higher concentrations, these conductile cells will begin to become involved in generation of high-frequency action potentials and, therefore, arrhythmias. A summary of the electrophysiological effects of digitalis is shown in Table 9–3. Factors known to increase digitalis toxicity include (1) hypokalemia, (2) hypercalcemia, (3) hypomagnesemia, (4) acid-base disturbances, (5) renal failure, (6) hypothyroidism, (7) hypoxemia, (8) age greater than 70, (9) history of cardiac arrhythmias, and (10) drug interactions (quinidine or verapamil). As each individual requires different concentrations of digitalis, it is particularly important to monitor for signs of toxicity.

Table 9–3. ACTIONS OF DIGITALIS ON CARDIAC ELECTRICAL FUNCTION*

Effect	Atria	Atrioventricular Node	Ventricles, Purkinje System
Direct	Shortens refractory period.	Increases refractory period.	Shortens refractory period, or no significant effect.
	No significant effect on conduction velocity.	Decreases conduction velocity.	Decreases conduction velocity.
	Decreases normal automaticity; increases abnormal automaticity.	Increases or decreases normal automaticity; increases abnormal automaticity.	Increases or decreases normal automaticity; *increases abnormal automaticity.*
Indirect (ANS)			
1. Vagal	*Shortens refractory period.*	*Increases refractory period.*	
	Decreases sinoatrial rate.	*Decreases conduction velocity.*	
2. Sympathetic (toxic doses)	Increases sinoatrial rate.	Shortens refractory period.	*Increases abnormal automaticity.*
		Junctional extrasystoles.	
Effect on ECG and rhythm			
Early	P wave changes.	*Lengthens PR interval.*	*ST depression, T wave inversion.*
Progressive toxicity	Premature atrial beats.	Second- or third-degree block.	*Ventricular premature depolarizations.*
	Atrial fibrillation.	Junctional tachycardia.	Bigeminy. Ventricular tachycardia. Ventricular fibrillation.

*Dominant effects appear in **boldface italics**.

From Katzung, BG and Parmley, WW: Cardiac glycosides and other drugs used in the treatment of congestive heart failure. In Katzung, BG (ed): Basic and Clinical Pharmacology, ed 3. Appleton & Lange, Norwalk, CT, 1987, p 142, with permission.

Another important aspect of the action of digitalis is stimulation of the parasympathetic nervous system, causing a slowing of the heart and a **depression of conduction through the AV node,** which appears as a lengthened P-R interval on the electrocardiogram. This action of digitalis is used in preventing the conduction of atrial arrhythmias into the ventricles, as was described in

**Table 9–4. USE OF VASODILATORS IN TREATMENT OF
CONGESTIVE HEART FAILURE**

	Indications
1. Arterial ($\downarrow$ afterload) Hydralazine Minoxidil Diazoxide	Fatigue due to low left ventricular output
2. Venous ($\downarrow$ preload) Isosorbide dinitrate Nitroglycerin	Dyspnea/pulmonary congestion
3. Arterial and venous Nitroprusside $\Big\}$ a$\cong$v Prazosin Nifedipine $\Big\}$ a$>$v Captopril	Severe, chronic congestive heart failure

a—arterial effects; v—venous effects.

the section on antiarrhythmic agents. While the increased vagal action might be beneficial in preventing most arrhythmias, the concomitant blockade of the Na^+ pump (and depolarization) in the muscle cells (the direct action of digitalis) leads to depolarization and arrhythmias. When arrhythmias occur, treatments include stopping administration of digitalis, increasing plasma K^+ back to the normal range (if it is low), treatment with other agents, notably lidocaine or phenytoin, which are effective against digitalis-induced arrhythmias, and digitalis antibodies.

Amrinone

The search for a replacement for digitalis, which has been in use for over 200 years, has recently been promising. Several potentially useful alternatives have been developed. **Amrinone** is a **phosphodiesterase inhibitor** that seems also to act to increase Ca^{2+} release by myocardial cells, but that unfortunately is toxic, causing hepatotoxicity, fever, and reversible thrombocytopenia. The mechanism of action of amrinone is not yet understood, but its ability to increase contractile function in some instances of congestive heart failure may be a signal that improved therapies are on the way.

Vasodilators

In consideration of other therapies, it is important to keep in mind that the afterload against which the heart pumps is one of the most important determinants of whether the heart can supply the necessary blood flow. In patients with congestive heart failure, it is especially important to consider the use of vasodilators (Table 9–4), which have been shown to be superior to digitalis glycosides in certain cases. These agents increase cardiac efficiency by reducing preload, afterload, or a combination of the two. Recent clinical and experimental evidence indicates that ACE inhibitors prolong life in patients with chronic congestive heart failure.

LIPID-LOWERING AGENTS

The hyperlipidemias comprise a heterogenous group of diseases of lipoprotein metabolism. Multiple genetic and acquired lesions have been associated with the various types of hyperlipidemias including defects in lipoprotein-receptor structure and in pathways of apoprotein synthesis. Specific treatment of these defects is not possible at this time and the therapy is directed at the sequelae of these defects, that is, elevated plasma lipoproteins (very low-density lipoproteins, low-density lipoproteins; or VLDL, LDL), resulting in increased cholesterol or plasma triglyceride levels or both.

The consequences of hyperlipidemia are both direct and indirect. Elevated triglyceride levels are directly associated with an increased risk of pancreatitis. In contrast, the complications related to chronic **hypercholesterolemia** are indirect, that is, elevated cholesterol levels predispose the individual to accelerated atherosclerosis and thus to an increased risk of coronary vascular disease as well as peripheral vascular disease. Isolated **hypertriglyceridemia** seems to be much less important as a risk factor for the development of atherosclerotic complications.

Benefits of Pharmacological Intervention

Despite the clear demonstration that elevated levels of plasma cholesterol predispose patients to an increased risk of atherosclerotic complications, it has been more difficult to prove that lowering plasma cholesterol levels pharmacologically results in a reduction in subsequent risk of atherosclerotic complications. The reason for these difficulties may be twofold. First, atherosclerotic disease occurs over decades. Therefore, trials of risk factor modification (i.e., lower plasma cholesterol) would be expected to require many years of follow-up and large numbers of subjects, both of which are difficult to achieve in conventional clinical trials. Second, it is unclear whether the atherosclerotic lesions that develop in hypercholesterolemic humans are reversible. If these lesions are irreversible, treatment of patients with hypercholesterolemia who already harbor atherosclerotic lesions may result in little benefit.

Despite these potential reservations, several trials have suggested benefit of pharmacological intervention in patients with hypercholesterolemia. The Lipid Research Clinic Coronary Prevention Trial was a multicenter, double-blind, randomized study of the efficacy of **cholestyramine** (see further on) in reducing the incidence of coronary artery disease in asymptomatic middle-aged men. These investigators demonstrated that with cholestyramine there was a 24 percent lower incidence of coronary artery disease–related deaths, as well as a 19 percent reduction in the incidence of coronary artery disease (i.e., coronary artery disease deaths and nonfatal myocardial infarction). However, it should be noted that overall mortality was not significantly different between treatment and control groups. A related compound, **colestipol hydrochloride,** has been similarly studied in a randomized, placebo-controlled, multicenter trial of 2278 hypercholesterolemic subjects followed for 3 years. Here the treatment group demonstrated a 74 percent reduction in coronary artery disease–related deaths in a comparable (but not significant; $p = 0.12$) reduction in total mortality. In contrast, however, it should be noted that cardiovascular death rates were not reduced in female subjects taking colestipol. These trials indicated that at least these two agents might be effective in reducing coronary artery atherosclerotic complications of hypercholesterolemia. More recently, a long-term follow-up of the Coronary Drug Project (conducted between 1966 and 1975) reported that niacin treatment resulted in an 11 percent lower mortality than placebo—a difference that remained significant almost 9 years after termination of the trial.

It must be emphasized, however, that the equation relating pharmacological reduction in plasma cholesterol with lowered cardiovascular mortality and morbidity may not hold universally. In fact, a multicenter trial of **clofibrate** (see further on) demonstrated that therapy resulted in an overall **increase** in "all cause mortality," particularly cancer. Because therapy of hypercholesterolemia must be viewed as prophylactic, that is, in expectation of preventing atherosclerotic complications, it would seem only prudent to prescribe those agents that have been demonstrated both to lower cholesterol and to reduce cardiovascular mortality/morbidity (if not overall mortality).

Pharmacology of Lipid-Lowering Agents

Cholestyramine and Colestipol

At present, these drugs are probably the therapies of choice for the treatment of hypercholesterolemia, judged on the basis of safety and efficacy. They are ion-exchange resins, which act in the GI tract to bind bile acids. They are thus associated with increased LDL catabolism. Neither cholestyramine nor colestipol is absorbed systemically, and their adverse effects are almost entirely gastrointestinal as would be anticipated. These include constipation, nausea, vomiting, cramping, and abdominal distention. As also might be expected, cholestyramine and colestipol may interfere with the absorption of many other drugs, including thyroxine and digoxin.

They are administered in powdered form and taken two to four times daily. Their unpalatability and frequent dosing regimen are the major significant drawbacks to patient enthusiasm about this form of therapy.

Nicotinic Acid

Nicotinic acid acts by inhibiting lipolysis in adipose tissue and decreased hepatic esterification of triglycerides in the liver and increased activity of lipoprotein lipases. It is effective in the treatment of both hypercholesterolemia and hypertriglyceridemia, which makes it very useful in the treatment of combined hyperlipidemias. Its use has, however, been limited by its unfavorable pattern of adverse effects including prominent flushing, pruritus, and GI symptoms.

Probucol

This agent is effective primarily in the therapy of hypercholesterolemia although its mechanism of effect is unclear. It is believed structurally to alter LDL, making them more susceptible to non–receptor-mediated clearance.

Although generally well tolerated, probucol is associated with GI tract side effects. A proarrhythmic effect noted in animal models has yet to be seen in humans.

Clofibrate

Clofibrate is widely used in the therapy of both hypercholesterolemia and hypertriglyceridemia, although as previously noted there is no evidence to suggest that it reduces the mortality and morbidity associated with elevated cholesterol levels. Therefore, it is generally reserved for treatment of combined hyperlipidemias. It acts primarily by reducing VLDLs and elevating the high-density lipoprotein (HDL) fraction. Clofibrate is associated with a number of adverse effects including myalgias, arthralgias, skin rash, and hepatitis, but more importantly it has been shown to be associated with an increased risk for cholecystitis, gall stones, and cancer deaths.

Gemfibrozil

Gemfibrozil is chemically and pharmacologically similar to clofibrate. Its mechanism of action is thought to relate to its ability to reduce VLDL levels and to increase HDL levels, although there may also be some variable effects in lowering LDLs. This agent's adverse effects parallel those of clofibrate.

Lovastatin

Lovastatin represents the first of a new class of lipid-lowering drugs that act primarily by inhibiting hydroxymethylglutaryl coenzyme-A (HMG Co-A) reductase, an enzyme catalyzing the conversion of HMG Co-A to mevolonate. This represents an early and rate-limiting step in cholesterol synthesis. In hepatocytes, this results in reduced intracellular cholesterol levels and the subsequent stimulation of LDL-receptor synthesis, resulting in increased LDL clearance systemically and hence to reduced plasma cholesterol levels. Lovastatin therapy results in marked reduction in LDL cholesterol with little effect on HDL cholesterol or triglycerides.

This class of agents promises to be much more effective and relatively free of side effects. It must be stressed, however, that at this time there is no evidence clearly demonstrating that lowering of plasma cholesterol by HMG Co-A reductase inhibitors actually lowers the risk of cardiovascular disease and reduces mortality, although these studies are now underway.

The only rare side effects reported for this class of drugs includes occasional elevations in liver enzymes, the significance of which is unclear at this time, and an increased risk of lens opacities.

THROMBOLYTIC AGENTS

Used in the acute management of thrombotic disorders, this class of drugs has been chiefly employed for acute clot-lysis in pulmonary emboli (and deep venous thrombosis) and, most importantly, for acute myocardial infarction. For therapy of pulmonary emboli and deep venous thrombosis, those subgroups of patients who definitely benefit from thrombolytic therapy have not yet been clearly identified. In the treatment of myocardial infarction, there is increasing evidence suggesting that, especially in high-risk patients and those with anterior myocardial infarctions, streptokinase is associated with a significant reduction in morbidity and early mortality.

Streptokinase/Urokinase

These agents both act by activating plasminogen and thereby enhancing fibrinolysis. They are effective in clot-lysis in both venous and arterial circulations. **Streptokinase** is a protein product of group C hemolytic streptococci. **Urokinase** is a naturally occurring plasminogen activator extracted from human urine. These agents are comparably effective. However, it is notable that most clinical studies documenting the efficacy of fibrinolytic therapy have used streptokinase. Both agents are administered intravenously and occasionally by an intracoronary route in the case of acute myocardial infarction. In general they are given over a short-term basis (less than 2 hours).

The major side effects of this therapy are bleeding complications, generally confined to sites of vascular puncture or recent surgical incisions. Streptokinase as a bacterial antigen is associated with occasional hypersensitivity reactions, and its use is generally confined to a single administration. In contrast, urokinase, a purified preparation, is nonantigenic and can be readministered.

Tissue-Type Plasminogen Activator (TPA)

This newer class of thrombolytic agents acts by converting plasminogen to plasmin most effectively on the fibrin surface of an already formed clot and may, at lower doses, have less systemic fibrinolytic effect. It is also administered intravenously over a 60- to 90-minute period, and to date the only significant adverse effects reported are hypofibrinogenemia and occasional bleeding complications including cerebral vascular hemorrhage.

Antiplatelet Agents

This class of compounds, which generally inhibit platelet adhesion and aggregation *in vitro*, has been used in various thromboembolic disorders in humans, including transient ischemic attacks of the cerebrovascular circulation, superficial venous thrombosis, and as adjunctive therapy to anticoagulants in prophylaxis of thromboembolic phenomena following insertion of prosthetic heart valves.

Aspirin

As previously described, aspirin acts as an irreversible inhibitor of prostaglandin synthesis, primarily through its effect on cyclo-oxygenase. It is used in the therapy of superficial deep venous thrombosis, has proven effective in reducing the frequency of transient ischemic attacks, and has been clearly demonstrated to reduce mortality when administered in the course of unstable angina.

Sulfinpyrazone

Sulfinpyrazone, a congener of phenylbutazone, is both a potent uricosuric agent and an inhibitor of platelet aggregation. Its use as an antiplatelet agent is, however, very limited. As demonstrated in clinical studies, it may have a marginal effect in reducing the incidence of sudden death over the first 6 months of therapy following a myocardial infarction.

Dipyridamole

Dipyridamole can be demonstrated to act *in vitro* to inhibit cyclic adenosine monophosphate (AMP) phosphodiesterase activity and hence to increase intracellular levels of cyclic AMP. *In vivo* it acts both as an inhibitor of platelet aggregation and as a vasodilator. By itself, it has little clinical efficacy in any thromboembolic disorder; however, it may further inhibit embolization from prosthetic heart valves when used with aspirin.

ANTICOAGULANT DRUGS

Heparin

Heparin in a naturally occurring anticogulant that acts primarily by activating antithrombin III which inactivates thrombin and neutralizes several activated clotting factors including XII, XI, X, IX, II, and XIII.

Heparin is used extensively in acute therapy of deep venous thrombosis and pulmonary embolism. At lower doses (which do not significantly elevate clinical indices of coagulation, i.e., the partial thromboplastin time, or PTT) it has been shown to be effective in reducing the risk of developing deep venous thromboses following a number of surgical procedures.

The administration of heparin is primarily intravenous or subcutaneous. Chief complications include hemorrhage and a thrombocytopenia syndrome related to both heparin-induced platelet aggregation and heparin-dependent antiplatelet antibody formation.

Warfarin

Warfarin (Coumadin) is the most commonly used oral anticoagulant. The other available anticoagulants (dicumarol and phenprocoumon) are essentially not used in clinical medicine in the United States. These agents act primarily as antagonists of vitamin K–dependent clotting factor synthesis and are used in the longer-term therapy following deep venous thromboses, pulmonary embolism, and implantation of prosthetic valves. Occasionally oral anticoagulants have been used in the therapy of patients who have had either myocardial infarction or transient ischemic attacks; however, the efficacy of therapy in these situations is controversial.

The adverse effects of these agents are primarily related to bleeding complications. A hypersensitivity reaction resulting in hemorrhagic infarction and necrosis of the skin (the so-called purple toe syndrome) may rarely occur. Of more clinical importance, warfarin is associated with multiple drug interactions. These relate to multiple mechanisms including (1) competition for plasma-binding sites (as seen with phenylbutazone), which will increase warfarin effect; (2) inhibition of warfarin metabolism (as seen with cimetidine), again leading to increased warfarin effect; (3) reduced absorption of warfarin (as seen with cholestyramine), resulting in a reduction in drug effect; and (4) accelerated metabolism resulting in increased clearance and a reduced effect (as seen with rifampicin and phenobarbital).

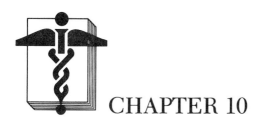

CHAPTER 10

Diuretics and Uricosuric Drugs

H. E. WILLIAMSON, Ph.D.

Diuretics are agents that increase solute excretion to increase the volume of urine. Principal uses of diuretic agents are in the treatment of diseases in which an excess of sodium (and consequently water) is present in the interstitial and plasma compartments of the extracellular space. Such conditions include edema of cardiac or renal origin, ascites of hepatic disease, and hypertension. Other uses for the increased urinary volume produced by diuretics include decreasing the irritation of substances on the urinary tract, increasing the excretion of a poisonous substance by the kidneys, preventing precipitation of agents with low solubility in the urinary tract, and maintaining a minimal level of excretion by diseased kidneys.

The primary function of the kidneys (the site of action of diuretics) is the maintenance of the extracellular compartment. It does so by regulating volume, acid-base balance, osmolality, and concentration of electrolytes, and by excreting metabolites and foreign compounds.

The extracellular space comprises about 20 percent of body weight; it can be subdivided into interstitial compartment (space between cells) and plasma compartment. Plasma proteins maintain the separation of plasma and interstitial spaces, whereas sodium (with its anions) maintains the volume of the extracellular space. The distribution of this cation is limited to the extracellular space by the enzyme system, sodium-potassium activated adenosine triphosphatase (Na^+, K^+-ATPase), which is present in cellular membranes. Na^+, K^+-ATPase transports potassium ions into cells and sodium ions out of cells and thus is responsible for the high cellular concentration of potassium and low cellular concentration of sodium. Because its distribution is limited to the extracellular compartment and because it is responsible for most of the osmotic pressure of the extracellular space, the quantity of sodium in the body determines the volume of the extracellular compartment. Thus, the kidneys, by regulating sodium reabsorption, are able to regulate the extracellular volume. If sodium is retained, water will be retained and extracellular volume increased. If sodium is lost, water will also be lost and extracellular volume decreased. The retention of sodium that occurs in various disease states is responsible for the development of edema and ascites.

RENAL TUBULAR HANDLING OF WATER AND ELECTROLYTES

The functional unit of the kidneys is the **nephron:** each human kidney contains approximately one million such units. Diuretic drugs act by altering the movement of electrolytes and water across membranes of the nephrons. Figure 10–1 is a diagram of a nephron and shows the sites involved in the handling of water and electrolytes as well as the principal sites of action of different diuretic drugs. The nephron consists of vascular and tubular epithelial elements. The vascular element includes afferent arteriole, glomerulus, ef-

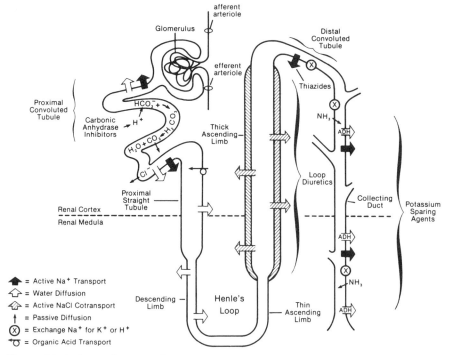

Figure 10–1. Sites of action of some renal drugs. (Modified from Roberts, RJ: Drug Therapy in Infants. W.B. Saunders, Philadelphia, 1984, with permission.)

ferent arteriole, peritubular capillary bed, and venule. The epithelial element includes Bowman's capsule, convoluted and straight segments of the proximal tubule, thin descending segment, thin ascending segment, medullary and cortical portions of the thick ascending segment, distal convoluted tubule, and collecting tubule. The epithelial structures that descend from the cortex into the medulla and back into the cortex are referred to as loops of Henle, and the segments involved are the straight segment of the proximal tubules, descending and ascending thin segments, and cortical and medullary thick segments.

In humans, approximately 100 to 120 ml of essentially protein-free fluid is filtered at the glomeruli each minute. About 99 percent of the water and sodium is usually reabsorbed along the tubules, although this can range from 85 to 99.9 percent depending on the needs for these substances. Daily urine volume averages 1.5 to 2 liters but depends on intake and thus varies markedly.

In the proximal tubules, about 70 percent (range 50 to 90 percent) of filtered sodium is reabsorbed by a combination of active and passive processes. Since this segment is involved in maintaining extracellular volume, the reabsorption of sodium varies to regulate the size of this compartment. A part of the reabsorption of sodium in this area is under the control of **atrial natriuretic factor** (ANF). This peptide hormone is synthesized in the atria (and probably in the ventricles) of the heart. It is released when extracellular volume is expanded and acts upon the kidneys to increase the excretion of sodium and water. Its actions include increasing glomerular filtration rate without altering renal blood flow to increase the load of sodium to the tubules and a partial inhibition of proximal and distal tubular reabsorption of sodium.

Either bicarbonate or chloride ions usually accompany the reabsorption of sodium. Bicarbonate reabsorption occurs in the first third of the proximal tubules and involves the enzyme carbonic anhydrase, whereas chloride reabsorption occurs in the last two thirds of this segment. The reabsorption of these anions is affected by the acid-base balance. In acidosis, bicarbonate reabsorption is favored, whereas chloride reabsorption is favored during alkalosis. Throughout the proximal tubules, the epithelium is freely permeable to water. Thus, as solutes are reabsorbed, water follows passively. Because of the free permeability to water, an osmotic gradient cannot be formed here. Hence, the same osmotic pressure (approximately 280 to 300 mOsm/kg H_2O) will be found in the tubular fluid as is present in the surrounding interstitial space.

The descending thin segment is also freely permeable to water. Since this segment passes through a section of the kidney that has a very high osmotic pressure in the interstitial space surrounding the tubules, fluid moves out of the thin descending segment. About 10 to 15 percent of filtered water is reabsorbed here, whereas sodium that is not reabsorbed becomes very concentrated.

In the ascending thin segment, permeability to water is markedly diminished so that little or no reabsorption of water occurs. The tubules have some permeability to sodium; because the concentration of sodium has been increased because of reabsorption of water from the descending limb, some passive reabsorption of sodium and chloride occurs here.

The medullary and cortical thick ascending segments (diluting segments) are also water impermeable. About 20 percent of filtered sodium chloride is reabsorbed here, but this percentage varies, partially because of the need for sodium to adjust the extracellular volume. This segment has considerable excess capacity; it can reabsorb a considerably larger fraction of the filtered sodium if delivery is increased. The active mechanism in the thick ascending limb of the loop of Henle is a sodium chloride cotransport pump. In the medullary portion, the reabsorption of sodium chloride is involved in the formation and maintenance of the elevated osmotic pressure of the interstitial space of the medulla. The reabsorption of substantial amounts of sodium chloride into an area in which blood supply is limited and in which blood equilibrates with concentration of sodium as it moves into and out of the medulla results in a system that is not very efficient in carrying away reabsorbed electrolytes.

The sodium that is retained results in the development of an increasing concentration of this cation with increasing depth in the medulla, and hence an increasing osmotic pressure. Whereas osmotic pressure is 280 to 300 mOsm per kg H_2O in the cortex, osmotic pressure can reach values of 1200 to 1500 mOsm per kg H_2O at the tip of the medulla. The increased osmotic pressure serves to remove water from the descending limb of the loop of Henle and from the medullary collecting tubules. Inasmuch as water is not reabsorbed from the lumen of the thick ascending segment, the fluid in the tubules becomes increasingly more dilute as it moves through this part of the nephron, and by the time it reaches the end of the segment and passes into the distal convoluted tubules it is much less concentrated than plasma. Thus a major part of the ability of the kidneys to excrete a dilute urine (osmotic pressure less than that of plasma) and hence eliminate excess water, to control osmotic pressure, is due to this segment.

In the distal convoluted tubules, sodium is actively reabsorbed and chloride passively follows. The first part of this segment is also impermeable to water, so that the reabsorption of sodium results in further dilution of the tubular contents. About 5 percent of filtered sodium is reabsorbed here.

In the collecting tubules, water reabsorption is dependent on the presence or absence of **antidiuretic hormone (ADH)**. In the presence of the hormone, tubular permeability is increased. Thus, water will move out of the tubule in response to the osmotic pressure in the surrounding areas. In the cortex, fluid will equilibrate at 280 to 300 mOsm per kg H_2O, whereas in the medullary segment of the collecting tubules, fluid will equilibrate at the higher osmotic pressures (e.g., 1200 to 1500 mOsm/kg H_2O) found in this area. Thus, in the presence of ADH, a very concentrated urine can be formed and water is conserved. In the absence of ADH, the dilute fluid formed in the thick ascending segments and distal convoluted tubules will pass through the collecting tubules and be excreted. In this case, excess water is excreted by the kidneys. In addition, there are exchange mechanisms for sodium in this segment of the tubules and about 5 percent of filtered sodium is handled in this manner. Sodium in the tubules is exchanged for either potassium or hydrogen ions of the tubular cells. Hydrogen ion exchange for sodium is favored in acidosis, whereas potassium for sodium exchange is favored in alkalosis. The exchange mechanisms are stimulated by the presence of sodium in the tubules, but they are also under the control of **aldosterone,** which serves as a fine regulator.

It is apparent that sodium and water are handled by different mechanisms as these substances pass along the tubular elements of the nephron. The importance of the different mechanisms to diuretic activity is related to the likelihood that inhibition of a particular segment will produce a meaningful loss of sodium. The proximal tubules are the least useful site for diuretic activity even though the greatest fraction of filtered sodium and water are reabsorbed here. This is because any sodium whose reabsorption is blocked here must still pass through other segments of the nephron. The thick ascending segment of the loop of Henle and the distal segment are usually able to reclaim most of the additional sodium so that very little will be excreted. The distal convoluted tubule and collecting tubule are useful sites, but the amount of sodium reaching these segments is limited and may be further curtailed in diseases in which these agents are used. Hence, only a limited increase in sodium excretion is possible. The site where the greatest effect on sodium excretion by diuretics is possible is the thick ascending segment. A sizable fraction of sodium is handled here, and if its reabsorption is inhibited the limited action of the later segments of the nephron is not sufficient to reclaim all of the sodium. Hence, marked losses of sodium can occur if reabsorption of sodium chloride is affected in the thick ascending segment of the nephron.

DIURETICS

Diuretic agents can also be referred to by other terms, which more definitively describe their action. These include **natriuretics** (i.e., agents that increase renal excretion of sodium) and **saluretics** (i.e., agents that increase the renal excretion of sodium and chloride).

Descriptions of the principal agents used as diuretics follow.

Carbonic Anhydrase Inhibitors

Acetazolamide (Diamox) (Fig. 10–2) is an example of a class of agents that increase the excretion of sodium by inhibiting **carbonic anhydrase** activity in the kidneys. Although agents of this type are not used to any great extent as diuretic agents today, they are worthy of discussion first because several of the most frequently used diuretics inhibit this enzyme in addition to their principal action on sodium reabsorption.

Excretion Pattern and Mechanism

Carbonic anhydrase is found in the proximal tubules as well as in the distal segments of the nephron. Inhibition of this enzyme results in an increase in the renal excretion of sodium, bicarbonate, and potassium ions, as well as water, whereas hydrogen ion and ammonia excretion are decreased. In the proximal tubules, carbonic anhydrase increases the formation of hydrogen ions that are exchanged for sodium ions present in the glomerular filtrate in the lumen (Fig. 10–3). The secreted hydrogen ion then interacts with bicarbonate ions in the lumen to form carbonic acid. Carbonic anhydrase in the brush border of the proximal tubules catalyzes the conversion of carbonic acid to carbon dioxide which is then absorbed. An inhibition of this enzyme decreases the

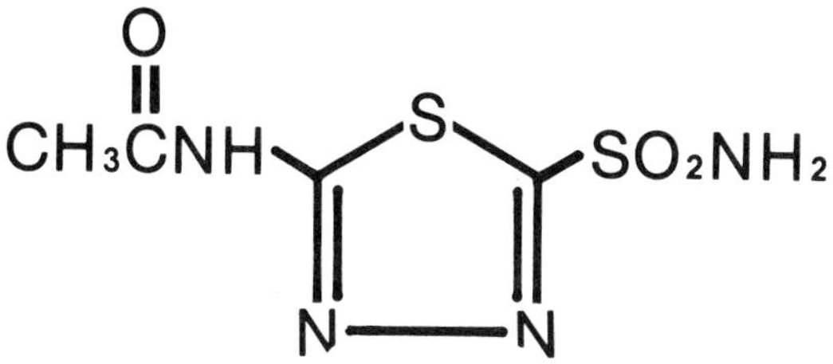

$$CH_3\overset{\displaystyle O}{\overset{\displaystyle \|}{C}}NH\text{—}\left\langle\begin{array}{c} S \\[-4pt] \\ N\text{——}N \end{array}\right\rangle\text{—}SO_2NH_2$$

Figure 10–2. Chemical structure of acetazolamide.

secretion of hydrogen ions and decreases the reabsorption of sodium and bicarbonate ions in the proximal tubules. The rejected sodium is not reabsorbed in the thick ascending segment of the loop of Henle, because it is accompanied by bicarbonate which is not reabsorbed in this segment.

In the distal nephron, carbonic anhydrase located in cells is involved in the formation of hydrogen ions, which compete with potassium ions in exchange for sodium ions in the lumen (see Fig. 10–3). Ammonia secreted by cells in the distal nephron serves to buffer the hydrogen ions as ammonium ions and thus allows secretion of hydrogen ions to continue. Inhibition of carbonic anhydrase here decreases the renal excretion of hydrogen ions as well as ammonia. The inhibition of hydrogen ions exchange for sodium ions results

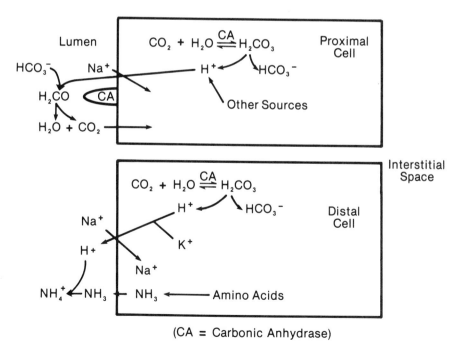

(CA = Carbonic Anhydrase)

Figure 10–3. Renal sites of carbonic anhydrase activity.

in an enhanced exchange of potassium for sodium ions. This increases the excretion of potassium and salvages some of the sodium ions. The increased quantity of sodium, potassium, and bicarbonate in the lumen serves to retain water and increase its excretion.

At maximally effective doses, only 5 percent of sodium reabsorption is affected by carbonic anhydrase inhibitors and the effect on sodium reabsorption is of short duration—just a few days. The short duration is due to the systemic acidosis produced by these agents as a result of the renal excretion of bicarbonate ions. The acidosis leads to an increased cellular uptake of hydrogen ions. In the kidney, this increased uptake can override the inhibition of carbonic anhydrase because the hydrogen ions taken up can enter into exchange for luminal sodium ions. Also, because of the acidosis, there is less bicarbonate in the blood and thus less is filtered. Since refractoriness develops within a few days, the usefulness of these agents as diuretics is severely limited.

Uses

Although seldom employed as a diuretic, these agents are used for other purposes. Because they also inhibit carbonic anhydrase activity in the eye, they decrease the formation of intraocular fluid; thus, they are useful in the treatment of **glaucoma**. They also are sometimes of value in the treatment of **epilepsy**. Their mechanism of action for this use is not clear but may be related to the systemic acidosis that they produce. More recently these agents have been found to be useful in the treatment of **acute mountain sickness**. The hyperventilation that occurs in patients with this condition leads to excessive loss of carbon dioxide and thus to the development of respiratory alkalosis. A carbonic anhydrase inhibitor helps to restore the normal ratio of bicarbonate to carbon dioxide by increasing the renal loss of bicarbonate. Restoration of the bicarbonate–to–carbon dioxide ratio, and hence plasma pH, relieves the symptoms related to the respiratory alkalosis. While these agents increase urinary pH and thus may increase renal excretion of weak organic acids, their use in poisonings is not advisable, because these agents produce a systemic acidosis that would decrease the ionization of weak organic acids and hence increase their volume of distribution. This would decrease their excretion but more importantly would increase cellular access, which could increase their toxicity.

Thiazide and Thiazide-Like Agents

Structurally, thiazide agents are derivatives of benzothiadiazine, and about a dozen such compounds have been marketed, such as **chlorothiazide** (Diuril) (Fig. 10–4) and **hydrochlorothiazide** (Hydro-Diuril, Esidrix). Compounds with other ring structures, however, exhibit similar activity. These

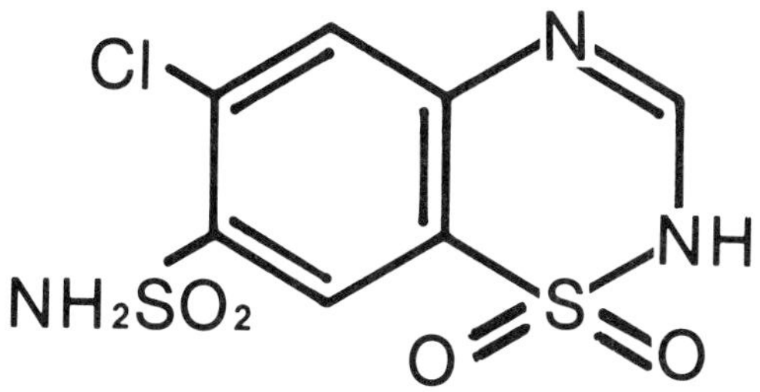

Figure 10–4. Chemical structure of chlorothiazide.

thiazide-like agents include a compound with a phthalimidine ring structure, e.g., **chlorthalidone** (Hygroton), as well as a quinazoline nucleus, e.g., **metolazone** (Diulo, Zaroxolyn).

Electrolyte Excretion Pattern

The thiazides increase the excretion of sodium ions, and these are matched by chloride ions. These agents also increase the excretion of potassium ions. The ions retain water in the lumen and thus increase urinary volume. As these compounds contain a sulfamyl group, they may also inhibit carbonic anhydrase. Thus, increases in the excretion of bicarbonate ions and decreases in the excretion of hydrogen ions and ammonia may also occur.

Site of Action

The primary site of action of these agents is on the luminal membrane of the distal convoluted tubules where they block the active reabsorption of sodium. This causes a decrease in the passive reabsorption of chloride ions. The increased quantity of sodium in the distal nephron stimulates the exchange mechanisms located here. Potassium for sodium exchange is usually stimulated most, as the carbonic anhydrase inhibitory activity of the compounds diminishes the exchange of hydrogen for sodium ions.

Comparison of Agents

All of the thiazide and thiazide-like agents are capable of inhibiting about the same fraction of sodium reabsorption (5 to 8 percent) at maximally effective doses. They differ markedly, however, in their dosage and duration of action. These differences appear to be related to their hydrophilic or lipophilic properties. Those agents with high water solubility (hydrophilic) are not absorbed as readily or as completely from the GI tract and thus require higher dosages. There is little metabolism of the thiazides, so that the rate of renal loss is the primary factor that determines their duration of action. Because these agents are highly bound to plasma proteins, glomerular filtration is not a major factor in their excretion. All of these agents are actively secreted by an organic anion transport system (*p*-aminohippurate system) located in the proximal tubules. Although all of the thiazide and thiazide-like agents are secreted by this system, they differ markedly as to whether they will remain in the tubules. The hydrophilic agents remain in the tubules and are excreted rapidly, whereas the lipophilic compounds diffuse out of the tubules and are eliminated very slowly. Thus, hydrophilic compounds such as chlorothiazide require greater dosages (500 to 1000 mg) and have short durations of action (6 to 8 hours), whereas lipophilic agents such as cyclothiazide require lesser dosages (1 to 2 mg) and have long durations of action (up to 2 days). All agents are marketed in oral forms; only a few are available for intravenous use.

Toxicity

Since these agents are relatively potent agents and may be used for many years, an appreciation of their toxicity is necessary in order to limit their adverse effects. An inspection of the toxicities of these agents reveals that many of the adverse effects are caused by excessive renal actions.

Excessive losses of sodium are capable of leading to too great a decrease in the extracellular space. With too great a decrease in plasma volume, hypotension and even shock can occur.

Thiazides can produce a systemic alkalosis, which is usually described as **contraction alkalosis**. This occurs because these drugs cause a loss of sodium and volume. Since the sodium loss is matched primarily with chloride ions, bicarbonate ions remaining in the extracellular space are now dissolved in a smaller volume. The concentration of bicarbonate is increased and this increases plasma pH.

Potassium excretion is increased by all of the thiazides and this produces a fall in the plasma level of this cation. By itself this change is asymptomatic if the concentration does not fall below 3 mEq per liter. Below this level, muscular weakness, as well as changes in the ECG, can occur. In certain individuals, however, even small decreases may be a problem. If a cardiac glycoside is also being used, decreases in the concentration of potassium in plasma will potentiate these compounds to produce intoxication. Recently the question has been raised as to the safety of the thiazides in individuals who are subject to arrhythmias. The Multiple Risk Factor Intervention Trial study found a higher mortality in this group of individuals when they were treated with a thiazide diuretic. It was suggested that the decreased concentration of potassium in plasma produced by the thiazides may have been involved. There are several different ways to prevent the decrease in the concentration of potassium. Potassium supplements may be given, or foods that are high in potassium (oranges, bananas, prunes) may be added to the diet. Another approach is to use a potassium-sparing diuretic agent with the thiazide. These drugs decrease the renal excretion of potassium and, with careful adjustment of dosages, enable maintenance of a normal plasma level of potassium. Still another approach is to decrease the amount of sodium in the diet. This allows a smaller dose of a thiazide to be employed, which in turn decreases the loss of potassium.

Since the thiazides are secreted by the organic anion transport system in the proximal tubules, they may displace other anions from this system. This occurs with uric acid with the result that the concentration of uric acid in plasma increases. Thiazides may also indirectly lead to an increase in the passive reabsorption of uric acid in the proximal tubules. As extracellular volume falls with chronic use of the thiazides, the proximal tubules are stimulated to increase the reabsorption of sodium and therefore water. As water is reabsorbed, it may carry a number of different substances, such as uric acid, with it. This process is termed bulk flow, and thiazides can also increase uric acid reabsorption in this manner. In most individuals, an increase in the plasma level of uric acid is of little consequence; in others, the level may already be elevated. Such individuals may be prone to develop gout, and a further increase in the concentration of uric acid in plasma could exceed the solubility of this substance and lead to its precipitation in tissue, and thus an acute attack of gout.

A number of different allergic responses to the thiazides have been reported. These range from mild reactions such as skin rashes to very serious problems such as agranulocytosis. Fortunately, the more serious problems are quite rare.

The thiazides have also been reported to alter the glucose tolerance curve and thus to induce diabetes mellitus. They are believed to act by decreasing the secretion of insulin, and stopping thiazide administration usually results in reversal of this condition. However, the fact that this condition occurred indicates that the patient is a borderline diabetic and is very likely to develop the disease in time.

Other toxicities that have been reported to occur with these agents include pancreatitis and nonocclusive intestinal infarction. It has been suggested that these toxicities may be related to excessive reduction of extracellular fluid. Severe reductions in plasma volume can lead to marked decreases in intestinal blood flow and consequently ischemia.

Advantages

When the thiazides first became available, they represented a major advance in diuretic therapy. They were effective by the oral route and furthermore could be used on a continuous basis without the patient becoming refractory to them. Although tolerance can develop, the agents will usually still continue to exert some activity if they are effective initially.

Limitations

Since their major site of action is on the distal convoluted tubules, their activity is limited to the amount of sodium that reaches this part of the nephron. In certain instances, particularly renal disease, the amount of sodium delivered to the distal nephron may be so reduced that no meaningful increase in loss can be attained. Attempts to increase the dose may be counterproductive because at higher doses the thiazides decrease renal blood flow.

Uses

The thiazides are useful in treating the **edema** of congestive heart failure as well as that of other causes. They are used with a cardiac glycoside in the treatment of congestive heart failure. Recently, however, they have been employed as the primary agent to treat congestive heart failure. Not only do they decrease plasma volume but more importantly they decrease preload to the heart.

All thiazide diuretics have relatively flat dose-response curves, which makes them relatively easy to handle. Thus, they are usually employed first in the treatment of edema. If, however, the response is not satisfactory, then a loop diuretic may be tried (see next section).

Another major use of these drugs is in the treatment of **hypertension,** and frequently thiazides will be the first drugs employed. The thiazides produce a modest decrease in blood pressure in hypertensive individuals, a response that is delayed in onset, usually taking a few days to occur. There appear to be two components to the decrease in pressure. Initially the increased loss of sodium results in a decrease in plasma volume, which contributes to the hypotensive effect. Within a few weeks the plasma volume is partially or totally restored, thus minimizing this component of the hypotensive action. In addition to reduction of plasma volume, it has been proposed that thiazides may alter electrolyte concentrations of blood vessels, making them less responsive to catecholamines or to stimulation by sympathetic nerves. It should also be noted that the hypotensive action of the thiazides is enhanced if they are used in conjunction with a low-sodium diet. Because the action of thiazides on blood pressure is modest, other agents must be given simultaneously to obtain a satisfactory response. The thiazides exhibit their greatest antihypertensive effectiveness when given along with other agents, whose action they potentiate. Thus, because other, more potent agents can be used in lower dosages, these agents produce fewer side effects. The potentiation is related to the reduction in plasma volume by the thiazides and to the prevention of sodium retention frequently produced by other agents.

Another use of the thiazides is to decrease the excretion of calcium ions to prevent **nephrolithiasis** caused by precipitation of calcium in the urinary tract. Thiazides may directly stimulate some calcium reabsorption in the distal nephron, but this effect on calcium excretion is not very marked. Usually, when thiazides are given, there is little change in the renal excretion of calcium ions initially. With chronic use, however, calcium excretion is decreased. This reduction in calcium excretion is due to an increase in the reabsorption of calcium ions in earlier segments of the tubules, and is related to the increase in the reabsorption of sodium induced by the thiazides. By increasing the excretion of sodium, thiazides cause a decrease in extracellular volume. This stimulates the early segments of the nephron to reabsorb a greater fraction of the filtered sodium. Since calcium reabsorption follows sodium reabsorption in the early segments (but not in the distal nephron), calcium reabsorption increases as sodium reabsorption increases. As long as a deficit of sodium in the body is maintained, calcium excretion will be diminished and presumably the frequency of calcium stones will be reduced.

Metolazone (Diulo, Zaroxolyn) is a thiazide-like agent that deserves special mention because some of its actions differ from those of the thiazides. It does not decrease renal blood flow, and in addition it appears to act on the proximal tubules to inhibit some reabsorption of sodium. For these reasons, unlike other thiazides, metolazone is more likely to be useful in the treatment of edema of renal origin. The inhibition of sodium reabsorption in the proximal tubules increases the delivery of sodium to the later segments of the tubule where the usual action of the thiazides occurs. Thus the compound acts to provide its own substrate. As the agent does not decrease renal blood flow, it does not limit its usefulness at higher dosages, as the other thiazides do.

Loop Diuretics

Agents that are called loop diuretics are also referred to as high-ceiling diuretics. The term "loop diuretics" is used because the primary site of action of these agents is on the thick ascending segments of the loop of Henle. They are also called "high-ceiling diuretics" because these agents can produce a greater excretion of sodium than other classes of diuretic agents. Agents in this class include furosemide (Lasix) (Fig. 10–5), bumetanide (Bumex), and ethacrynic acid (Edecrin) (Fig. 10–6). While structurally quite different, these agents have very similar effects on the kidneys.

Electrolyte Excretion Pattern

Loop diuretics increase the excretion of sodium, chloride, and water and at maximally effective doses are capable of inhibiting about 20 percent of the reabsorption of these substances. Potassium excretion is also increased by these agents. Because furosemide is also an inhibitor of carbonic anhydrase, this agent increases the excretion of bicarbonate ions and decreases the excretion of hydrogen ions and ammonia.

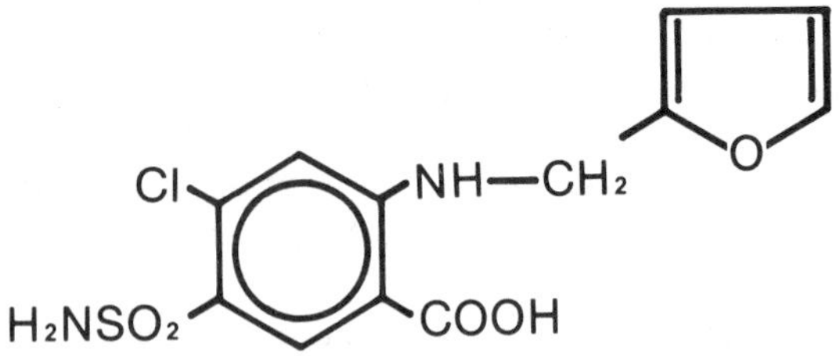

Figure 10–5. Chemical structure of furosemide.

Site of Action

The loop diuretics inhibit the cotransport of sodium chloride in the thick ascending segment of the loop of Henle by an action on the luminal membrane. Inhibition of the reabsorption of sodium and chloride in this segment leads to a dissipation of the elevated osmotic pressure of the medullary portion of the kidney. This occurs because the elevated sodium chloride concentration in this area must be continually replaced or it will be removed by blood flow to the medulla. As the elevated osmotic gradient is removed, the ability of the kidneys to form a concentrated urine (i.e., a urine with an osmotic pressure greater than that of plasma) is lost. In addition, because of the loss of the gradient, the water that is normally reabsorbed from the thin descending segment of the loop of Henle will remain in the tubules and be excreted. Furthermore, the lack of reabsorption of sodium and chloride in the thick ascending segment compromises the ability of the kidneys to form a dilute urine. This occurs because sodium and chloride are normally reabsorbed in this segment while water is not, thus leading to the formation of a dilute fluid. With sodium and chloride reabsorption inhibited, an isosmotic fluid leaves this segment. While dilution can still occur in the later segments of the nephron, the dilutional process is severely limited when reabsorption of sodium chloride is inhibited in this segment. The increased delivery of sodium ions to the distal nephron stimulates the exchange mechanisms, which salvages some of the sodium. With all loop diuretics, there is an increased exchange of potassium for sodium. With ethacrynic acid, which is not an inhibitor of carbonic anhydrase, an increased exchange of hydrogen ions for sodium ions also occurs; thus, it causes urine to become acidic. With furosemide, urinary pH increases because of the increased excretion of bicarbonate.

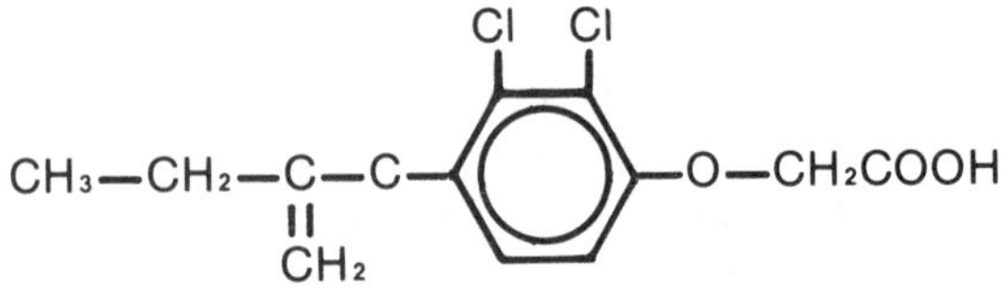

Figure 10–6. Chemical structure of ethacrynic acid.

The loop diuretics possess cardiovascular actions also. They are capable of increasing renal blood flow by a mechanism that involves an increase in the synthesis and release of vasodilatory eicosanoids by the kidney. These agents also increase venous capacitance by a mechanism involving eicosanoids. Both of these actions add to the clinical usefulness of the loop diuretics.

Disposition

Loop diuretics act within an hour after oral administration and within minutes after intravenous administration. All have a duration of action of approximately 4 to 6 hours. Metabolism plays little part in terminating their action. The short duration of action is due to rapid renal excretion. All of the agents are secreted by the organic anion transport system and, as they are hydrophilic compounds, they remain in the tubules and are excreted. With ethacrynic acid, conversion to a cysteine adduct by the kidneys is essential since this is the active form of this diuretic.

Toxicity

As with the thiazides, most of the toxicity of loop diuretics is related to excessive renal actions due to overuse or overdosage. Furthermore, the toxicities of the loop diuretics are very similar to those seen with the thiazides.

Because loop diuretics are more efficacious than the thiazides, volume depletion can occur faster and be more severe.

Contraction alkalosis also occurs with these agents. As with the thiazides, sodium loss is not balanced by a loss of chloride and bicarbonate ions in the same ratio as they are present in plasma. The greater loss of sodium with chloride ions leaves bicarbonate ions behind, but now dissolved in a smaller volume of water; this increases the pH.

Potassium excretion increases as sodium excretion increases. Thus, with loop diuretics, potassium losses may be greater and similar problems (as discussed in the section on thiazide agents) will occur.

Because these agents are secreted by the organic anion transport system in the proximal tubules, they can displace other anions handled by this system (such as uric acid). Uric acid reabsorption may be increased with loop diuretics—just as with the thiazides—by increasing bulk flow in the proximal tubules. Hence, these agents can produce gout in susceptible individuals.

Diabetes mellitus, pancreatitis, and nonocclusive intestinal infarction also can occur with these agents. As with the thiazides, it has been suggested that excessive depletion of extracellular volume may play a role in the development of these toxicities.

Loss of hearing has been reported with all loop diuretics. Usually this is temporary, but occasionally a permanent loss occurs. This form of **ototoxicity** is dose-related; it is usually seen only with very large doses. The concurrent use of other ototoxic agents (e.g., aminoglycoside antibiotics) increases the frequency of this toxicity. Of the three agents discussed, bumetanide may be the least ototoxic. Although probably as toxic as furosemide on a molar basis, bumetanide is 40 times as active as a diuretic on a molar basis; thus, it is less likely to produce ototoxicity when employed at similar diuretic dosages.

Although some gastric symptoms are reported on occasion with all of the loop diuretics, ethacrynic acid is particularly prone to produce marked **gastric distress**. This occurs with both oral and intravenous administration.

A variety of allergic responses have been reported, but their frequency is not high. If an allergy does develop to a thiazide or to one of the sulfamyl-containing loop diuretics, ethacrynic acid may be substituted. Since it is so different structurally, overlapping allergenicity is unlikely.

Uses

These agents are useful in the treatment of most types of edema. Not only are they more efficacious than other diuretics, but also they are more likely to be effective. Whereas the thiazides are reported to be useful in approximately 80 to 85 percent of patients for whom diuretics are indicated, the loop diuretics are reported to be useful in approximately 95 percent of such patients.

The thiazides are usually tried first in cardiac edema, but loop diuretic agents are also effective. Furthermore, they are apt to be more effective than the thiazides when used as the primary agent in the treatment of congestive heart failure.

Spironolactone is usually employed first in the treatment of the ascites of hepatic disease, but loop diuretics may be added if spironolactone alone is not effective. However, extreme caution must be employed. In hepatic cirrhosis, plasma volume is decreased owing to a decrease in the concentration of albumin. A potent diuretic such as a loop agent may cause too great a loss of sodium, thus decreasing both interstitial and plasma volumes. With plasma volume already decreased, any further decrease could result in inadequate circulating volume and lead to hypotension or shock. This could precipitate hepatorenal syndrome (the addition of severe renal failure to hepatic disease). The cause is unknown, but it has been hypothesized that nephrotoxic substances previously inactivated by the liver increase in concentration. In addition, vasoconstrictor substances may be increased, which could suppress renal blood flow.

Other problems can also occur with these agents in the treatment of hepatic disease. The concentration of aldosterone is increased because it is not metabolized as efficiently in hepatic disease and also because of enhanced secretion due to decreased effective plasma volumes. The increased levels of this hormone enhance renal loss of potassium; consequently, the concentration of potassium in plasma is already decreased, and the loop diuretics will add to this. Another problem relates to the production of alkalosis produced by these agents and the resultant decrease in the excretion of ammonia by the kidneys. Because ammonia metabolism by the diseased liver is decreased, reductions in renal loss can cause plasma levels to increase; such changes can lead to the development of hepatic coma.

If renal disease is present, loop agents are the preferred diuretics. Their ability to increase renal blood flow adds to their usefulness. Also, since they act in an earlier segment of the nephron than the thiazides, they are more likely to produce a loss of sodium. If no response is obtained with usual doses of these agents, the dosage may be increased until a response is obtained. Regimens for dosages of 4 g per day for furosemide, compared with the usual dose of 40 mg per day, have been published. Increasing the dose to these levels is possible, as most of the toxic effects of these agents are caused by excessive renal actions. The use of other agents that act in the proximal tubules to block sodium reabsorption may potentiate the action loop diuretics by delivering more sodium to the ascending limb of the loops of Henle. Thus, metolazone may be combined with a loop diuretic agent to produce a greater response.

The use of a loop diuretic such as furosemide may be lifesaving in the treatment of pulmonary edema. Although useful for reducing plasma volume by their diuretic action, these agents produce an improvement in the symptoms of pulmonary edema prior to or in the absence of diuresis. This latter action is due to their ability to increase venous capacitance, which causes a shift of fluid from the pulmonary circuit to the systemic circuit, and hence the beneficial effect. For treatment of pulmonary edema the intravenous forms of these drugs are indicated.

In addition to these actions, these drugs are also useful in a number of nonedematous conditions such as hypertension. In this regard, however, they do not appear to be as useful as the thiazide diuretics. Although their natriuretic action decreases plasma volume, loop diuretics do not appear to affect the arterioles, whereas the thiazides do. If hypertension is associated with renal disease, however, the loop diuretics are preferred.

Another use of loop agents is to increase the excretion of calcium ions. In the thick ascending limb of the loop of Henle, calcium is reabsorbed and this occurs in association with sodium reabsorption. Thus, when sodium chloride reabsorption is inhibited by a loop diuretic, calcium reabsorption is also inhibited. This action is useful in the treatment of the hypercalcemia of hyperparathyroidism.

Potassium-Sparing Diuretics

Agents in this category decrease the excretion of potassium, while increasing the excretion of sodium. They are frequently used with diuretics that increase potassium excretion in order to offset this loss. There are two classes of these agents: (1) competitive antagonists of aldosterone and (2) inhibitors of the permeability of the distal nephron to sodium.

Spironolactone (Aldactone)

This agent is a competitive antagonist of aldosterone and thus exerts a very modest effect on sodium reabsorption, inhibiting at most only 2 percent of sodium reabsorption. Because the compound inhibits aldosterone, it is effective only in the presence of this hormone. In addition to increasing sodium excretion and decreasing potassium excretion, increases in chloride and bicarbonate ions and water excretion are produced while potassium and hydrogen ion excretion are decreased.

Site and Mechanism of Action. The tubular sites of action of spironolactone are the cortical and medullary collecting tubules. Here spironolactone competes with aldosterone for receptor sites on an endoplasmic transport protein. While the inhibition occurs within minutes after administration, the onset of changes in renal excretion of electrolytes takes several hours to occur. This is because aldosterone acts by stimulating the synthesis of a peptide which then acts to stimulate exchange of potassium or hydrogen ions for sodium ions. The delay in onset of action of spironolactone is due to the time required for catabolism of previously synthesized peptide.

Toxicity. Spironolactone can cause sodium depletion, but it is not likely to be as severe or as fast in onset as with more potent natriuretic agents.

With spironolactone, retention of potassium can occur, which can lead to muscular weakness as well as serious cardiac arrhythmias. If this agent is used to offset the loss of potassium induced by a potassium-losing diuretic, it should not be used in conjunction with potassium supplements or a high-potassium diet, as this would result in excessive retention of potassium. If potassium retention occurs, then spironolactone will inhibit the activity of the cardiac glycosides. Thus, an individual who is well regulated on a cardiac glycoside could slip out of control and into cardiac decompensation.

Spironolactone also possesses weak **androgenic activity**. In females and children this can result in masculinizing effects, whereas in males this weak androgen competes with the more potent androgen, testosterone, to produce feminizing effects.

On the basis of animal studies, the compound is considered to be carcinogenic. Thus, it should probably not be used for long-term therapy.

Uses. Spironolactone is available for oral administration and is used primarily to offset the excretion of potassium produced by the thiazides and loop diuretics, especially when these agents are used concurrently with a cardiac glycoside. It is also used as the initial diuretic in the treatment of the ascites of hepatic disease, since aldosterone levels are elevated here.

Triamterene (Dyrenium) and Amiloride (Midamor)

These agents act on the distal nephron to decrease its permeability to sodium. This results in an increase in the excretion of sodium, chloride, and bicarbonate ions. The decrease in the reabsorption of sodium decreases the exchange for potassium and hydrogen ions and thus decreases their excretion. Unlike spironolactone, these potassium-sparing agents are effective in the absence of aldosterone. Furthermore, they are more efficacious, being capable of inhibiting as much as 5 percent of sodium reabsorption at maximally effective doses. They have an onset of action within 1 to 2 hours following oral administration, and peak activity occurs at 6 to 8 hours.

Toxicity. Sodium depletion is again possible with these agents but less likely than with the more efficacious thiazide and loop diuretics.

Potassium retention is more apt to be a problem, as these agents cause a greater decrease in the excretion of potassium than spironolactone causes. They should not be used in combination with potassium supplements or a high-potassium diet.

The chief drawback in the use of these agents is gastric distress. Even when taken with meals, these drugs are intolerable for many patients.

Uses. These agents, like spironolactone, are used primarily with the thiazides or loop diuretics to offset the potassium losses induced by the more potent agents. Although they have opposite effects on potassium, their effects on sodium are additive.

Osmotic Diuretics

Osmotic diuretics are used when there is a need to increase urinary volume but not to increase loss of sodium. Agents that are useful as osmotic agents are substances that are very hydrophilic and thus do not cross cellular membranes very readily. Such substances, when filtered at the glomeruli, will remain in the tubular lumen. In the proximal tubules when an osmotic gradient cannot be established, these agents decrease the reabsorption of water. This occurs because these agents themselves are not reabsorbed and exert an osmotic effect, holding water in the tubules. They also decrease water reabsorption from the descending segment of the loop of Henle because of their osmotic action. Thus, they increase the volume remaining in the tubules, which leads to an increase in urinary volume.

Osmotic diuretics have a fast onset but short duration of action. Most of the substances must be given intravenously, as they are too hydrophilic to be absorbed from the GI tract in amounts sufficient to be effective. Osmotic agents include mannitol and urea, which are infused intravenously in hyperosmotic solutions.

Uses

Osmotic diuretics have several uses.

1. They can increase the excretion of a poisonous substance.
2. Surgically, they can prevent deterioration of or restore renal function.
3. In neurosurgery, because they do not penetrate the blood-brain barrier, their osmotic pressure causes water to move out of the CNS, thus decreasing cerebral edema and affording the surgeon more working space.
4. They can also be used as a last resort to treat the edema of renal disease: If no other agent exerts any effect, these agents could cause some increase in urinary volume and thus could help to increase the loss of water and other substances.

ANTIDIURETIC AGENTS

Antidiuretic agents are used in the treatment of diabetes insipidus. This condition may be of CNS or renal origin. If of CNS origin, there is a decrease in the secretion of **ADH (vasopressin)** by the posterior pituitary. If of renal origin, the renal tubules, because of disease, no longer respond to ADH. The net effect in diabetes insipidus of either CNS or renal origin is the same. Water entering the collection tubules will remain in the tubules and be excreted. This can amount to as much as 20 liters of fluid per day.

To treat diabetes insipidus of CNS origin, replacement therapy with ADH is indicated. There are a number of preparations available, including synthetic compounds as well as the purified hormone obtained from hogs and cattle. The hormone found in cattle is arginine vasopressin, the same as human ADH, whereas the hormone found in hogs is lysine vasopressin, which differs by one amino acid from human ADH. Synthetic **lysine vasopressin** and a synthetic analog of lysine vasopressin, **desmopressin,** are available. Because ADH is a peptide, it is destroyed in the GI tract following oral administration. Previous therapy consisted of giving ADH parenterally, usually subcutaneously. Giving vasopressin in oil or as a tannate salt in oil delays its absorption from injection sites and hence prolongs duration of action. More recently a number of preparations have become available that allow ADH to be given intranasally, as absorption across nasal mucosa occurs without destruction of the peptide. For this route of administration, nose drops, nasal sprays, and powders for insufflation are available.

To treat diabetes insipidus of renal origin, other forms of therapy had to be developed, as administering ADH is of no value: indeed, in this condition, there is an elevated concentration of ADH in plasma. The only drugs that have been found to be useful are the more potent diuretics—the thiazides and the loop diuretics. These agents decrease the extracellular volume by increasing the excretion of sodium. By inducing a decrease in extracellular volume, the proximal segments of the kidneys are stimulated to increase the reabsorption of sodium and water to replace the volume lost. The increase in the reabsorption of water in the proximal segments of the nephron results in less water getting to more distal segments. Thus, if less water gets to the collecting ducts, then less water will be available for loss. As long as the diuretic is given and a deficit of sodium maintained, this form of therapy will result in a decrease in the daily urine volumes of these patients. The effect is not the same as that obtained with ADH. Whereas the hormone is capable of decreasing urinary volume and increasing urinary osmostic pressure to values of 1200 mOsm per kg water, the use of a diuretic causes a decrease in urinary volume but does not result in excretion of a concentrated urine. Osmotic pressures will be no greater than plasma osmotic pressure. With this form of therapy only about a 50 percent decrease in urinary volume is possible.

ANTAGONISTS OF ANTIDIURETIC HORMONE

There is a need for antagonists of ADH in the treatment of inappropriate secretion of ADH (SIADH). In this condition, ADH continues to be secreted, even though plasma osmolality is diminished. A useful agent in the treatment of water intoxication due to SIADH is **demeclocycline,** a tetracycline antibiotic. Lithium carbonate has also been employed. Both agents inhibit the action of ADH on the renal tubules. The mechanism by which these agents act has not been established. Several peptide-competitive antagonists are currently under study and may soon be available.

URICOSURIC DRUGS

These agents increase the urinary excretion of uric acid. Their primary use is in the treatment of **gout.** In this condition, there is an increase in the concentration of uric acid in plasma to the point at which solubility is exceeded and uric acid precipitates. When deposits occur in the joints (as in an acute attack), there is a great deal of pain. The body's response to the crystals is to encapsulate them. These enlarged areas, called **tophi,** can result in a loss of mobility of the affected joints.

One form of therapy in the treatment of gout is to increase the renal excretion of uric acid. If excretion is increased, the concentration of uric acid in plasma will fall and uric acid previously precipitated will, in time, go back into solution. Thus, it is possible to cause the tophi to decrease in size and to restore mobility of the joints.

Uric acid is handled by the kidneys by several processes. It is filtered at the glomeruli, secreted by the organic anion transport system in the proximal tubules, and actively reabsorbed. Useful uricosuric drugs include **probenecid (Benemid)** and **sulfinpyrazone (Anturane)**. These agents affect both transport mechanisms for uric acid. Because the drugs are organic acids they are secreted by the organic anion transport system and, having a higher affinity than uric acid for the transport system, they readily displace uric acid. This effect occurs first, and thus uric acid levels may increase initially and may produce an acute attack of gout. As levels of the drugs increase, they will inhibit the reabsorption of uric acid, and thus increase the renal excretion of uric acid. When uric acid excretion is increased, it is possible that its solubility may be exceeded and it will precipitate out in the urinary tract. Alkalinization of the urine by administration of sodium bicarbonate increases the solubility of uric acid and thus minimizes this problem. Increasing fluid intake is also advisable.

Other drugs may also be used in the management of gout, including **allopurinol (Zyloprim)**, which inhibits xanthine oxidase and thus decreases the synthesis of uric acid, and **colchicine**, which exerts an anti-inflammatory effect during acute attacks (see Chapter 12, Anti-Inflammatory Drugs).

CHAPTER 11
Endocrine Drugs

P. MICHAEL CONN, Ph.D.

Endocrine pharmacology is one of the least complicated areas in pharmacology. Most clinical problems can readily be explained in the majority of cases; they originate from too much or too little availability of a hormone. In other cases the blood levels are correct, but they are incorrectly sensed by target cell **receptors**. In the event that too little hormone is available, the problem is corrected by replacement therapy or by stimulation of endogenous release. In the event the problem results from too much hormone, therapy is directed toward inhibition of synthesis, inhibition of release, or blockade of action at the level of the target cell. In some cases the release pattern is abnormal. An understanding of endocrine pharmacology requires knowledge of the methods by which hormones are stored, synthesized, and released as well as the means by which circulating levels are sensed. Hormones are also useful for testing components of integrated systems (e.g., testing the ability of the pituitary to release thyroid-stimulating hormone in response to its releasing hormone) and for controlling cell regulatory processes in order to relieve non-endocrine disease states (e.g., preventing inflammation with glucocorticoids). Accordingly, the major developmental work in endocrine pharmacology has been directed toward identification, isolation, and synthesis of biologically active compounds and toward preparation of agonistic and antagonistic derivatives that may be administered conveniently.

PITUITARY AND HYPOTHALAMIC HORMONES

The pituitary produces a number of protein hormones (some are glycoproteins) that have as targets plasma membrane receptors in peripheral tissues (Fig. 11–1). Hormones released include growth hormone, prolactin, adreno-

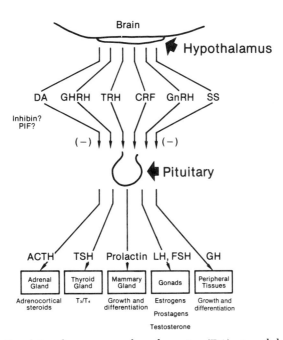

Figure 11–1. Regulatory hormones such as dopamine (DA), growth hormone-releasing hormone (GHRH), thyrotropin-releasing hormone (TRH), corticotropin-releasing factor (CRF), gonadotropin-releasing hormone (GnRH), and somatostatin (SS) act on the pituitary gland to release (or inhibit the release of) trophic hormones that act on distal tissues. These trophic hormones include adrenocorticotropic hormone (ACTH), thyroid-stimulating hormone (TSH), prolactin, luteinizing hormone (LH), follicle-stimulating hormone (FSH), and growth hormone (GH) and provoke both growth and metabolic alterations at sites distal to the pituitary gland. The existence of prolactin-inhibiting factor (PIF) and inhibin remain in question.

corticotropic hormone, luteinizing hormone, follicle-stimulating hormone, and thyroid-stimulating hormone. These are released by chemical mediators that are synthesized in the median eminence of the hypothalamus and carried to the pituitary (adenohypophysis) by the portal system, which traverses the stock and forms sinusoids in the anterior pituitary. These are peptides and proteins themselves and may range from 3 to 42 or more amino acids. Some of these are available as synthetic products, and there is considerable interest in these compounds for their therapeutic potential (for causing release of endogenous hormones and in testing pituitary responsiveness).

Anterior Lobe Pituitary Hormones

Growth Hormone (GH, Somatotropin)

This is the best stored of all the pituitary hormones; therefore, initial preparations were from cadaver material. This hormone has been extensively purified. There appears to be some cross-species homology, although animal-derived GH does not produce good efficacy when used in human treatment. Accordingly, human-derived material is needed for replacement. There is enhanced activity associated with some fragments of this molecule. It is a protein and therefore is destroyed in the GI tract; accordingly, oral administration of growth hormone is of little value. *In vivo* this hormone stimulates protein synthesis and growth in bone, skin, muscle, and viscera; many actions of GH are indirect, being mediated by somatomedin. Adenoma leads to **gigantism** if levels of this hormone are enhanced prior to puberty. It leads to **acromegaly** (tissue overgrowth) if elevation occurs after epiphyseal closure. This compound is now available for some experimental use although its general availability has been limited because of the difficulty of obtaining large quantities of this hormone. GH has major anti-insulin actions including increased gluconeogenesis, increased lipolysis, increased ketogenesis, and decreased lipogenesis.

At the time of preparation of this volume, concern arose that patients receiving some batches of GH developed Jakob-Creutzfeldt disease, a fatal dementia, suggesting potential contamination with slow virus-like agents. Material prepared by genetic engineering is now available and will likely supplant the need. Hypothalamic releasing hormones that release endogenous growth hormone may prove to be useful in the near future, but these can be used only when the existing pituitary gland is capable of synthesizing and releasing GH.

Prolactin

This compound is chemically similar to growth hormone, and purification of prolactin from growth hormone has been difficult. It stimulates the production of milk (an action that is antagonized by estrogens). High levels of prolactin inhibit ovulation; the mechanism for this is not clear, although it is now apparent that gonadal binding sites exist for this pituitary hormone. Prolactin is released constitutively by the pituitary gland, and regulation of this hormone appears to be by inhibition of release. Although a **prolactin-inhibiting factor** (PIF) has not yet been identified with certainty, several laboratories are making major efforts in this area; other laboratories feel that dopamine may fulfill the requirements of a PIF. The placenta produces human chorionic somatomammotropin (human placental lactogen, hPL), which is a prolactin-growth hormone-like material.

Adrenocorticotropic Hormone (ACTH)

ACTH stimulates cortisol, androstenedione, and transiently, aldosterone production by the adrenal gland. Animal-derived preparations of this material that are bioactive are available. Pituitary tumors (of the corticotrope cell) may produce symptoms identical to overproduction of cortisol in the adrenal gland, as adrenal cortisol is stimulated by high levels of ACTH (Cushing's disease). Chronic increases in ACTH result in adrenal cortex hyperplasia. ACTH is released in times of stress in response to corticotropin releasing factor (40 amino acid protein released from the hypothalamus). ACTH release is inhibited by cortisol. ACTH replacement, in the case of a destroyed pituitary gland, is a significant use of this hormone.

Gonadotropins (LH, FSH)

Luteinizing hormone (LH, sometimes called interstitial cell–stimulating hormone, or ICSH, in the male) and follicle-stimulating hormone (FSH) are present in both sexes. LH regulates gonadal steroidogenesis and provokes ovulation. FSH regulates growth of the Graafian follicle and sperm production. The administration of LH and FSH, along with clomiphene, induces ovulation. Release of LH and FSH are stimulated by a decapeptide released from the hypothalamus (GnRH) by a calcium-dependent mechanism. By some as yet unclear means, regulation of LH and FSH appears to be differentially controlled (possibly due to altered effects of these hormones or due to "inhibin"). GnRH is useful in treatment of some forms of infertility states, cryptorchidism, and precocious puberty. It can be used as a contraceptive as well as a means of producing chemical castration for the treatment of hormone-dependent neoplasia. In 1985 the first GnRH analog (Leuprolide) received FDA clearance in the United States; others are currently in use in Europe. A nonpituitary compound (human chorionic gonadotropin, HCG) is released from the placenta. It is LH-like in its actions and important in diagnosis of pregnancy.

Thyroid-Stimulating Hormone (TSH, Thyrotropin)

TSH normally stimulates events associated with the production and release of thyroid hormones. These include increased growth and vascularity of the thyroid, enhanced iodide uptake, and increased synthesis release of thyroid hormones (T_4 and T_3). Lack of sufficient TSH leads to thyroid gland atrophy and hypothyroidism. TSH itself is released in response to that of hypothalamic **thyrotropin-releasing hormone** (TRH) from the hypothalamus. Altered levels of TRH are released in response to environmental temperature changes or other physiological stresses (such as starvation). Because TRH is a small molecule (tripeptide) it can be synthesized inexpensively and with high purity. Consequently it is extremely useful for testing components of the hypothalamic-pituitary-thyroid axis. Infusion of TRH should be followed by a prompt elevation of serum TSH, unless the pituitary is not functional or has been suppressed by elevated levels of thyroid hormones.

TSH is sometimes used to enhance radioiodine uptake during thyroid ablation in patients with hyperthyroidism. Antibodies often appear when bovine TSH is administered; TSH should not be used when angina pectoris is present following a recent myocardial infarction or in congestive heart failure. Side effects include swelling of the thyroid gland, arrhythmias, atrial fibrillation, tachycardia, nausea, and vomiting.

Intermediate Lobe Pituitary Hormones

α- and β-Melanocyte–Stimulating Hormone (MSH)

Hormones present in the intermediate lobe include α- and β-melanocyte–stimulating hormone (MSH). The role of these hormones in humans remains unclear (in amphibia, they appear to regulate pigmentation). Because of the chemical similarity between MSH and ACTH, the hyperpigmentation observed with elevated ACTH (Addison's syndrome) may be mediated by cross-reaction at MSH receptors in the skin. Hyperpigmentation may also be due to cleavage of ACTH into α-MSH and cosynthesis of ACTH and β-MSH (derived from the same precursor).

Posterior (Neural) Lobe Pituitary Hormones

Vasopressin (Antidiuretic Hormone, ADH)

Vasopressin, or antidiuretic hormone (ADH), is made in nerve cells of the supraoptic and paraventricular nuclei in the hypothalamus. Vasopressin is stored in the posterior lobe and released, at least in part, owing to the actions of osmoceptors and volume receptors. Secretion of this hormone is inhibited by alcohol, leading to diuresis. Vasopressin binds to renal tissues, activates cyclic adenosine monophosphate (AMP) production, and leads to water retention. Side effects in its use include nausea, vomiting, and uterine cramps; this compound also may provoke angina due to coronary restriction in patients with coronary atherosclerosis. Recent studies suggest that elevation of vasopressin leads to release of atrial natriuretic factor from heart tissue, suggesting a role for this peptide in volume regulation (see further on). Vasopressin is an effective treatment of diabetes insipidus, reducing urine produced to normal levels.

Oxytocin

Oxytocin is also produced in the neural lobe. This compound stimulates uterine smooth muscle contraction following conditioning of the uterus by gonadal steroids. It stimulates mammary smooth muscle contraction (the milk "let-down" phenomenon). It is frequently used in humans to induce labor, although its use is contraindicated if the pelvis is too small or the patient has had recent uterine surgery, as it is associated with a significant incidence of uterine rupture in such patients.

THYROID HORMONES (T_3, T_4) AND ANTITHYROID AGENTS

Biosynthesis of T_3 and T_4

Circulating levels of iodide are low; for this reason the first event in the production of **thyroid hormones** is the active concentration of this ion in the thyroid gland. Inborn errors in iodide uptake lead to the formation of a **goiter**. Because accumulation of iodide occurs against a concentration gradient, energy must be used. In a healthy individual the ratio of iodide in the thyroid gland to iodide in the plasma is in the range of 20:1 to 200:1. More than 95 percent of the body's iodide is located in the thyroid gland. After transport into the thyroid gland, iodide is "activated" to a form that can react with tyrosine residues on the high molecular weight protein thyroglobulin. **Monoiodotyrosine** (MIT) and **diiodotyrosine** (DIT) are thereby formed on the **thyroglobulin**. Two molecules of DIT, while still attached to the thyroglobulin, interact to form one molecule of T_4 (3,5,3'5' tetraiodothyronine) (Fig. 11–2). One molecule of MIT plus one molecule of DIT interact to form one molecule of T_3 (3,5,3'-triiodothyronine) (although this is not the only source of T_3 in the circulation, since it can also arise from the deiodination of T_4). MIT is preferentially formed in cases of iodide deficiency. In cases of severe iodide deficiency, no active products whatever are formed. In response to **thyroid stimulating hormone** (TSH) thyroglobulin is proteolyzed and T_3 and T_4 are released to the circulation. For this reason proteolysis is an important regulatory step in the release of thyroid hormones.

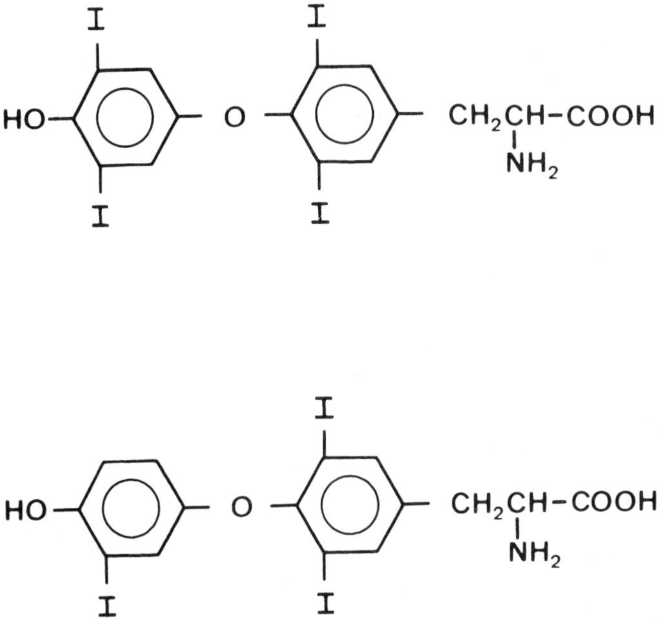

Figure 11–2. Structure of thyroid hormones T_4 and T_3.

While T_3 and T_4 are both active principles of thyroid hormone they differ markedly in the amount released daily, the rate of degradation, the amount in the circulation, their state in the circulation, and their origin. T_3 is approximately three times more potent than T_4. This information is summarized in Table 11–1.

General Metabolic Actions of T_3 and T_4

T_3 and T_4 are important regulators of growth and development. In fact, thyroid hormones are required to maintain most mammalian cells in culture. A characteristic action of T_3 and T_4 is enhancement of the metabolic rate. This is evidenced by enhanced heat production, enhanced oxygen consumption (except in pituitary tissue), enhanced cardiac output, enhanced gastrointestinal motility, enhanced bone turnover, and nervous system irritability.

Thyroid Disorders

Hypothyroidism. Restriction of dietary iodide (as is available in fish, for example) leads to the formation of goiter. Kelp is an excellent source of iodide, but this is not a common element of diets outside the Orient. While it is generally believed that other vegetables are an excellent source of iodide, this is not so, as it would take approximately 15 pounds of vegetables daily to provide

Table 11–1. COMPARISON OF T_4 AND T_3

	T_4	T_3
Daily release	75 μg	25 μg
Degradation	$t_{1/2} = 6-7$ days	Fivefold faster (note: hypothyroid state slows degradation)
Normal level	5–12 μg%	0.1–0.15 μg%
State in circu-lation*	85% bound to acid glycoprotein 15% bound to prealbumin Small fraction free	Binds less well to carriers
Source	Synthesized in thyroid	Half from T_4

*Note that the binding proteins are increased by estrogens and decreased by androgens or by loss in nephrotic syndrome. Binding is inhibited by phenytoin, aspirin, dinitrophenol.

the 100 to 200 μg daily adult requirement for iodide. In the United States iodide deficiency is very rare because of the widespread use of iodized salt. Diseases of hypothyroidism include **athyrotic cretinism** (failure of the thyroid to develop), defects in synthesis and release of thyroid hormones, or failure of sufficient thyroid hormone to be released as a defect secondary to the lack of TSH availability from the pituitary gland. Congenital **hypothyroidism** is called **cretinism**. Individuals suffering from this disease have a characteristic puffy, expressionless face, shortened extremities, poor appetite, and low body temperature and pulse rate. If hypothyroidism occurs during childhood, growth is greatly retarded. Hypothyroidism occurring in adults leads to **myxedema,** which is characterized by retardation of mental and physical activities, dry and sparse hair, dry pale skin, anemia, constipation, and cold intolerance. A common cause of hypothyroidism (especially among women) is an immune disorder, Hashimoto's thyroiditis, exhibiting antibodies directed against the thyroid gland.

Hyperthyroidism. This disorder is occasionally neoplastic but is usually seen as a **thyrotoxic goiter (Graves' disease)** resulting from the accumulation of an immunoglobulin in the serum. This immunoglobulin, variously called LATS (**long-acting thyroid stimulator**) or TSI (**thyroid-stimulating immuno-globulin**), is actually an antibody to the TSH receptor. It is able to mimic the actions of TSH and to stimulate the thyroid gland to produce T_3 and T_4. It is an excellent example of a newly understood class of diseases wherein antibodies to receptors are able to stimulate hormone-like actions. In other cases, hormone actions may be either blocked or stimulated by similar antibodies.

Thyroid Hormone Preparations

A number of different preparations are available. These include powders from animal thyroid glands (which are disadvantageous in that they vary

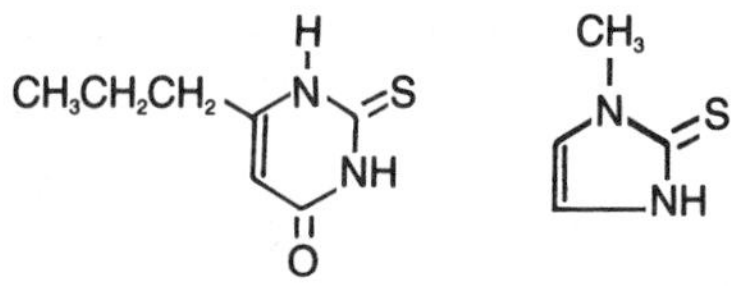

Propylthiouracil   Methimazole

Figure 11-3. Thiocarbamides.

widely in potency and T_4:T_3 proportions), thyroglobulin itself (which must be proteolyzed prior to being active), synthetic and pure T_3 (Liothyronine) and T_4 (Levothyroxine), or combinations of these hormones mixed together in a fixed ratio (Liotrix). Specific indications for use of these agents are TSH, T_3, or T_4 insufficiency; however, their use is contraindicated in heart disease as they may provoke congestive heart failure or coronary insufficiency. Overtreatment with these agents is characterized by signs of excessive metabolic stimulation, hypertension, arrhythmias, and nervousness.

Antithyroid Agents

A number of different antithyroid agents are also available. Such compounds interfere with the production of thyroid hormones, modify the actions of these hormones at target tissues, or result in partial destruction of the thyroid gland. **Thiocarbamides** (also called thioamides, such as **propylthiouracil** and **methimazole,** shown in Fig. 11-3) interfere with the uptake and (possibly) coupling of iodide to thyroglobulin and are used to treat hyperthyroidism. Thiocyanates, nitrates, and perchlorates inhibit the uptake of iodide. Very high levels of iodide in the diet will itself lead to (paradoxical) goiter formation. Radioactive iodide (^{131}I) may be used to ablate the thyroid. This is used in patients over 40 years of age but is typically avoided in young patients, and is specifically contraindicated in pregnancy, since it is potentially dangerous to expose a developing fetus to high levels of radioactivity. Moreover, because the fetal thyroid gland can concentrate iodide, ^{131}I administration may ablate the fetal thyroid and lead to cretinism.

PARATHYROID HORMONE (Pth), CALCITONIN, AND VITAMIN D

Parathyroid Hormone and Regulation of Serum Calcium and Phosphate

Calcium is an abundant element in living systems; it is found largely in bones and teeth. Additionally, it has a role in blood coagulation and serves as a second messenger for the action of many hormone systems. It is also involved in contractility of cardiac and skeletal muscle and in nerve excitability. The **parathyroid gland** is under control of negative feedback and is regulated by the concentration of calcium in the fluid (serum) bathing the gland. As blood calcium drops, parathyroid hormone (Pth) is released. Pth mobilizes bone calcium and enhances intestinal absorption of calcium. The action on intestinal calcium absorption is likely to be indirect and based on enhanced conversion of calcifediol (25-hydroxy vitamin D-3) to calcitriol (1,25-dihydroxy vitamin D-3) in the kidneys, which in turn promotes intestinal absorption of calcium. Other actions of Pth include increased calcium reabsorption and decreased phosphate reabsorption in the kidney. Hypertrophy of the gland occurs in response to hypocalcemia. Involution of the gland occurs in response to **hypercalcemia.** Pth is not well stored; it is a protein consisting of 84 amino acids, and its synthesis and secretion fluctuate rapidly. The half-life (t½) of this hormone is less than 30 minutes. There is now some evidence that the active forms may be a family of chemically different parathyroid hormones rather than a single molecule.

Parathyroid Disorders

Hyperparathyroidism. This disorder usually results from excessive secretion from the parathyroid gland. Similar symptoms may result from other disorders, resulting in a negative calcium balance. Chronic elevated levels of Pth can lead to osteitis fibrosa cystica generalisata, but this is not typical. More commonly seen is the development of renal calculi or nephrocalcinosis due to excretion of calcium and phosphate.

Hypoparathyroidism. This disease state is usually caused by accidental damage to the parathyroid gland, typically occurring during removal or surgery of the thyroid gland, which is located nearby. There is another recently appreciated disease state, called **pseudohypoparathyroidism,** in which Pth levels in the blood may be normal (or even elevated); however, because of a defect in the second messenger system, the bone does not respond appropriately to the actions of this hormone.

Calcitonin

This hormone is released by foregut-derived cells in the thyroid gland and promotes hypocalcemia. It is a protein with a t½ of 5 to 10 minutes in blood. **Calcitonin** inhibits bone resorption in response to Pth or to vitamin D; chronic use of calcitonin leads to increased bone mass. Compared with Pth and vitamin D, calcitonin plays a minor role in regulating serum Ca^{2+}. Because calcitonin causes hypocalcemia it may prove useful in the treatment of hypercalcemia.

Vitamin D

In recent years it has become obvious that this hormone has a molecular mechanism of action very much like a steroid hormone. Both its receptor and the means by which the receptor ligand complex activates the target system appear similar for steroid hormones and for vitamin D. Vitamin D is synthesized in the skin in response to ultraviolet light or derived from diet and converted to the active form 1,25-dihydroxy vitamin D (Fig. 11–4). It is deficient in patients with rickets, to whom a supplement must be given. Vitamin D stimulates intestinal absorption of calcium and phosphate, and decreases renal loss of these ions. Vitamin D also mobilizes Ca^{2+} and phosphate from bone (enhanced bone resorption).

Alterations in Serum Calcium

Hypocalcemia

This disorder is characterized by neuromuscular excitability and tetanic muscular contractions. It may be treated by fusion of calcium ions, as either the chloride or the gluconate form. Hormonal manipulations are usually too slow to assist in the management of severe onset of hypocalcemia.

Hypercalcemia

This is often seen in connection with malignant tumors of the breast or vitamin D intoxication. It can also be caused by hyperparathyroidism. Chela-

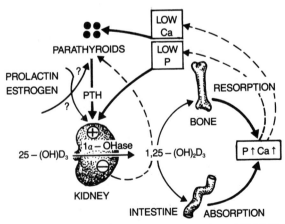

Figure 11–4. Model for regulation of the biosynthesis of 1,25-$(OH)_2D_3$. *Solid arrows* indicate a positive effect; *broken arrows*, negative feedback. (Modified from Haussler, MR and McCain, TA: Basic and clinical concepts related to vitamin D metabolism and action. N Engl J Med 297:974, 1977.)

tors of calcium, such as ethylenediaminetetraacetic acid (EDTA), may drop the free calcium in the blood very rapidly and are therefore dangerous, not being useful in treatment of this disorder. Other treatments helpful in treating hypercalcemia include mithramycin, phosphate, or forced diuresis with saline and a loop diuretic.

INSULIN, GLUCAGON, AND ORAL HYPOGLYCEMIC AGENTS

Insulin

Biosynthesis, Secretion, and Cellular Site of Action of Insulin

Insulin is a small protein consisting of two amino acid chains that are held in position by disulfide bonds. Insulin and glucagon (a single chain) are produced from the β and α cells of the pancreas, respectively. Both are processed from larger precursor molecules that are single chains. It is by this means that the coordinated synthesis of the two chains of insulin is afforded. Enhanced blood levels of metabolizable sugars (such as glucose) or vagal stimulation stimulate insulin release. In the circulation insulin is bound to serum globulins; even so, the t½ of insulin is relatively short (approximately 10 to 15 minutes). Once initiated, however, the action of insulin in target cells may last for many hours after the hormone itself has been degraded by the liver. Antibodies to insulin, which can occur as a result of long-term therapy, may also alter its effects on target tissues.

Antibodies directed against the insulin receptor have also been reported; such antibodies may either mimic or inhibit the actions of insulin. Insulin is retained by most tissues. As in the case of glucocorticoids and thyroid hormones, cells in culture frequently require insulin for growth and development. The initial site of insulin interaction with the cell is a plasma membrane receptor; although intracellular receptors have been reported, their functional significance remains unknown.

Effects of Insulin

Generally, insulin promotes use of glucose as an energy source—it promotes storage of sugars in muscle and adipose tissues. Its actions are both anabolic (increased glycogen synthesis in liver and muscle; increased lipogenesis in liver and adipose tissue; increased protein synthesis in muscle; enhanced glucose, potassium, and phosphate uptake in adipose tissue and muscle; and enhanced amino acid uptake in muscle) and anticatabolic (decreased glycogenolysis in liver and muscle, decreased gluconeogenesis and ketogenesis in liver, decreased lipolysis in adipose tissue, and diminished protein breakdown in muscle). Because glucose uptake is the rate-limiting step in sugar metabolism, insulin may be thought of as a key regulator, as it controls the availability of glucose to cells. Additionally, in adipose cells, insulin inhibits the lipase that breaks down triglycerides to glycerol and fatty acids. It also promotes synthesis of triglycerides from fatty acids. In the liver, glucose uptake is **not** regulated by insulin (this is an exception to the general rule); rather, uptake is regulated by the concentration of glucose in portal plasma.

Insulin Deficiency: Diabetes Mellitus. When sufficient insulin is not available, glycogen is converted to glucose, protein is degraded to amino acids and subsequently transaminated to glucose. Triglycerides are converted to acetylcoenzyme A, resulting in ketosis. During glucocorticoid therapy, glucocorticoid levels are high (therefore, glucose in the blood is high) and insulin action is antagonized. Insulin levels may be "textbook normal" although functionally insufficient to handle this added burden.

Diabetes mellitus is a heritable disorder characterized by insulin deficiency. Because fats and proteins are degraded and used as an energy source, diabetes mellitus is characterized by azoturia, ketonemia, and hyperlipidemia. Severe and uncontrolled diabetes leads to ketoacidosis. The buildup of (nonutilizable) sugars in the blood leads to hyperglycemia. Diabetes may be classified as type 1 (insulin-requiring, sometimes called "juvenile onset," diabetes) or type 2 (non–insulin-dependent, or "adult onset," diabetes). Less common types are drug-induced diabetes and diabetes occurring secondary to disease or certain heritable disorders. There is a strong genetic component in diabetes mellitus type 2, but this plays a lesser role in type 1.

Clinical Use of Insulin

Insulin is a protein, so the oral route is not useful. The so-called **oral insulins** are not insulin as such but stimulate the release of endogenous insulin. Insulin itself must be given by injection and is indicated for replacement therapy in patients with diabetes mellitus.

The type and dose of insulin must be determined and individualized for each patient. This is often related to the patient's diet, characteristic amount of exercise, and amount of endogenous insulin available. Adverse reactions to insulin (**hyperinsulinism**) may occur through overdose or tumors of the islet cells; this may occur in prediabetic individuals. Symptoms begin to appear as blood glucose falls. Such symptoms may include a feeling of hunger and weakness, lightheadedness, sweating, tachycardia, numbness, tingling, anxiety, and tremor. When symptoms are due to "long-acting" insulin, these may include mental, motor, and emotional disturbances. A number of different insulin preparations are available (Table 11–2), ranging from crystallin insulin to insulin that has been complexed with erythrocyte globulin, precipitated acid pHs, or protamine. Recently, genetic engineering has provided us with a form of insulin synthesized by bacteria from human gene templates.

Table 11–2. COMPARATIVE DATA FOR INSULIN
PREPARATIONS

Class	Name	Onset (hours)	Peak (hours)	Duration (hours)
Fast Acting	Injection (crystalline)	1	2–4	8
Intermediate	Prompt (semilente)	1	2–8	14
	Isophane	2	6–12	24
	Insulin suspension (zinc, lente)	2	7–15	24
Long Acting	Protamine	4	14–24	36
	Extended insulin (ultralente)	4	14–24	36

Oral Hypoglycemic Agents

These compounds are associated with increased patient compliance because they may be given orally. As mentioned earlier, though they are sometimes called "oral insulin" they are not truly insulin or insulin products, but rather cause a release of pancreatic insulin. Consequently, the patient must have releasable insulin available if these compounds are to work. Individuals who have diminished levels of pancreatic insulin or refractory target cells do not benefit from oral hypoglycemics. Accordingly, oral hypoglycemic agents have no efficacy in juvenile onset diabetes. The oral hypoglycemic agents (Fig. 11–5) include the **sulfonylureas.** Such compounds are promptly absorbed following oral administration and are distributed throughout the extracellular fluid. They travel in the circulation bound to serum proteins. Included among these compounds are tolbutamide, acetohexamide, chlorpropamide, and tolazamide. These range from short acting (i.e., less than half an hour to peak of action) to long acting (i.e., several days' duration of action). With some long-acting agents (especially chlorpropamide) there is added risk of severe, prolonged hypoglycemia with overdose. The oral hypoglycemics are generally reserved for older patients for which insulin therapy or compliance is difficult. Even so, some patients experience heartburn, abdominal pain, and diarrhea as a result of these compounds. Cholestatic jaundice and blood dyscrasias are also reported. The action of these compounds is antagonized by corticosteroids, thyroxine, and oral contraceptives. Patients receiving oral hypoglycemics are also frequently intolerant to alcohol. More recently developed oral hypoglycemics include glipizide and glyburide. Major characteristics of oral hypoglycemic agents are summarized in Table 11–3.

The **biguanides** are also oral hypoglycemics. These are no longer in use in

Table 11-3. ORAL HYPOGLYCEMIC AGENTS (SULFONYLUREAS)

Name	Dosage	Onset	Duration	Peak	Side Effects	Contraindications and Precautions
First-Generation Sulfonylureas						
Tolbutamide (Orinase)	0.5–3 g (divided doses)	30 min–1 hr	6–12 hr	3–5 hr	Hypoglycemia, GI disturbances (anorexia, nausea, vomiting, diarrhea), blood dyscrasias, hemolytic anemia, allergic skin reactions, headache. Hyperglycemia if not adequate to control diabetes. Some research has indicated a higher incidence of cardiovascular complications (myocardial infarction, strokes).	Withhold if patient is hypoglycemic or unable to take food. Not for use in insulin-dependent diabetics or pregnant or lactating women. Use with caution in renal insufficiency or allergy to sulfa preparations.
Acetohexamide (Dymelor)	0.25–1.5 g in single or divided doses	30 min–1 hr	12–24 hr	6 hr	Same as above.	Same as above, plus: Use with caution in hepatic disease.

Drug	Dose			Adverse Effects	Contraindications/Cautions
Chlorpropamide (Diabinese)	0.1–0.5 g in a single dose	1 hr	36–90 hr	12 hr	Same as above.	Same as above. Also contraindicated in thyroid dysfunction. Use with caution in patients with kidney disease and in the elderly. May cause water retention and dilutional hyponatremia.
Tolazamide (Tolinase)	0.1–1 g in single or divided doses	4–6 hr	12–24 hr	6 hr	Same as above, plus: Altered liver function tests.	Same as above, plus: Use with caution in any other endocrine disease.
Second-Generation Sulfonylureas						
Glyburide (Micronase, DiaBeta)	1.25–20 mg daily in 1 or 2 doses	2–4 hr	12–24 hr	6 hr	Skin reactions, GI distress. Cholestatic jaundice necessitates stoppage.	Same as above, plus: If gain clearly outweighs risk, and it is used during pregnancy, discontinue 2 weeks before delivery since it can cause severe hypoglycemia in neonate.

Adapted from Mathewson, MK: Pharmacotherapeutics: A Nursing Process Approach. FA Davis, Philadelphia, 1986, pp 826–827, with permission.

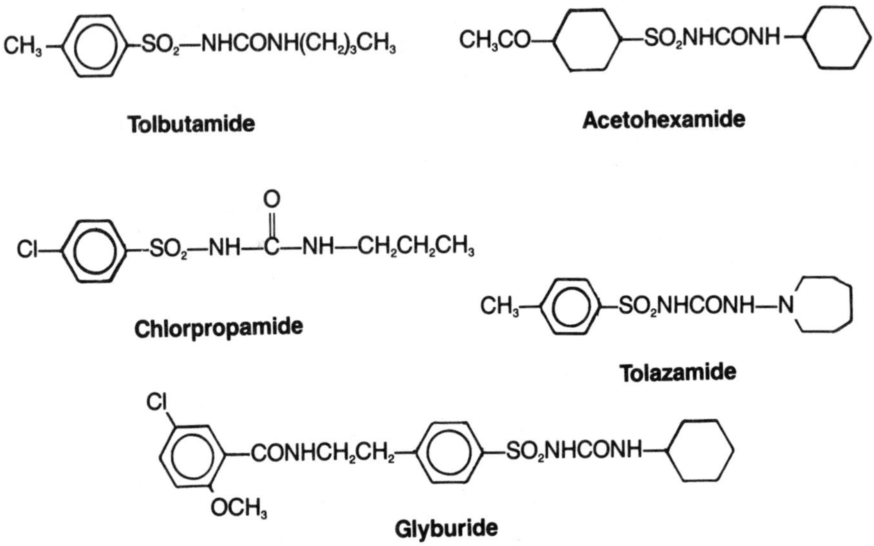

Figure 11-5. Sulfonylurea oral hypoglycemic agents.

the United States because they are associated with increased blood pressure, increased heart rate, and cardiovascular problems.

Hyperglycemic Agents

These compounds are useful in acute shock. Glucose is the most common of these, although glucagon is administered occasionally, as this compound leads to glycogen breakdown in elevated serum glucose levels. Glucagon is produced by the α cells of the pancreas and promotes hyperglycemia and glycogenolysis and is useful in acute insulin shock. **Alloxan** and streptozocin destroy insulin-secreting (β) islet cells of the pancreas. Both drugs are used experimentally in animals to induce diabetes mellitus; streptozocin is also used clinically in treating malignant pancreatic islet cell tumors.

ADRENOCORTICAL STEROIDS AND THEIR ANTAGONISTS

Adrenocortical hormones are steroids released in response to pituitary ACTH (adrenocorticotropic hormone) (Fig. 11–6). Adrenocortical steroids may be divided into three categories. First of all, **glucocorticoid** hormones (primarily cortisol in humans) regulate intermediary metabolism. Second, **mineralocorticoids** (aldosterone) regulate salt-retaining activity. Third, the adrenal gland also releases small amounts of **androgens** and **estrogens**. It is significant

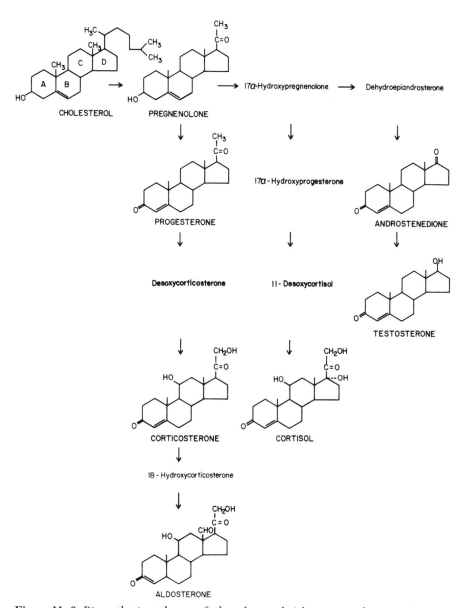

Figure 11–6. Biosynthetic pathways of adrenal steroids (glucocorticoids, mineralocorticoids, and androgens).

to note, in considering steroids in general, that the distinctions in classifications is not absolute. For example, a compound classified as a glucocorticoid may also have some mineralocorticoid-like action.

Glucocorticoids

Biosynthesis, Secretion, and Transport of Glucocorticoids

In humans **cortisone** is the major glucocorticoid (in rats the major glucocorticoid is corticosterone). Cortisone is made in the zona fasciculata and the zona reticularis. Smaller amounts of a more potent agent, **cortisol,** are also made. Glucocorticoids are released in a rhythmic pattern during the day. A peak is reached shortly prior to noon and a nadir about 3 A.M. for normal individuals. It is carried in the circulation by binding globulins. The majority of this steroid circulates in a bound form and the remainder, the small percentage that is metabolically active, is unbound. Glucocorticoids and other steroids may also be in the circulation bound to albumin.

Effects of Glucocorticoids

Glucocorticoids act permissively to allow many normal cellular reactions to occur. Such reactions do not occur at significant rates in the absence of glucocorticoids. As was noted previously, thyroid hormone is required for many mammalian cell cultures. Similarly, many cell cultures have a requirement for glucocorticoids. These hormones stimulate the production of glucose from proteins. The anti-insulin actions of cortisol result in increased gluconeogenesis, protein catabolism, and decreased glucose uptake. This results in hyperglycemia and glucose intolerance. The increased blood glucose stimulates insulin release and fat deposition in the trunk, face, and other areas of the body. Glucocorticoids and **ACTH,** which releases glucocorticoids, are important for their actions as anti-inflammatory agents. They are rapidly and completely absorbed if taken orally. Large doses of these compounds can stimulate ulcer formation. Glucocorticoids are associated with the relief of inflammation of allergic reactions; even so there is no evidence that these compounds diminish antibody formation when administered at pharmacological doses, nor that they interfere with the development of acquired immunity. Adrenocortical steroids inhibit homograft rejection and can be used in the diagnosis of disturbed adrenal function. The effects of glucocorticoids are summarized in Table 11–4.

Diagnostic and Therapeutic Uses of Glucocorticoids

Glucocorticoids such as dexamethasone are commonly used to suppress the production of ACTH and therefore identify whether a particular secretion

Table 11-4. COMPARATIVE DATA FOR
GLUCOCORTICOIDS

	Relative Anti-inflammatory Potency	Relative Mineralo-corticoid Potency	Duration of Action	Dosage (mg)
Betamethasone	25.0	0	Long	0.75
Cortisol	1.0	1.0	Short	20.00
Cortisone	0.8	0.8	Short	25.00
Dexamethasone	25.0	0	Long	0.75
Prednisone	4.0	0.8	Intermediate	5.0
6α-Methylprednisone	5.0	0.5	Intermediate	4.0
Triamcinolone	5.0	0	Intermediate	4.0

is influenced by ACTH. For example, a high dose of dexamethasone (8 mg) can be used to distinguish elevated cortisol due to elevated pituitary release of ACTH (Cushing's disease), in which suppression occurs, from ectopic or adrenal tumor-derived ACTH, in which suppression does not occur. For such ACTH suppression tests one frequently uses glucocorticoid analogs because these have high potencies and therefore may be administered in small quantities that do not interfere in specific radioimmunoassays directed against the endogenous hormones.

Cortisol is also used to treat a number of diseases that are not caused by altered adrenal function; this use is based on the ability of these compounds to suppress inflammatory and immune responses. In most cases this is, of course, a symptomatic treatment and not a cure. The diet of such patients should be high in potassium and low in sodium to prevent electrolyte imbalances. Protein should be adequate in diet to make up for the loss of endogenous protein to gluconeogenesis. Antacids are typically used in such patients because of the tendency of glucocorticoids to cause formation of peptic ulcers. Symptoms of diseases such as gout, asthma, rheumatoid arthritis, or rheumatic fever can be treated with glucocorticoids. These steroids are also useful for immunosuppression following tissue transplant.

The physician should be aware of a number of adverse reactions to steroids; for example, administration of high levels of cortisol daily for as little as 2 weeks can result in **iatrogenic Cushing's syndrome**. In addition, such patients are prone to ulcers, development of psychosis during long-term use, and related problems. Following suppression of the immune system by glucocorticoids, insufficiency may last for 2 or more months. The immune-suppressed individual will likely require supplemental steroids in case of surgery or other trauma. It is significant to note that it may require more than 6 months to withdraw a patient from glucocorticoids; abrupt withdrawal may lead to an addisonian crisis in long-term immune-suppressed individuals. Contraindications include psychosis, diabetes, osteoporosis, glaucoma, or known ulcers. Glucocorticoids are preferred over ACTH, as with the former cortisol levels can be set more easily and specific steroids may be elevated. In the case of ACTH remember that **all** steroids from adrenal origin will be elevated (including androgens and aldosterone, although elevation of the latter is transient), whereas the administration of cortisol allows selective elevation of individual steroids. Steroid creams are particularly useful and are sold by prescription and now over the counter. The main use of ACTH is that of a diagnostic tool (measuring the glucocorticoid response, as in adrenal insufficiency).

Mineralocorticoids and Mineralocorticoid Antagonists

The primary **mineralocorticoid** in humans is **aldosterone**. Its release is regulated by a reduction in the blood volume. A drop in the renal arterial pressure results in renin release from the juxtaglomerular apparatus. This enzyme proteolyzes α_2 globulin producing angiotensin I. Additional proteolysis results in the production of angiotensin II, which stimulates the synthesis and release of aldosterone. Conversion of angiotensin I to angiotensin II is inhibited by the drug **captopril** and this is part of the basis of the hypotensive action of this agent. **Deoxycorticosterone** is also released at significant levels. These mineralocorticoids induce reabsorption of sodium by the renal tubules in exchange for potassium and hydronium ion. This action occurs at the distal tubule of the kidney. Compounds such as **spironolactone** are aldosterone antagonists, which block the sodium-retaining and the other effects of aldosterone. **Amphenone** inhibits aldosterone synthesis and is, therefore, a useful antagonist.

Androgens and Estrogens

The primary androgen secreted by the adrenal cortex is dehydroepiandrosterone (DHEA), a weak androgen. Lesser quantities of androstenedione (another weak androgen) and testosterone, and possibly small quantities of estrogens, are produced. In peripheral tissues, some of the adrenal androstenedione undergoes aromatization to form estrone.

Diseases of the Adrenal Cortex

Addison's Disease (Adrenocortical Insufficiency)

This disorder is characterized by hyperpigmentation of the skin and an easily fatigued patient. Hypotension and weight loss are also common. Minor trauma or infection may produce acute adrenal insufficiency and cause death in **Addison's disease** patients. Accordingly, this disorder is commonly treated by the administration of cortisol as replacement therapy. A salt-retaining hormone (mineralocorticoid) is also typically given.

Congenital Adrenal Hyperplasia

Patients with **congenital adrenal hyperplasia** display defects in cortisol synthesis. This results in decreased serum cortisol and a resultant increase in pituitary release of ACTH. Since the pituitary is relieved of feedback inhibition by the steroid, the result is the normalization of serum cortisol. However, other steroids (especially androgens) are released at excessive levels; this event leads to virilization. The liver metabolism of these excess levels of steroids results in the formation of pregnanetriol, which is the basis for a diagnostic test when assayed in the urine of these patients.

Cushing's Syndrome and Cushing's Disease

Cushing's syndrome is a disorder caused by excess glucocorticoids, whether from an endogenous source or from administered steroids. The syndrome is characterized by fatty deposits in the face and trunk, accounting for the so-called moon-face. Patients exhibit trunk obesity as well as protein and muscle loss. Fat deposition at the base of the neck is sometimes referred to as "buffalo hump." These patients are characterized by a high degree of bruisability and poor wound healing, as well as mental disorders, hypertension, and diabetes. Typical interventions include surgical or other means (irradiation) to decrease the tumor size. The patient must be supported by cortisol to prevent rapid withdrawal from the endogenous hormone.

Bilateral adrenal hyperplasia occurs when there is increased ACTH from the pituitary gland (as in **Cushing's disease,** or secondary hypercortisolism) or from another ectopic site.

Hyperaldosteronism (Conn's Syndrome)

This disorder is caused by the primary hyperproduction of aldosterone resulting from adrenal adenoma or carcinoma. It is characterized by hypokalemia, which leads to muscle weakness, and by hypernatremia, contributing to hypertension, polyuria, and polydipsia. Treatment is typically administration of spironolactone (Aldactone; an aldosterone antagonist).

Inhibitors of Adrenocortical Steroid Synthesis

Metyrapone (Metopirone) inhibits 11β-hydroxylation of steroids and results in the accumulation of an intermediate (11-desoxycortisol), which **does**

not feedback on the pituitary gland to inhibit ACTH release. Accordingly, ACTH and steroidal precursors of cortisol are elevated in the serum along with the steroid intermediate which appears in the urine. In individuals with **Cushing's disease** (increased pituitary ACTH secretion) this response is exaggerated. Interpretation of metyrapone data requires the prior demonstration that the adrenals respond normally to ACTH. Metyrapone can produce acute adrenal insufficiency.

Aminoglutethimide blocks side chain cleavage enzyme and is consequently an effective antagonist of the synthesis of most steroids from cholesterol. This compound is frequently used with dexamethasone to reduce or eliminate estrogen and androgen production by the breast. Aminoglutethimide is presently in use to treat adrenal tumors that release steroids. With metyrapone it is used in treatment of pituitary Cushing's syndrome.

GONADAL HORMONES AND THEIR ANTAGONISTS

Estrogens

Large amounts of estrogens (Fig. 11–7) are found in the ovary. In the circulation these compounds are frequently complexed to **testosterone-estrogen binding globulin** (TEBG) or to albumin. Only about 1 percent of gonadal steroids circulate freely. This is the active fraction, as free steroid may diffuse into cells whereas that bound to carriers or albumin cannot. For excretion steroids are conjugated to glucuronides. Ovarian steroid disturbances are common. In women the major circulating forms are estradiol-17β (E_2), estriol (E_3), and estrone. Estradiol is the primary secretory product produced by the ovary; in the liver E_2 is oxidized to estrone and hydrated to estriol. In the initial part of the menstrual cycle estrogens are produced by the Graafian follicles and by thecal cells. Following ovulation the estrogens as well as the progestins are synthesized in the granulosa cells of the corpus luteum. In pregnancy the fetus and placenta coordinate their estrogen production, and the measure of circulating estriol in the mother is a good indication of fetal well-being.

Estrogens are required for normal maturation in females; they stimulate vaginal, uterine, fallopian, and endometrial lining development. They are involved in breast development and ductal growth in the female at puberty. In addition, they are a signal for epiphyseal closure to additional bone growth. These compounds also decrease resorption of bones and are therefore antagonistic to parathyroid hormone. They decrease motility of the bowel, increase glucocorticoid binding proteins, enhance coagulability of the blood, increase α-lipoprotein, and influence libido.

Because steroid hormones are easy to synthesize, many synthetic estro-

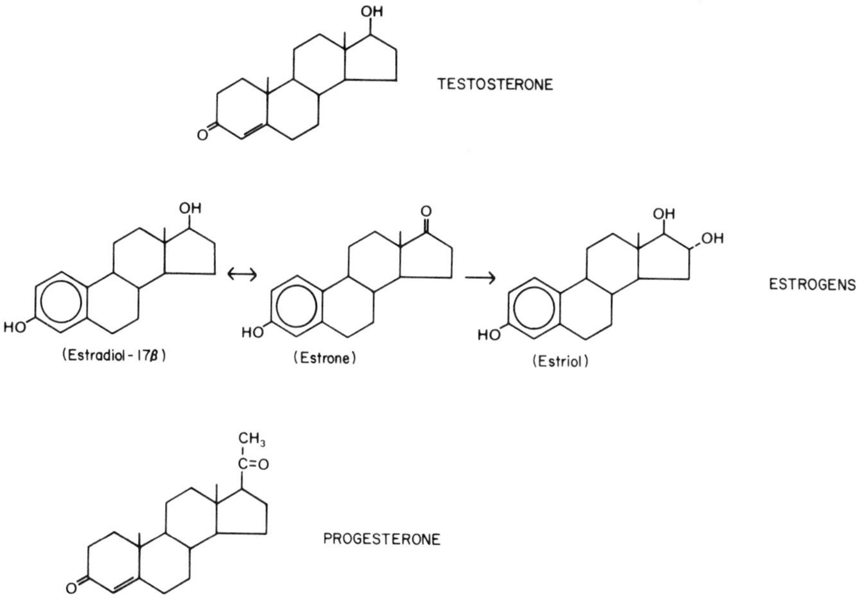

Figure 11–7. Structure of androgen (testosterone), estrogens (estradiol-17β, estrone, estriol) and a progestin (progesterone).

gens (some of which are not rigorously chemical steroids) have been designed that have increased oral efficacy.

Estrogens are commonly used for replacement in deficiencies such as failure of the ovaries, castration, or menopause. Ethinyl estradiol is active when taken orally and is slowly inactivated in the liver and elsewhere; accordingly, single daily doses usually suffice. Estrogens, in fact, are generally given cyclically when the uterus is present to avoid hyperplasia of the endometrium. They are used in menopause for relief from hot flashes, sweating, and atrophic vaginitis. When begun promptly after onset of menopause, estrogen therapy has potential use in prevention of osteoporosis, as these compounds oppose the action of Pth. Because they themselves do not increase bone formation, however, extant damage cannot be reversed.

Adverse effects of estrogens include bleeding in postmenopausal women, nausea (the most common), breast tenderness, migraine headaches, cholestasis, hypertension, and increased endometrial cancer risk. When the estrogen diethylstilbestrol (DES) was given to pregnant women to prevent miscarriage, an increased risk of vaginal cancer was found in female offspring resulting from such pregnancies.

Because **estrogen receptors** are widely distributed in tissues, estrogens cannot be considered to be specifically acting drugs. Use of estrogen therapy is contraindicated in patients with estrogen-dependent neoplasia, undiagnosed genital bleeding, liver disease, or thromboembolic disorders. These compounds should be used with caution in postmenopausal women. Such patients should be examined at 6-month intervals or more frequently. They should be used with caution also in patients with epilepsy, migraine headaches, asthma, depression, and cardiac or renal failure. Estrogen therapy may exacerbate symptoms in porphyria (elevated blood porphyrins) and may activate endometriosis. Many diverse formulations and derivatives of gonadal steroids are available and it is essential to weigh the benefits against the risks for each patient.

Progestins

Progestins (see Fig. 11–7) are the chemical precursors to estrogens, androgens, and adrenocortical steroids. In the ovary these are produced in the corpus luteum mostly during the second half (luteal phase) of the cycle. They are produced in larger quantities in females than in males. When administered as drugs these are rapidly absorbed by virtually all routes. For excretion they are conjugated in the liver, forming pregnanediol glucuronide. This is often taken as an index of progesterone secretion. Progestins can compete with aldosterone at the renal tubule, therefore, decreasing sodium reabsorption. This is an example of cross-reactivity of steroid hormone receptors for different steroids. Progestins mediate the so-called pyrogenic effect, which is often used as a measure of ovulation, and thereby constitutes a crude form of birth control. Many diverse formulations and derivatives of these compounds are available. They are used for contraception and for ovarian suppression (useful in the treatment of dysmenorrhea, endometriosis, hirsutism, and bleeding disorders involving estrogens). They also form the basis of the useful diagnostic test for estrogen secretion (progestin is given for several days, then withdrawn; withdrawal bleeding occurs only if the endometrium was estrogen primed). Progestins are involved in initiation of the secretory phase of the endometrium and maintenance of the endometrial lining. They are believed to play a role in glandular development of the breasts and, because they inhibit uterine contractions, progestins play a significant role in pregnancy.

Relaxin

Relaxin is an ovarian polypeptide of minimal therapeutic use that causes relaxation of pelvic ligaments and softening of the uterine cervix at the time of parturition.

Oral Contraceptives

The development of oral contraceptives provides a complex yet interesting history. At present "**combination**" pills (an estrogen plus a progestin) are in common use with nearly 100 percent effectiveness. **"Sequential"** pills (estrogen for 2 weeks, then an estrogen plus a progestin) have been dropped in the United States because of apparent increased occurrence of endometrial tumors. A **"mini-pill"** of medroxyprogesterone only is also available (>95 percent effective), as is a postcoital pill of an estrogen only. While effective, the latter is particularly undesirable and potentially dangerous. Developmental work has continued on injectable and implant forms of steroids. Some progesterone antagonists, notably mifepristone (RU-486) may have efficacy as a contraceptive or abortifacient. Side effects of oral contraceptives include nausea, dizziness, headaches, breast discomfort, weight gain, depression, as well as increased risk for thromboembolism, thrombophlebitis, benign hepatomas, cholestatic jaundice, and cholelithiasis.

Ovulation-Inducing Agents and Antiestrogens

Steroids are usually orally active. The major compound of use is clomiphene citrate (Clomid), which elevates luteinizing hormone (LH) and therefore increases the probability of ovulation. Although usually classed as an antiestrogen, clomiphene has estrogenic activity. It binds to the receptor and enhances the production of gonadotropins from the pituitary gland and therefore gonadal estrogens. It stimulates ovulation in women with amenorrhea and other ovulatory disorders. It may somehow block the inhibitory effects of the estrogens in the pituitary gland, and requires an intact pituitary gland in order to work. Side effects during use include hot flashes (although these are usually mild and may disappear with withdrawal) and prolongation of afterimages in the eye (accordingly night driving may be difficult); also, multiple pregnancies occur in 10 percent of patients in whom clomiphene is used. It should not be used in patients with enlarged ovaries and should be discontinued if abdominal pain is reported.

Tamoxifen, nafoxidine, and a nonsteroidal agent chlorotrianisene are other antiestrogens. It is a consensus view that these agents act by occupying the estrogen receptor and blocking the negative feedback on gonadotropin release at the pituitary and hypothalamus. Tamoxifen is often used as palliative therapy in advanced breast carcinoma (especially if the tumor has estrogen receptors) in postmenopausal women.

Androgens

Androgens (see Fig. 11–7) are produced in the testes, ovary, and adrenal cortex. The primary androgen is **testosterone,** which is metabolically active in some tissues only after conversion to **5α-dihydrotestosterone** (DHT). Its synthesis and release is controlled by pituitary LH (although some literature refers to this hormone as interstitial cell–stimulating hormone, ICSH, when discussed in the male). Androgens are responsible for the onset of puberty and generalized masculinization. This includes hair growth, increases in muscle mass, activation of sebaceous glands, lower-pitched voice due to action on the vocal chords and larynx, behavioral changes, and bone epiphysis closure. Androgens are active orally and rapidly absorbed as methyl testosterone and fluoxymesterone. The anabolic effects of these compounds is sometimes abused, particularly in sports. Oral long-acting preparations are useful in replacement therapy, although full maturation may not be achieved if therapy has begun long after puberty. Administered in combination with estrogens, these compounds are also useful in treatment of osteoporosis. Danazol is a weak androgen that suppresses spermatogenesis in the male. Androgens are contraindicated in pregnant women or in men who may have carcinoma of the prostate, and are generally avoided in children or patients with renal or cardiac diseases.

Antiandrogens

Cyproterone is a primary antiandrogen and inhibits testosterone action in target tissues. This area has not been developed to a marked degree.

SOMATOMEDINS

Growth hormone (somatotropin) induces its actions in bone by intermediary agents (previously referred to as sulfation factor) known as the somatomedins. Somatomedins are produced in the kidney, liver, muscle, and elsewhere and are also active in adipocytes, where they stimulate enhanced lipid and protein synthesis in muscle. The clinical significance of this compound will probably be developed in the near future. There is a similarity regarding structure and physiological effects of somatomedins and of insulin.

ATRIAL NATRIURETIC FACTOR

A newly appreciated endocrine organ is the heart. The cardiac atria respond to changes in blood pressure and volume by releasing atrial natriuretic factor (ANF). This agent enters the circulation and promotes natriuresis and diuresis. Neurons containing ANF are found in the CNS and may also be important in regulation of blood volume. ANF has been purified and its amino acids sequenced. Although not yet used clinically, this agent will likely become important because of its profound diuretic, natriuretic, and antihypertensive actions.

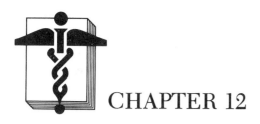

CHAPTER 12

Anti-Inflammatory Drugs

THOMAS K. SHIRES, Ph.D.

Inflammation is the process of response to tissue injury, regardless of cause, and is precursory to tissue healing. Characteristics of its **acute phase** include (1) mobilization and activation of leukocytes; (2) regional vasodilation resulting in increased blood flow in the vicinity of affected tissue; (3) contraction of nonvascular smooth muscle; and (4) bulk movement of fluid and serum constituents from vascular to tissue compartments in inflamed tissue. General **chronic inflammation** tends to present monocytic infiltrations of affected regions, sometimes mixed with various degrees of fibroplasia. Some swelling, pain, and tissue destruction accompany all inflammations. Ordinarily, in-

303

flammation can be regarded as restorative and desirable, an unpleasant process to be endured for the sake of healing. In other situations, however, inflammation results in significant morbidity.

Chemotherapy of inflammation is multifaceted. It may intercept the process at its beginning, for instance, by interdiction of pathogenic organisms with antimicrobial agents. It may target particularly salient features of the ongoing inflammatory process for suppression as, for instance, in certain forms of arthritis with immunosuppressive drugs. It may aim to palliate troublesome symptoms of inflammation, such as pharyngeal oversecretion, bronchospasm, or pain. Antibiotics, immunosuppressive agents, antihistaminics, and smooth muscle relaxants are not customarily categorized as anti-inflammatory agents. This designation is usually reserved for two groups of drugs: the anti-inflammatory steroids and the nonsteroidal (or aspirin-like) anti-inflammatory agents. They are **indicated** for a restricted number of inflammatory conditions, most of which are chronic forms of the process: rheumatoid arthritis, degenerative joint disease, systemic lupus erythematosus and polyarteritis, gout, multiple sclerosis, ulcerative colitis, dermatomyositis, psoriasis, and, on occasion, severe contact dermatitis. However, many of the nonsteroidal agents are widely, and not incorrectly, used for palliation of symptoms accompanying inflammation—particularly pain and hyperpyrexia.

THE INFLAMMATORY PROCESS

Underlying inflammation constitutes a diverse group of interrelated systems. Prominent aspects of the inflammatory response to injury are the effects on the microcirculation and blood elements. Activation of **serum factor XII (Hageman factor)** initiates production of the **kinins,** fibrin clots (via the extrinsic **coagulation pathway**), and fibrinolytic **plasmin** (Fig. 12–1). The kininogen peptide products **kallidin** and **bradykinin** appear to have special importance in inflammation. Both increase small vessel permeability, relax vascular smooth muscle, and stimulate sensory nerve endings. The **kininogen precursors,** including both the high molecular weight form II and a low molecular weight form I, occur as circulating plasma α-globulins that are proteolytically converted to kinins by **kallikrein.** Prekallikreins are found in plasma and in extravascular locations. Because the kinins are quickly inactivated by kininases or other proteolytic enzymes (half-life of approximately 30 seconds), sustainment of their effects requires their continuous generation. **Plasmin, kallikrein,** and physical tissue damage all serve to activate factor XII and this may have a multiplicative effect in stimulating kinin formation.

In addition to kinin formation, **factor XII** activation stimulates both the clotting and fibrinolytic systems (see Fig. 12–1). Tissue **thromboplastin,** generated through the extrinsic clotting pathway, will reinforce **factor XII** stimulation of **fibrin** formation *via* the intrinsic pathway. **Thrombin,** generated in

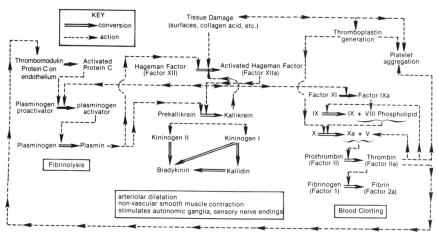

Figure 12–1. Interrelationship of the pathways for clotting, kinin activation, and fibrinolysis.

the clotting cascade, not only converts fibrinogen to fibrin but also enhances (1) activity of the modulatory **factors V and VII**, (2) platelet aggregation, (3) **thrombomodulin**-dependent activation of protein C, and (4) proliferative activity among some types of connective tissue cells for which thrombin is mitogenic. The **antithrombin III** protein (whose high affinity for **heparin** leads to its inactivation) would, of course, antagonize all of these actions of thrombin. Overall, the direct and indirect effects of **factor XII** in stimulating clotting and thrombolysis may explain the sometimes observed slowing of capillary blood flow in central regions of inflamed tissues, along with the dilatation of precapillary vessels, possibly through the action of the kinins.

Histamine

Histamine causes vasodilation and increased vascular permeability, stimulates contraction of most types of nonvascular smooth muscle (except that in the bladder, ureter, iris, and gallbladder), and stimulates peripheral sensory nerve terminals, producing pain. Unlike the kinins, **histamine** inhibits the chemotactic response of neutrophils and basophils, stimulates chemotaxis of eosinophils, and stimulates the release of lysosomal enzymes from neutrophils. It is synthesized in mast cells (where it is stored as a complex with heparin or chondroitin sulfate) and in the gastric mucosa, skin, neurons, and regenerating tissues. Its role in inflammation is most assured when hypersensitive IgE-mediated mast cell secretion is involved, but histamine also appears in chronic inflammatory exudates, suggesting its possible role in longstanding inflammatory tissue injury.

Arachidonic Acid and Phospholipid Derivatives

On release from phospholipid in cell membranes, **arachidonic acid** (C-20:4) undergoes rapid and complex metabolism to a variety of derivatives collectively termed eicosanoids (Fig. 12–2). Conversion of C-20:4 to the endoperoxides PGG2 and PGH2 by cyclooxygenase initiates production of the **prostanoid** group of metabolites; conversion of C-20:4 to 5-hydroperoxyeicosatetraenoic acid (5-HPETE) initiates the **leukotriene** pathway (see Fig. 12–2). Release of C-20:4 from phospholipid requires activation of either of two enzymes that cleave the C-20:4 acyl esters, **phospholipase C** or **phospholipase A2**. Ca^{2+} is a possible trigger for phospholipase A2 activation; both enzymes are stimulated by thrombin, angiotensin II, histamine, the kinins, and serotonin.

Synthesis of the different types of **prostanoids** depends on the tissue distributions of particular prostanoid synthetic enzymes. The first enzyme in the prostanoid synthetic pathway, **cyclooxygenase,** appears to occur in most tissues. Prostacyclin synthase is particularly associated with endothelial cells, thromboxane synthase with platelets; endoperoxide isomerase (for D_2), endoperoxide reductase (for $F_{2\alpha}$), and prostaglandin E isomerase (for E_2) occur in a number of tissues. Catabolic rates for the major functional prostanoids are rapid, the half-lives for thromboxane and prostacyclin being less than 60 seconds and for prostaglandins D_2, $F_{2\alpha}$, and E_2 several minutes.

Collectively the prostanoids have a variety of effects on vascular and non-

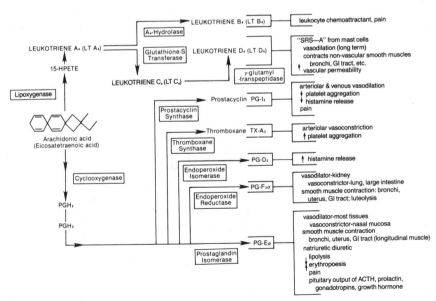

Figure 12–2. Pathways of eicosanoid activation: prostanoid and leukotriene synthesis.

vascular smooth muscle, sensory nerve endings, permeability, and platelet aggregation (see Fig. 12–2). Prostanoids are released from the membranes and must diffuse to receptor sites on target cells in order to act. Different prostanoids may antagonize the effects of other prostanoids and mediators of inflammation. $PG-I_2$ and $PG-E_2$ oppose histamine released by $PG-D_2$. Platelet aggregation stimulated by $TX-A_2$ is antagonized by $PG-I_2$. In some vascular beds (e.g., lung) $PG-F_{2\alpha}$ reverses vascular relaxation caused by $PG-E_2$. In other effects, prostanoids may reinforce each other, as with arteriolar dilatation caused by E_2, $F_{2\alpha}$, and I_2, with bronchiolar constriction by E_2 and $F_{2\alpha}$, and with pain by E_2 and I_2. The association of E_2 and I_2 with pain seems to involve their enhancement of the sensitivity of sensory nerve terminals **to kinin** and perhaps **histamine** stimulation.

The **leukotriene** products of the **lipoxygenase** pathway are most notable for their action on smooth muscle. Vascular smooth muscle responds to leukotrienes initially with transient constriction followed by the characteristically prolonged relaxation. The leukotrienes are roughly 1000-fold more potent than histamine in increasing vascular permeability, and their duration of action greatly outlasts histamine (hours versus minutes).

Besides being the source of free C-20:4, membrane phospholipids may be metabolized to **platelet activating factor** (**PAF**), a β-acetyl form of lecithin. Major producers of PAF are neutrophils, monocytes, and mast cells, and it occurs at detectable levels in serum. **PAF** causes vascular permeability, vasodilatation, bronchospasm, and aggregation of platelets. Its release from mast cells accompanies the release of histamine, heparin, and prostaglandin stimulated by IgE antibodies in hypersensitivity reactions.

The Immune System and Complement

Inflammations are likely to involve (1) the introduction of foreign protein into the body, (2) the release of antigens to which the body is or will be sensitized, or (3) the exposure or unmasking of previously sequestered "self" antigens. Some inflammatory diseases may arise wholly or to a major degree from an unremitting or unmodulated immune response localized in particular tissues. In the sensitization phases of immune response, during macrophage processing and presentation of antigen, and the activation and differentiation of lymphocytes, a number of soluble factors are released that mediate cell actions (Table 12–1). These factors, the **interleukins** and the **lymphokines,** influence sensitized-lymphocyte functions as well as the functions of macrophages, fibroblasts, and osteoclasts, thereby contributing to the overall picture of the inflamed tissue.

Immune complexes of antigen and antibody initiate a series of reactions that also figure in the character of an inflammatory response: **complement** activation (Fig. 12–3). The **complement** cascade can be triggered either with **C1**

Table 12–1. SOME LYMPHOCYTE MEDIATORS

Factor	Source	Action
Interleukin I (IL-1)	Macrophages Leukocytes	Stimulates release of IL-2; stimulates proliferation of fibroblasts, endothelial and mesangial cells; increases release of lysosomal enzymes and collagenase from neutrophils and fibroblasts; causes hyperpyrexia; acts as a calcium ionophore; increases muscle proteolysis, stimulates gluconeogenesis and the acute-phase response
Interleukin II (IL-2)	T helper cells	Stimulate growth and differentiation of newly sensitized T or B cells
Macrophage inhibitory factor (MIF)	Activated T cells	Inhibits migration of macrophages
Macrophage activation factor (MAF)	Activated T cells	Activates macrophages
Chemotactic factors	Activated T cells	Stimulates movement of macrophages toward point of lymphokine release
Lymphotoxin (LT)	Activated T cells	Cytotoxic factor for certain types of lymphocytes
Osteoclastic factor (OAF)	Activated T cells	Activates osteoclasts to destroy bone matrix
Immunoglobulin-binding factor (IBF)	Activated T cells	Promotes binding of immunoglobulins to cell surfaces

activation or with **C3** activation. A number of bacterial products and various venoms may accomplish the latter. **C3** is by far the most abundant of the complement proteins circulating in the plasma, and its activation, once started, can be quantitatively magnified by a separate protease cascade (involving proteins B, D, and so on—not shown in Figure 12–3). Activated complement spills out a family of anaphylactoid (**C3a, C5a**) and chemotactic (C5a) peptides, as well as activated complement aggregates (e.g., **C6, 7, 8, 9**) that are capable of lysing cells.

Inflammatory Cells

Accumulation of tissue and blood **monocytes** and **neutrophils** and on occasion **eosinophils** in sites of inflammation is the result of the chemotactic actions on injury-related eicosanoids and activated complement components. Blood neutrophil and monocyte adhesion to vessel walls is enhanced by **TX-A$_2$** and possibly by platelets. Diapedesis of these cells across vessel walls

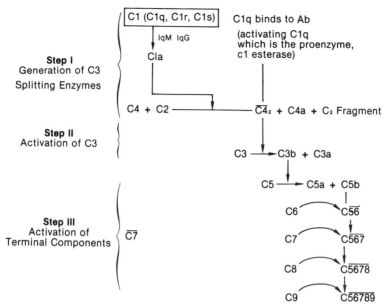

Figure 12–3. Activation of complement. Biologic activities of the complement system. $\overline{C42}$, Enhanced vascular permeability. C3a, Releases histamine, leukotrienes, prostanoids, and so on from mast cells and basophils. Causes smooth muscle contraction. C3b, Stimulates phagocytic activity of leukocytes and tissue macrophages. C5a, Same activities as C3a. Strong chemotaxin for neutrophils and monocytes. $\overline{C567}$, Binds to any nearby membrane preparatory to formation of terminal complement complexes. $\overline{C56789}$ Cytolytic: forms a transmembrane channel for ions and water that leads to osmotic lysis.

to regions of inflammation is governed by (1) factors that increase random cell movements (chemokinesis), as, for example, by $LT-B_4$ or $PG-F_{2\alpha}$; (2) an increase in directed cell movement (chemotaxis), as seen with **C5a;** and (3) inhibitors of macrophage movement (the MIF lymphokine, for example) that keep already accumulated macrophages in the tissue vicinity of inflammation.

During phagocytic activity, **macrophages** and leukocytes release a number of deleterious agents into the extracellular space. **Hydrolases** of both the acidic and the neutral types (optimal at pH 3 to 6 and pH 7.0, respectively) are released by leakage of the enzymes from phagocytic vesicles during engulfment, by true secretion from lysosomal stores, or by lysis of the phagocyte. Acidic hydrolases include a number of proteases, nucleases, and glycosidases, and the neutral group includes collagenase and elastase. Collectively, these enzymes digest most biological material inside the phagocytic vesicle, but when free in the interstitial compartment, they can attack both cells and extracellular structures. Also released from phagocytizing cells are several strong **oxidizing agents,** hydrogen peroxide [H_2O_2], the superoxide anion [O_2^-], hypochlorous acid [HOCl], and possibly singlet oxygen and the hydroxyl radical. These are generated inside the phagocytic vesicle by an NADPH-dependent oxidase system that univalently reduces the oxygen molecule. As with the hydrolases, oxygen radicals not only attack internalized material caught up in the phagocytic vesicle but also appear to leak from these vesicles to attack nearby cells and interstitial materials. Langerhans' cells of the skin, dendritic cells of the spleen, and glial cells of the brain seem to respond and function in the inflammatory process in much the same way as macrophages and leukocytes.

Macrophages and leukocytes also secrete, as part of their participation in immune response, **interleukin I** (IL-I), a polypeptide lymphokine. The actions of IL-I (listed in Table 12–1) take place at local targets close to the site of release (e.g., mitosis, lysosomal enzyme secretion) or are systemic (e.g., hyperpyrexia). In inflamed or traumatized tissue, disruption of blood supply causes regional ischemia, hypoxia, and a shift to **anaerobic glycolysis** as the major metabolic source of ATP. Anaerobic cells are critically dependent on a continuous supply of glucose. IL-I stimulates **gluconeogenesis,** particularly in the liver, and the so-called **hypercatabolic state** affecting skeletal muscle in which muscle protein is converted to amino acids at a greatly increased rate. In the liver these amino acids are metabolized to pyruvate as the initial step in hepatic sugar formation. Also in the liver, IL-I stimulates the **acute-phase response** (AP). In AP, the synthesis and secretion of 15 or more groups of enzymes (AP proteins) is induced. The activities of individual proteins in some of these groups include proteinase inhibition (e.g., α-1 proteinase inhibitor), blood-clotting and fibrinolysis (e.g., fibrinogen, α-2 antiplasmin), removal of foreign material from the body (e.g., serum amyloid, C-reactive protein), modulation of immunological responses (e.g., α-1 acid glycoprotein), and the binding and transport of metals (e.g., haptoglobin, ceruloplasm). AP proteins tend to restore host homeostasis after its disturbance by inflammation.

ANTI-INFLAMMATORY STEROIDS

Natural and synthetic **glucocorticoids** (Table 12–2) are capable of a range of actions that ameliorate the intensity of tissue inflammation. Anti-inflammatory steroid actions primarily involve phagocytic cells and possibly lymphocytes. They reduce the chemotactic responses and ameboid movements of neutrophils, monocytes, and macrophages, and depress the mobilization of these cells into a focus of inflamed tissue. Phagocytized material is less well inactivated and degraded, and the release of lytic enzymes and chemotactic agents from actively phagocytizing cells is diminished. Corticosteroids act in part through their inhibition of **phospholipase A₂**, thus antagonizing eicosanoid production. Inhibition is dependent on the steroids' stimulation of the synthesis within target cells of proteins that directly depress the intramem-

Table 12–2. NATURAL AND SYNTHETIC ANTI-INFLAMMATORY STEROIDS

Natural Adrenocortical Steroids	Relative Anti-inflam. Potency	Relative Na⁺ Retaining potency	Biological Half-life
Cortisol (hydrocortisone)	1	1	8-12 hrs.
Cortisone	0.8	0.8	

Synthetic Steroids			
Prednisone	4	0.8	12-36 hrs.
Prednisolone	4	0.8	
Methyl-prednisolone	5	0.5	
Triamcinolone	5	0	
Paramethasone	10	0	36-72 hrs.
Betamethasone	25	0	
Dexamethasone	25	0	

brane A_2 enzyme. Two such proteins have been identified: **lipomodulin** from neutrophils and **macrocortin** from macrophages.

An additional mechanism of steroids involves their depression of **interleukin I** released from macrophages. This reduces release of **interleukin II** from activated T lymphocyte helper cells and inhibits the proliferation of newly sensitized lymphocytes. Lymphocytic release of lymphokines—especially macrophage inhibitory factor (MIF)—is inhibited. Reduced levels of MIF decrease the cueing of macrophages to remain in inflamed foci.

Glucocorticoids may be lytic for some subpopulations of lymphocytes of thymic origin. Thymic involution is observed in young animals as a consequence of administering these steroids. In humans, the lympholytic effects have not been observed. However, glucocorticoids are toxic to tumor cells in human lymphomas and lymphocytic leukemias and are used in chemotherapy of these neoplasms, particularly in combination with other agents whose antitumor actions are enhanced by the steroids.

The acute-phase response of the liver in inflammation is also dependent on corticosteroids, but it is unclear whether exogenously administered antiinflammatory steroids actually heighten AP response. The anti-inflammatory steroids seem to have little direct effect on vascular permeability and the formation of edema, and have little utility in treatment of acute inflammation.

Systemic employment of natural glucocorticoids like **cortisol** or **cortisone** for their anti-inflammatory properties is compromised by their renal effects, which overlap with those of the primary mineralocorticoid, aldosterone. Systematic chemical modification of glucocorticoid structure has resulted in a series of steroid derivatives having diminished mineralocorticoid activity and enhanced anti-inflammatory activity. Major differences among the **synthetic glucocorticoids** involve their relative anti-inflammatory potency and the duration of their action, crudely indicated in Table 12–2 as biological half-life. Overall, significant qualitative differences among the different synthetic antiinflammatory steroids are minimal.

All glucocorticoids are well absorbed from the GI tract and skin but may be usefully administered by intravenous or subcutaneous routes. Plasma binding is extensive; two plasma proteins, albumin and a serum globulin, are responsible. Difference in the residence time in the body of the various glucocorticoids may relate to affinities for these proteins. Glucocorticoids are metabolically inactivated by reductions of double bonds, keto groups, or hydroxyl groups at hepatic and nonhepatic sites. Conjugation of metabolized or nonmetabolized corticoids with glucuronide or sulfate occurs largely in the liver and to a lesser extent in the kidney. Virtually all of the altered steroid is excreted through the kidney.

The frequent employment of **synthetic glucocorticoids** in prolonged highdose regimens inevitably elicits undesirable side effects. These include truncal obesity and cushingoid features, gastrointestinal toxicity (peptic ulcers), hypertension, hyperglycemia, blood dyscrasias (leukocytosis, lymphocytopenia), insomnia, depression, immunosuppression, musculoskeletal changes (myopathy, osteoporosis, growth reduction), and fluid and electrolyte disturbances (Na^+ retention, K^+ loss).

NONSTEROIDAL ANTI-INFLAMMATORY DRUGS

The nonsteroidal anti-inflammatory drugs (NSAIDs) are aspirin-like oral agents that share a common ability to **inhibit prostanoid synthesis**. Sixteen useful NSAIDs occur in seven different chemical classes: salicylates, pyrazolons, chlorthenoxazins, fenamates, propionic acid derivatives, tolmetins, and piroxicams. Although NSAIDs influence a range of different biochemical and physiological systems, their common inhibition of **cyclooxygenase** underlies their main effect, suppression of all prostanoid synthesis (see Fig. 12–2). Unlike steroids, NSAIDs do not influence leukotriene formation. NSAIDs have three main effects: analgesia, antipyresis, and anti-inflammation. To be discussed along with the NSAIDs are acetaminophen and phenacetin, which share analgesic and antipyretic properties with the NSAIDs but which have no effects on the inflammatory process itself.

Salicylates

The salicylates (Fig. 12–4)—**sodium salicylate, aspirin** (acetylsalicylic acid), **diflunisal** (difluorophenyl salicylic acid), and **salsalate** (salicylsalicylic acid)—reduce fever (antipyresis) and are analgesic, in addition to their anti-inflammatory properties. **Prostanoid synthesis inhibition** can be linked to all three of these therapeutic properties. Pyrogens released from active granulocytes act on the preoptic hypothalamic thermoregulatory center in a mechanism that involves $PG-E_2$. Salicylates may moderate **hyperthermia** by reducing hypothalamic production of this prostaglandin. The **analgesia** obtained with salicylates may stem from their inhibiting the production of $PG-E_2$, $PG-F_{2\alpha}$, and/or $PG-I_2$. These prostanoids are proposed to increase the sensitivity of peripheral sensory nerve terminals for kinins. Nociceptive C fiber sensitivity to histamine may also be enhanced by these prostanoids and reduced through salicylate inhibition of the synthesis of E_2, I_2, or $F_{2\alpha}$. Not all types of pain are abatable with salicylates, however, visceral pain being a notable and unexplained example. The anti-inflammatory effects of salicylates are dependent on their depressing the prostanoid network of effects linked with tissue response to injury. All salicylates accomplish this by inhibiting the enzyme **cyclooxygenase** (see Fig. 12–2).

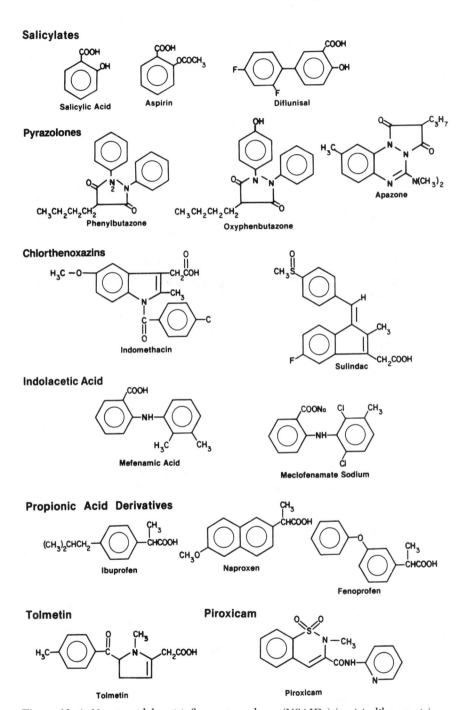

Figure 12–4. Nonsteroidal anti-inflammatory drugs (NSAIDs) (aspirin-like agents).

Aspirin

It has been said that if aspirin were introduced as a new drug today it might not be assigned its present over-the-counter status. **Aspirin** is an agent with complex effects and an important **toxicology**. Although aspirin has a place as a useful antiarthritic agent, its popular uses generally ignore the drug as an anti-inflammatory agent, preferring it solely as an inexpensive, readily available, effective analgesic or antipyretic agent.

The absorption of aspirin takes place in the stomach and is dependent on gastric acidity. Passage across the gastric epithelium occurs most readily when the drug is in a **non-ionized** state. Since aspirin is a weak acid with a pKa of 3.5, most of the drug will be non-ionized in a gastric lumen whose pH approaches 1.0. Once having crossed the gastric epithelium, the drug encounters a plasma environment whose pH is 7.4 where it becomes predominantly ionized. Ionization discourages antigrade movement back to the lumen. An increase of two pH units above the pKa of a compound will shift it completely to an ionized state. Thus, an increase in gastric lumenal pH to pH 5 to 6, which may occur in conditions such as atrophic gastritis, will inhibit aspirin absorption. The presence of food in the stomach also markedly decreases aspirin absorption. Uptake under less than optimal conditions (e.g., from a rectal suppository) can nonetheless be therapeutically sufficient given a large enough dose and enough time.

Once absorbed, **aspirin** is converted relatively quickly and spontaneously to **salicylic acid** (Fig. 12–5). A half-life of only about 15 minutes for the parent compound is not unusual (Table 12–3). Salicylic acid (itself a *bona fide* NSAID) is extensively **bound to plasma proteins** (80 to 90 percent) but eventually distributes throughout most tissues of the body and placenta. Concentrations in brain and CSF are low because of poor passage across the blood-brain barrier and an active transport system in the choroid plexus that exports the agent (Table 12–3). Many tissues, especially the liver, **conjugate salicylic acid** with either glucuronic acid or glycine (see Fig. 12–5). A small portion of salicylate

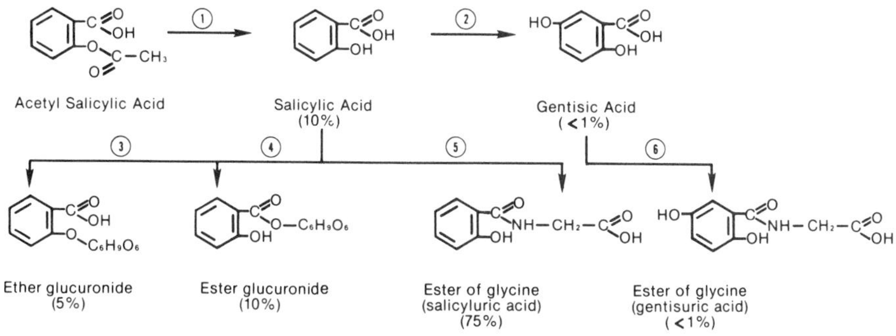

Figure 12–5. Metabolism of acetylsalicylic acid. Numbers in parentheses represent the percentages of original oral aspirin dose that are recovered from urine.

Table 12–3. CHARACTERISTICS OF NONSTEROIDAL ANTI-INFLAMMATORY AGENTS

	Antipyretic	Analgestic	Anti-inflammatory	Uricosuric	Serum Protein Binding (%)	$T_{1/2}$ (hr)	Excretion	Inhibitory Platelet Aggregation
Salicylic acid	+	+	+ decr.	+	80–95%	2–30	R	–
Acetylsalicylic acid (aspirin)	+	+	+	+	50–90%	0.25	R	+
Salsalate	+	+	+	+	80–85%	0.5	R	–
Diflunisal	–	+	+ incr.	+	99%	8–12	R	+
Phenylbutazone	+	+ decr.	+ incr.	+ decr.	98%	56–170	R (60%), F	+
Oxyphenylbutazone	+	+ decr.	+ incr.	+ decr.	99%	72	R	+
Azapropazone (apazone)	+	+	+	+ incr.	95%		R (65%), F	+
Indomethacin	+	+	+ incr.	+	90%	2–3	R (60%), F	+
Sulindac	+	+	+	+	93%	7	R (50%), F	+
Mefenamic acid (Ponstel)	+	+	+	–	?	2	R (75%), F	+
Meclofenamate (Meclomen)	+	+	+	–	?	2	R (66%), F	+
Ibuprofen	+	+	+	–	99%	2	R (70%), F	+ decr.
Naproxen	+	+	+ incr.	–	99%	14	R	+
Fenoprofen	+	+	+	–	99%	3	R	+
Tolmetin	+	+	+ incr.	–	90%	5	R	+
Piroxicam	+	+	+ incr.	+	~90%	30–86 (50 mean)	R (60%), F	+
Phenacetin	+	+	–	–	33%	1	R	–
Acetaminophen (paracetamol)	+	+	–	–	25%	2	R	–

+ or – = relative clinically useful effect
incr. or decr. = effect relative to that of aspirin
$T_{1/2}$ (hr) = approximate plasma half-life
Excretion by the kidney (R) or in feces (F) is shown in some cases with a percent total excretion drug.

316

is metabolized to gentisic acid. The kidney excretes virtually all metabolites of aspirin by glomerular filtration or secretion (see Table 12–3). The rate of excretion of free salicylate is dependent on urinary pH (higher at higher pHs), whereas excretion of the conjugated forms is independent of pH.

The enzymes responsible for the formation of the two main excreted metabolites of aspirin (salicyluric acid and ester glucuronide; see Fig. 12–3) are **saturated** by relatively low levels of substrate. Overloading of these steps occurs at quite low therapeutic doses of aspirin and results in an **increase in the plasma half-life** of salicylic acid. The minimal half-life of salicylate is 2 to 3 hours, but after repeated administration of the highest tolerated therapeutic doses its half-life increases to 15 to 30 hours.

The **biochemical effects of aspirin** on the body are diverse.

1. The spontaneous loss of acetyl groups from acetylsalicylic acid may involve the transfer of these groups to proteins and nucleic acids. These **acetylations** appear unimportant except with regard to the enzyme cyclooxygenase. Acetylation of the hydroxy group of serine that occurs at the catalytic site of this enzyme is important in aspirin's inhibition of its activity.
2. **Cyclooxygenase inhibition** by aspirin is also affected by the drug's metabolite, salicylic acid. In non-nucleated cells such as platelets, inhibition occurs with low doses of the drug and lasts the life of the cell. Salicyclate inhibition is reversible and by itself weaker than aspirin's.
3. Mitochondrial **oxidative phosphorylation** is uncoupled by aspirin. The mechanism is not understood. In decreasing cellular respiratory rates, both oxygen consumption and CO_2 evolution are increased and levels of ATP are decreased along with activities of ATP-dependent enzymes.

A number of physiologic changes can be detected in patients ingesting therapeutic levels of aspirin.

1. The systemic **elevation in CO_2 production** is sufficient to stimulate the respiratory center in the medulla and increase respiratory rate and alveolar ventilation. No elevation of plasma P_{CO_2} is observed unless a drug that depresses the medullary respiratory center (e.g., an opioid or barbiturate) has been administered concomitantly.
2. In the gastric mucosa, endogenous $PG-E_2$ and $PG-I_2$ maintain gastric secretion and synthesis of the protective mucous coating of the GI tract lumen. Thus, through its antiprostanoid effects, aspirin may cause **occult fecal blood loss** and **ulceration** of the gastric epithelium.
3. A modest **prolongation of bleeding time** and inhibition of platelet aggregation is tied to aspirin's inhibition of platelet $TX-A_2$ formation and endothelial $PG-E_2$ and $PG-I_2$. Low doses of aspirin (325 mg/day) selectively decrease platelet formation of $TX-A_2$, a vasoconstrictor pro-

stanoid and stimulator of platelet aggregation. Higher doses (2 to 4 g/day) also inhibit endothelial production of prostacyclin, a vasodilator and an inhibitor of platelet aggregation, in addition to TX-A$_2$ production. Low-dose aspirin therapy is prophylactic for coronary artery disease, myocardial infarction, and deep venous thrombosis. Bleeding time alteration may also contribute to occult fecal blood loss.

4. Renal **excretion of uric acid** is decreased by low doses of aspirin (2 g/day) and increased by higher therapeutic doses (4 g/day). With 4 g per day, tubular secretion and reabsorption of uric acid are reduced, resulting in a decline in serum uric acid levels.

Aspirin **toxicity** shows three patterns. The first, **chronic aspirin toxicity**, involves a prolonged period of continuous medication (years) during which the drug has been taken in more or less therapeutic doses; the second is simple **intolerance** to the drug; and the third is **acute aspirin overdose**.

Chronic aspirin toxicity leads to a heightened incidence of GI ulcers, renal disease, and possibly hepatic dysfunction. In the kidney, endogenous PG-E$_2$, from medullary interstitial cells, enhances the flow of blood through the renal medulla and increases net renal blood flow. PG-E$_2$ apparently acts antagonistically to antidiuretic hormone (ADH). Inhibition of PG-E$_2$ synthesis may restrict medullary flow to such a degree that ischemia develops. **Papillary necrosis,** presumably arising from medullary ischemia, is the earliest pathological change observed with chronic aspirin toxicity. Progression to chronic **interstitial nephritis** and end-stage renal failure may then follow. Another postulated function of renal PG-E$_2$ is to decrease tubular absorption of chloride anion. The formation of **edema** with aspirin abuse may be linked to the consequent sodium retention. A probably related phenomenon is the interference of aspirin with the action of furosemide-like diuretics.

Simple **intolerance** to aspirin appears in the absence of any form of drug abuse. Gastric distress following even a single dose may be a routine and self-limiting experience of patients with aspirin intolerance. Others in such a group who try using aspirin more regularly are more prone than the general population to develop GI ulceration, chronic blood loss, and rarely, hypochromic anemia. Milder manifestations of aspirin toxicity, collectively known as **salicylism,** include headache, vertigo, tinnitus, vomiting, and sweating. Also to be included in this pattern of simple intolerance to aspirin is aspirin allergy. Urticaria, angioedema, and other symptoms typical of anaphylactoid hypersensitivity may be observed, as well as the precipitation of acute attacks in asthmatic patients.

Acute overingestion of aspirin produces dose-dependent toxicity. In the cell, toxic levels of aspirin act to reduce **lipid synthesis** and enhance **fatty acid oxidation. Hexose metabolism** is altered. Hyperglycemia (especially in young children), glucosuria, and mobilization of glycogen accompany a reduced rate of glycolysis. Increased levels of the drug in the CNS produce general disturbances that include drowsiness, confusion, excitement, and ultimately progress to hallucinations, convulsions, and coma. Tinnitus is the result of the drug's effects on cortical auditory regions. Effects on the hypothalamus, *via* the pituitary, end up stimulating corticosteroid release from the adrenal. Strong evidence dissociates this action from anti-inflammatory actions of aspirin at nontoxic doses. Excess levels of salicylate are thought to be directly toxic to hepatic parenchymal cells. **Hepatocellular damage,** signaled by rising concentrations of hepatic enzymes in the serum, may be sufficient to produce hypoprothrombinemia.

Acute aspirin intoxication is marked by acid-base disturbance. Early in the course of toxicity, while aspirin levels are still low, the stimulation of the hindbrain respiratory center and the resultant hyperventilation produces a **respiratory alkalosis.** As drug levels rise above toxic levels, the medullary center is depressed, while CO_2 produced by the salicylate's mitochondrial effects continues to rise, causing a shift to **respiratory acidosis.** Three factors then combine to cause a further shift to a **metabolic acidosis:** (1) the accumulation of pyruvate, lactate, and acetoacetate as a result of aspirin's impairment of carbohydrate metabolism; (2) the acid load of the aspirin itself; and (3) impaired renal excretion of sulfuric and phosphoric acids. This later effect may in part be modulated by the aspirin effects on renal PG-E_2.

The aspirin **toxicity** of any pattern is aggravated by **codosage with other NSAIDs** or with the analgesics acetaminophen or phenacetin. The shared mechanisms of the NSAIDs apparently underlie their mutual exacerbation of each other's side effects. Aspirin has also been implicated in the occurrence of **Reye's syndrome** in children. Evidence suggests that widespread use of aspirin may carry a significant age-dependent risk for this disease.

In addition to the use of aspirin at low doses for various vascular and cardiac diseases, mentioned earlier, the drug is used in high doses (4 or more g/day) for its anti-inflammatory (and analgesic) effects in severe rheumatoid arthritis, spondylitis, bursitis, and other forms of rheumatic disease. Mid-range doses (about 1.3 g/day) are used for relief of pain, discomfort, and fever of a wide range of medical and dental afflictions.

Phenylbutazone and Other Pyrazolons

Phenylbutazone (Butazolidin) (see Fig. 12–4), like other NSAIDs, is an oral drug that is extensively bound to serum proteins and has analgesic, antipyretic, anti-inflammatory, and mild uricosuric actions. It is metabolized to oxyphenylbutazone and two hydroxylated forms, which are in part converted to glucuronides. About two thirds of the drug is **excreted by the kidney**—1 percent as unchanged phenylbutazone, 40 percent as glucuronidated phenylbutazone, 10 percent as unconjugated metabolite, and 12 percent as conjugated metabolites. The drug is effective for **acute gouty arthritis, rheumatoid**

arthritis, ankylosing spondylitis, degenerative hip disease, and bursitis. While its anti-inflammatory potency is superior to aspirin, its analgesic and uricosuric actions are inferior (see Table 12–3). Phenylbutazone, however, is associated with a wide range of unwanted side effects that require attention during use. The drug is most notorious for aplastic anemia, although actual incidence is less than 1 percent (with 2.2 to 6.5 deaths per 10^5 patients). Other marrow effects, particularly neutropenia, are encountered more frequently. Because of its therapeutic setting, its use is often prolonged, raising the risk for the full panoply of toxic effects. For elderly patients, it is contraindicated. Oxyphenylbutazone is accredited for use as an oral drug for dysmenorrhea but has many of the same problems as phenylbutazone. Apazone is a new pyrazolon that is reportedly less toxic than the other pyrazolons (see Table 12–3).

Indomethacin and Other Indoleacetic Acids

Indomethacin (Indocin; see Fig. 12–4) is among the most potent inhibitors of cyclooxygenase of all the NSAIDs. Like phenylbutazone, it is a drug with many undesirable side effects. Approximately 30 to 50 percent of those medicated with the drug experience some form of toxicity, compared with as high as 45 percent of patients treated with phenylbutazone. The most frequent problems (>1 in 1000) are GI disturbances, CNS difficulties (such as severe headaches, mild dizziness, lethargy, confusion), and tinnitus, but GI ulceration, prolonged bleeding time, and renal and hepatic dysfunction also occur. For patients who can tolerate the drug, it is very useful. In arthritis, joint swelling and morning stiffness are decreased and the number of joints involved diminishes. Mobility and functional capability are increased. Moderate to severe rheumatoid arthritis, osteoarthritis, spondylitis, acute gouty arthritis, and acute bursitis may be treated with oral indomethacin three times a day. In neonates, closure of persistent patent ductus arteriosus can be achieved with indomethacin in not quite three quarters of cases. One third of the drug is excreted in the feces after an extensive enterohepatic recycling, but considerable variation may be observed. Three quarters of the drug is metabolized to desmethyl or desbenzoyl forms. As with all NSAIDs, the drug is very extensively bound to serum protein.

Sulindac (Clinoril; see Fig. 12–4) has a somewhat longer serum half-life than indomethacin (see Table 12–3) and a reduced overall incidence of side effects at therapeutic dosage (about 26 percent). The drug is initially oxidized to a sulfone, which, in turn, is reduced to a sulfide derivative. Most of the anti-inflammatory, analgesic, and antipyretic activities of the drug are due to this sulfide metabolite. Sulindac is used in the same clinical situations as indomethacin. The analgesic and anti-inflammatory potency of sulindac is about equal to that of phenylbutazone, one-third that of indomethacin, and 10 times that of aspirin.

The Fenamates

The fenamate group of anti-inflammatory NSAIDs is represented by **mefenamic acid** (Ponstel) and **meclofenamic acid** (Meclomen; see Table 12–3 and Fig. 12–4). They are about half as potent as phenylbutazone. The overall incidence of **side effects** of fenamates at therapeutic dosage is about 25 percent. Diarrhea is a common and sometimes severe side effect of fenamate usage. Like salsalate (and unlike the other NSAIDs), the fenamates do **not** significantly **inhibit platelet aggregation**. After oral administration, meclofenamate is taken up more rapidly than is mefenamic acid, but both have similar serum half-lives. The use of mefenamic acid is for relief of moderate pain such as **dysmenorrhea**, whereas meclofenamate may be used for acute or chronic forms of **rheumatoid** and **osteoarthritis**.

Ibuprofen and Other Propionic Acid Derivatives

The propionic acid group of NSAIDs includes **naproxen** (Naprosyn) and **fenoprofen** (Nalfon) in addition to **ibuprofen** (see Fig. 12–4). Although all share the same unwanted **general side effects** with other NSAIDs, GI disturbances are said to be less severe with this group. Naproxen is about 20 percent **more potent than aspirin** as an inhibitor of prostanoid synthesis, and ibuprofen and fenoprofen are about **equivalent in potency to aspirin**. All three are poorly soluble in water at low pHs (as are other NSAIDs) and are rapidly absorbed from the stomach and upper intestine. Ibuprofen plasma level peaks occur 1 to 2 hours after oral administration, naproxen in 2 to 4 hours, and fenoprofen in 2 hours. Serum half-life for ibuprofen and fenoprofen is 2 to 3 hours, whereas it is 14 hours for naproxen (see Table 12–3). **Ibuprofen** is marketed as a prescription drug (Motrin, Rufin) in 200 to 600 mg tablets or as a **nonprescription preparation** (Advil, Nuprin) in 200 mg tablets. The overall incidence of **GI side effects** of ibuprofen is 5 to 15 percent, most being mild in nature: nausea, epigastric, or abdominal discomfort. An advantage of ibuprofen over aspirin is its **reduced inhibition of platelet aggregation**. Ibuprofen's major metabolites, involving carboxylation of the propyl side chain or hydroxymethylation, are largely excreted through the kidney, either free or glucuronidated. Ibuprofen's very high binding to serum protein (99 percent) may influence expected activities of other drugs that share this characteristic, such as other NSAIDs (see Table 12–3) and the warfarin (Coumadin) group of agents. Concurrent use of ibuprofen (or most other NSAIDs) with anticoagulants of the warfarin type may unexpectedly intensify **prolongation of prothrombin times** and, in the face of the antiplatelet action of most NSAIDs, lead to potentially **significant bleeding problems**. However, ibuprofen combined with warfarin drugs is said to be less likely than most other NSAIDs to alter coagulation effects. Combined administration of pairs of NSAIDs is inadvisable both because of the higher risk of toxicity and because of questionable therapeutic benefit. The combination of ibuprofen and aspirin, for instance, is known to cause a net **decrease** in anti-inflammatory activity of the two.

Ibuprofen is about **equal to aspirin** in efficacy against **rheumatoid arthritis** and **osteoarthritis**. While the drug gives adequate analgesia with many forms of pain, it is perhaps more useful than most NSAIDs for **dysmenorrhea**. Dysmenorrhea appears to arise from a release of E series prostaglandins associated with some menstrual phases of the uterine cycle.

Naproxen is a drug amenable to long-term treatment of **osteoarthritis**, **rheumatoid arthritis**, **spondylitis**, and **gouty arthritis**. As with most NSAIDs, absorption from an oral dose is retarded by the presence of food in the stomach. Only about one third of the drug is metabolized (by 6-demethylation). Both unchanged and metabolized naproxen are excreted by the kidney either free or conjugated with glucuronic acid (see Table 12–3). The drug inhibits the natriuretic effect of furosemide, the clearance of lithium in the kidney, and the renal tubular secretion of methotrexate.

Fenoprofen, like ibuprofen, is administered orally four times a day, compared with twice a day for naproxen. Nearly all (90 percent) fenoprofen is 4'-hydroxylated, conjugated with glucuronide, and excreted through the kidney. The **toxicity** of the drug includes the complete spectrum of problems observed with NSAIDs in general, but side effects of therapeutic dosage are tolerable for most users of the drug. Patients who have **arthritis** have reported **fenoprofen** to be **superior** to **ibuprofen** but less effective than naproxen in analgesia and palliation of morning stiffness.

Tolmetin and Piroxicam

Tolmetin (Tolectin) and **piroxicam** (Feldene) are chemically dissimilar drugs (see Fig. 12–4) having analgesic, antipyretic, and anti-inflammatory actions in common. **Tolmetin** is regarded as a somewhat more effective anti-inflammatory agent than aspirin, but not as strong as indomethacin. It is approved for use in **juvenile rheumatoid arthritis**. Piroxicam is claimed to be on a par with indomethacin or naproxen and **better tolerated** by some patients **than aspirin**. The advantage of piroxicam is a relatively long serum half-life (30 to 80 hours; see Table 12–3), which allows single daily doses.

ACETAMINOPHEN AND OTHER ANALGESIC AMINOPHENOLS

These compounds are **nonprescription analgesic and antipyretic agents** with no anti-inflammatory action (see Table 12–3). Although not NSAIDs, they are included in a discussion of the group because of their close association with anti-inflammatory therapeutics. **Phenacetin** (acetophenetidin), **acet-anilid,** and **acetaminophen** (paracetamol) have been employed as analgesics since the 19th century. The toxicity of acetanilid through some of its metabolites (Fig. 12–6)—plus the discovery that the active form of both acetanilid and phenacetin was acetaminophen—led to the discontinuation of both of the former and the more extensive use of acetaminophen. The **analgesic mechanism** of action of acetaminophen is obscure. In contrast to aspirin, the antipyretic action of acetaminophen principally takes place in the thermoregulatory region of the hypothalamus.

Acetaminophen is well absorbed from the intestinal tract and is relatively evenly distributed to all body fluids, including the CSF. About 80 percent of the drug is converted to conjugates of glucuronic acid, sulfuric acid (35 percent) or cysteine (3 percent) (see Fig. 12–6), and virtually all of an oral dose is recovered in the urine. Acetaminophen is free of many of the side effects and toxic reactions of aspirin, including acid-base and respiratory alterations, platelet aggregation, GI bleeding, and gastric irritation. There is no potentiation of warfarin anticoagulation through acetaminophen displacement of warfarin serum protein binding. With acetaminophen, blood dyscrasias in general are very infrequent.

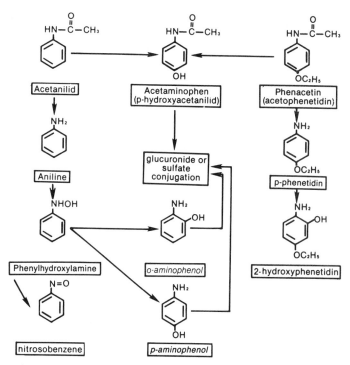

Figure 12–6. Metabolism of acetaminophen and phenacetin.

Acute overdosing with acetaminophen is potentially lethal at ingested levels >500 mg per kg. Hepatic necrosis and failure is the most likely of the serious consequences of intoxication. Ketolic metabolites of unconjugated drug, the apparent toxic intermediates, accumulate to high intracellular levels in overdosage. Their avid binding to glutathione causes a marked depletion of this important coenzyme. Initial symptoms of intoxication are nausea, vomiting, and abdominal cramping. Elevations in serum transaminase and bilirubin plus prolongation of prothrombin time, all manifestations of hepatotoxicity, are delayed 2 to 4 days after the overdose episode. Administration of N-acetylcysteine (Mucocyst) within 24 hours of drug ingestion will prevent hepatotoxicity, restoring hepatic glutathione levels possibly by competing with glutathione for binding of drug metabolites. Treatment of acetaminophen poisoning should also include immediate induction of vomiting or gastric lavage plus oral administration of activated charcoal. Approximately one tenth of the severely intoxicated patients who do not receive antidote go on to develop significant liver damage, and of those who suffer hepatotoxicity, as high as one fifth die of hepatic failure. Other serious consequences of acute acetaminophen overdosage are renal tubular necrosis and hypoglycemic coma. Like hepatotoxicity, the occurrence of renal pathology is dependent on glutathione depletion and is preventable with timely use of N-acetylcysteine.

The toxicity of acetaminophen taken over long periods of time but roughly at therapeutic levels is most notable when the drug is used concomitantly with aspirin. With prolonged use, the pair is associated with papillary necrosis and interstitial nephritis at a greater incidence than that found with comparable exposures to aspirin or acetaminophen alone. The reason for this apparent potentiation of salicylate renal toxicity by acetaminophen is not understood, but its observation has led some countries to prohibit the compounding of nonprescription preparations containing these two agents. Other NSAIDs appear to provoke papillary necrosis at a lower incidence than aspirin, but a definitive picture of the effects of acetaminophen combination with NSAIDs with respect to renal toxicity is not clear.

MISCELLANEOUS ANTI-INFLAMMATORY AGENTS

Gold

Gold, attached to sulfur on **glucose (aurothioglucose)**, **maleate (gold sodium thiomalate)**, or **trialkylphosphine (Auranofin)**, effectively arrests the progress of rheumatoid arthritis. Chrysotherapy is **not analgesic** or **antipyretic** and causes only a gradual reduction in the signs and symptoms of the rheumatoid disease. Best used for active cases of **rheumatoid arthritis** that have not responded well to NSAID treatment, *bona fide* remissions may be observed in 15 percent of persons with the disease, with improvement in most other cases. Improvements include a decrease in the erythrocyte sedimentation rate, decreases in circulating rheumatoid factor and fibrinogen, improvement in joint function, and prevention of extension of the disease to other joints. The mechanism of gold action is unknown. Aurothioglucose and sodium gold thiomalate are administered intramuscularly, their absorption in the GI tract being highly erratic. Auranofin may be given orally. Plasma half-lives of gold compounds are about 7 hours following single doses of 50 mg, and increase to several weeks with repeated subsequent injections. Excretion by the fecal route is only half that *via* the kidney. After cessation of prolonged therapy, removal of all gold from the body may not be complete for up to a year. Initially after administration the gold compounds bind to albumin and collect in erythrocytes. Later they are found deposited in tissue macrophages throughout the body. With prolonged administration, the drugs' concentrations in synovial fluids of inflamed joints will exceed that in unaffected tissues by severalfold.

The **side effects of chrysotherapy** include mucocutaneous lesions (15 percent—stomatitis, pharyngitis, gastritis, colitis, erythema, and so on), gold-induced nephrosis (5 to 8 percent), and blood dyscrasias (1 percent—leukopenia, agranulocytosis). Auranofin is more hydrophobic than the other two gold compounds and is almost completely excreted *via* the feces. Auranofin is not accumulated to the same concentration in body tissues as gold thioglucose or thiomalate; otherwise all three drugs appear comparable.

A number of miscellaneous compounds have empirically proven to be effective against rheumatoid arthritis in addition to those containing gold, including **penicillamine, levamisole,** and **aminoquinoline antimalarial drugs**. The last of these, especially chloroquine, have achieved a recognized place in the treatment of rheumatoid arthritis or other arthritic conditions such as Sjögren's disease. The basis for its effectiveness is not known.

Colchicine

Colchicine is a drug of plant origin whose clinical significance is limited to the prophylaxis and palliation of acute inflammatory episodes (flare-ups) of gout. Gout is a disease of purine catabolism, apparently inherited, characterized by serum concentrations of uric acid chronically in excess of solubility. Urate deposits tend to accumulate as tophi in articular cartilages, synovial membranes of joints and bursae, and in the cartilage of the outer ear. In the kidney, deposits in the form of calculi or tophi cause interstitial fibrosis, obstruction, and ultimately renal failure. Colchicine binds to microtubular protein dimers, inhibiting their polymerization and obstructing microtubular function, including (1) cell division, (2) secretion, and (3) cell locomotion. At therapeutic doses, inflammatory macrophages are particularly responsive to colchicine. The drug inhibits their migration into affected tissues and their secretion possibly of such substances as interleukin I, interferons, and lysosomal enzymes. The swelling, pain, and redness of gouty joints is relieved by colchicine, administered either as needed or in anticipation of episodic flare-ups. The drug is well absorbed after oral administration, concentrating in the spleen, liver, kidney, and GI epithelium. Vomiting, diarrhea, and abdominal pain may occur several hours after administration. Long-term use of the drug (months to years) carries the risk of neutropenia, anemia, alopecia, and azospermia. Indomethacin can effectively replace colchicine.

Allopurinol

Allopurinol (Zyloprim) is another agent of value for the treatment of gout. An analog of hypoxanthine, allopurinol inhibits xanthine oxidase and the conversion of hypoxanthine to uric acid, the last catabolic step in the degradation of purines. Therapeutic levels of allopurinol ameliorate the hyperuricemia of the patient with gout, reducing levels sufficiently so that all the serum urate is in solution. Long-term use of allopurinol (months to years) promotes gradual resorption of tophi. Like colchicine, allopurinol may alleviate the acute episodes of pain and swelling but without colchicine's side effects. Aside from occasional incidence of allergy, allopurinol may be used in prolonged therapy with virtually no toxicity. Besides gout, potentially pathogenic hyperuricemia occurs in polycythemia vera, myeloid metaplasia, and following treatment of malignancy with either chemotherapy or radiation. In such situations, allopurinol is employed to control blood levels of uric acid to forestall its unwanted deposition in tissue.

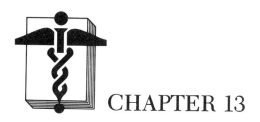

CHAPTER 13

Allergy and Asthma Drugs

H. E. WILLIAMSON, Ph.D.

ALLERGY

Allergies are a common clinical problem that can be manifested in a number of different ways, including skin conditions such as hives or eczema, sinus-nasal conditions such as hay fever, or pulmonary disorders such as asthma. All of these represent some type of disruption of the immunoinflammatory system. Causes of allergies may be pollens, venoms, foods, drugs, or a host of other substances. Contact with these substances, in sensitive individuals, can lead to the release of histamine as well as a number of different agents.

Histamine

Histamine is found throughout the body. Highest concentrations occur in the lungs, nasal mucosa, gastrointestinal (GI) tract, blood, and skin. Usually the histamine exists in a bound form in granules of mast cells in tissues or of basophils in blood. It is also found in platelets. Various stimuli are capable of releasing histamine, including injury to tissue, some drugs, and some amines. Immunological release occurs if storage cells are sensitized by attachment of IgE antibodies. Exposure to a specific antigen then results in release of histamine and other substances. The released histamine plays a major role in immediate hypersensitivity reactions. Excessive release can lead to anaphylactic shock.

The role of histamine in immunological responses is only partly understood. Its release results in local vasodilation and entry of various components of blood (e.g., antibodies, inflammatory cells) into affected tissue to exert their actions. In addition, histamine blocks release of lysosomal contents and inhibits some lymphocyte functions.

Histamine acts on two different receptors to produce its actions. These are referred to as H_1 and H_2 receptors. Some recent studies indicate that there may be a third receptor, H_3, in the brain. Responses of organs and tissues to histamine and the receptors involved are listed in Table 13–1.

Table 13–1. EFFECTS OF HISTAMINE AND RECEPTOR TYPES

System	Tissue and Response	Receptor H_1	H_2
Cardiovascular	Blood vessels (small)		
	Vasodilation	× (mostly)	× (some)
	Increase permeability	×	
	Blood vessels (large)		
	Contraction	×	
	Heart—increase force of contraction		×
	SA node—increase rate		×
Gastrointestinal	Smooth muscle—contraction	×	
	Stomach—stimulation of HCl secretion		×
Pulmonary	Bronchiolar smooth muscle contraction	×	
Nervous	Nerve endings for pain and itching—stimulation	×	
	CNS—arousal, emesis	×	×? (H_3)
Skin	Induce wheal and flare reaction	×	

Antihistamines: Uses and Effects

Since histamine is responsible for many of the signs and symptoms of allergies, drugs that decrease its actions (antihistamines) can decrease the severity of an allergic response.

H_1-Receptor Antagonists

Most of the effects of histamine in allergies are due to the stimulation of H_1 receptors. The method most frequently used to block these actions is the administration of an H_1-receptor antagonist. There are numerous antagonists (antihistamines) available, of several different chemical classes. All are competitive inhibitors. Some of the more frequently used compounds are listed in Table 13–2. The usefulness of these antihistamines is limited to the antagonism of the signs and symptoms of the allergic response, which are mediated by the release of histamine. Because other substances are involved, as well as activation of H_2 receptors in an allergic reaction, the H_1-receptor antagonists are not capable of suppressing all of the effects of an allergic response.

Other Actions. In addition to antihistaminic responses, the H_1-receptor antagonists also exert a number of other actions. These vary with the type of chemical derivative.

Table 13–2. H_1-RECEPTOR ANTAGONISTS

Compound	Sedative Action
Ethanolamine Derivatives	
Dimenhydrinate (Dramamine)	+ + +
Diphenhydramine (Benadryl)	+ + +
Doxylamine (Decapryn)	+ + +
Ethylenediamine Derivatives	
Pyrilamine (Neo-Antergan)	+ +
Tripelennamine (Pyribenzamine)	+ +
Piperazine Derivatives	
Cyclizine (Marezine)	+
Meclizine (Bonine)	+
Alkylamine Derivatives	
Chlorpheniramine (Chlor-Trimeton)	+
Phenothiazine Derivatives	
Promethazine (Phenergan)	+ + +
Piperidine Derivatives	
Terfenadine (Seldane)	0

Sedation is a very frequent side effect. The severity of this action for the various compounds is noted in Table 13–2. In some individuals, the effect can be so pronounced that they are unable to stay awake. Patients should be warned to avoid driving or the use of machinery. Because this action is so prominent, some of these compounds (**diphenhydramine and doxylamine**) have also been marketed as sleep aids. The lack of sedative action in some of the newer antihistamines (e.g., terfenadine) is due to the inability of these compounds to cross the blood-brain barrier.

Prevention of the nausea and vomiting of motion sickness is a useful action of some antihistamines. Agents used for this purpose include **dimenhydrinate, cyclizine,** and **meclizine.**

Several of the classes of H_1-receptor antagonists have anticholinergic activity. This probably explains the ability of these agents to decrease nasal secretions when they are used in the treatment of colds.

Antihistamines may also possess local anesthetic activity. Some of the benefits of topical application of antihistamines may be related to this action.

Toxicity. The undesirable effect of antihistamines most frequently reported is its sedative action. The sedative action is additive with that of other agents (e.g., alcohol). With the recent availability of agents that do not cross the blood-brain barrier, sedation will probably become less of a problem.

Dry mouth is a frequent side effect with the H_1 antihistamines, and when they are taken in excessive amounts, anticholinergic actions become very prominent. CNS stimulation can occur, especially in children. This can include hallucinations, excitement, and convulsions of intermittent tonic-clonic type.

Drug allergies can also be produced by these agents; these are seen most frequently after topical application.

H_2-Receptor Antagonists

Compounds are also available that are capable of blocking the actions of histamine at H_2 receptors. Such agents can suppress secretion of hydrochloric acid by the stomach and are useful in the treatment of peptic ulcers (see Chapter 14, on gastrointestinal drugs).

ASTHMA

Asthma is a disease in which there is an episodic and reversible increase in resistance to air flow in intrapulmonary airways, and the increase in resistance is characterized by wide variation over short periods of time. It is a condition in which wheezing or difficulty in breathing may occur. Such events are believed to be an overreaction to various stimuli, including allergens, viruses, stress, exercise, sleep, cold weather, drugs (aspirin and other NSAIDS), and nonspecific irritants. The responses to these stimuli include one or more of the following: bronchospasm (contraction of bronchial muscle), inflammation (edema of airway lining), or increased production of mucous secretions.

Bronchial smooth muscle that is innervated by vagal efferents is contracted by stimulation of the parasympathetic nervous system. In asthma, however, enhanced activity of this system does not appear to play a major role. Consequently, anticholinergic agents are only occasionally of value in therapy. The mast cells that are present in the bronchioles do appear to play an important part in asthma. These cells are capable of releasing several substances that can contract bronchial smooth muscle or produce inflammation or both. Substances that can be released include histamine, leukotrienes (slow-reacting substance), eosinophil chemotactic factor (ECT), neutrophil chemotactic factor (NCF), heparin, and proteases. Stimulation of mast cells triggers the release of these substances. Furthermore, mast cells may be sensitized by prior exposure to an antigen; thus, contents are released when the antigen reacts with IgE on mast cell surfaces.

Agents Useful in Asthma Treatment

A number of agents are useful in the treatment of asthma. These include sympathomimetics, methylxanthines, cromolyn, glucocorticoids, and anticholinergics. The sympathomimetics and methylxanthines dilate bronchial smooth muscles to relieve symptoms, whereas cromolyn is useful prophylactically to prevent attacks by preventing release of mediators from mast cells, and glucocorticoids relieve inflammation. Anticholinergics block bronchial smooth muscle contraction caused by parasympathetic nerve stimulation.

Sympathomimetics

Bronchial smooth muscle is dilated by β_2-adrenoceptor agonists (Fig. 13–1). Although there are no sympathetic nerves to bronchial smooth muscle, β_2 adrenoceptors are present. Stimulation of these is believed to result in an increased synthesis of cyclic adenosine monophosphate (AMP), by stimulating activity of adenylate cyclase. This in turn is involved in dilation of bronchial smooth muscle and inhibition of release of mediators from mast cells. Newer agents are more selective for β_2 adrenoceptors. They stimulate β_1 or α adrenoceptors only at very high doses; thus, side effects related to these receptors are limited. **Albuterol** (Salbutamol) and **terbutaline** (Brethine) are agents in this class. They may be given orally or used as an inhaler preparation. With oral use, the major side effect is tremors, which tend to diminish after several days of therapy. Other sympathomimetic agents that are useful for bronchospasm but that are not β_2-selective adrenoceptor agonists are isoproterenol (Isuprel) and epinephrine. When inhaled, their action is primarily local

HOCH₂
HO—⟨⟩—CHCH₂NHC(CH₃)₃
           |
           OH

Albuterol

[HO
    ⟨⟩—CHCH₂NHC(CH₃)₃
   HO   OH   ]₂ • H₂SO₄

Terbutaline

HO—⟨⟩—CH—CH₂—NHCH(CH₃)₂ • HCl
HO |
          OH

Isoproterenol

                    OH
                    |
HO—⟨⟩—C—CH₂NHCH₃
HO |
          H

Epinephrine

Figure 13–1. Sympathomimetics used in the treatment of asthma.

and they produce bronchodilation. In addition, epinephrine, by virtue of its α-adrenoceptor agonist activity, constricts blood vessels of the bronchial mucosa and aids in reducing edema; this further relieves asthmatic symptoms. In severe asthmatic attacks, injectable forms of sympathomimetics (epinephrine or terbutaline) may be used.

Methylxanthines

Methylxanthines (Fig. 13–2) include **theophylline, caffeine,** and **theobromine** and are found in a number of plant products such as tea (theophylline), coffee (caffeine), and cocoa (theobromine), as well as in a number of cola beverages (caffeine). Of the various methylxanthines, theophylline has gained wide usage in the treatment of asthma. It is capable of dilating bronchial smooth muscle by a direct action, the mechanism of which is not understood. Previously, it was proposed that it decreased the breakdown and hence increased the cellular concentration of cyclic AMP, which is believed to be in-

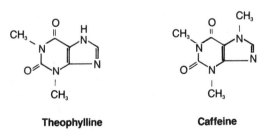

Theophylline   **Caffeine**

Figure 13–2. Methylxanthines.

volved in bronchodilation. Although theophylline can inhibit the activity of phosphodiesterase, the enzyme that converts cyclic AMP to 5'-AMP *in vitro*, it does not achieve sufficient concentration *in vivo* to inhibit this enzyme. Some recent evidence sugests that methylxanthines can block adenosine receptors, although it is not clear if this is the mechanism involved in bronchiolar smooth muscle relaxation.

Unfortunately, theophylline also exerts a number of other actions. Stimulation of the CNS can occur and nervousness and insomnia are seen with lower dosages; convulsions may be produced with higher dosages. These may also occur without prior signs of CNS stimulation. Theophylline is also a mild diuretic, producing an increase in renal blood flow and partially blocking sodium reabsorption in the proximal tubules of the nephrons. Refractoriness usually develops to the diuretic action of theophylline, however. Cardiac muscle is stimulated, resulting in an increase in force of contraction and in heart rate. Blood vessels are dilated by these agents. At higher doses and especially when given rapidly intravenously, cardiac arrhythmias and hypotension occur. In addition, theophylline is irritating to the GI tract and nausea and vomiting may occur.

Because the difference between therapeutic and toxic levels of theophylline is small, plasma concentrations must be determined and monitored continually. Blood levels of 10 to 20 μg per ml are optimal. It should also be noted that many drugs (cimetidine, erythromycin, and furosemide) can decrease the metabolism of theophylline, thus increasing blood levels of theophylline and producing toxicity. Conditions such as congestive heart failure, liver disease, and acute viral infections also decrease metabolism of theophylline. Faster metabolism occurs in smokers, however, so that higher doses are necessary in such persons. Metabolism of theophylline also varies with age, being low in infants but higher in young children than in adults.

Theophylline is usually given orally and is available in a number of forms. With the use of oral slow-release preparations, it is possible to reduce dosing to two to three times a day. Rectal suppository forms are available, but they can be very irritating. Absorption of theophylline from the suppository is erratic; absorption from solutions are more predictable.

Aminophylline is a form of theophylline that contains an equimolar amount of ethylenediamine. Supposedly this chemical aids in the dissolution of theophylline. However, the presence of ethylenediamine is not necessary, as the use of microcrystalline forms of theophylline has markedly increased its solubility. Furthermore, ethylenediamine can be a source of severe allergic responses such as Stevens-Johnson syndrome.

Because the toxicity of theophylline can be severe, it is essential that plasma levels of this agent be monitored. If the concentration of theophylline is maintained between 10 and 20 μg per ml, it can be a safe and useful agent for the management of chronic asthma.

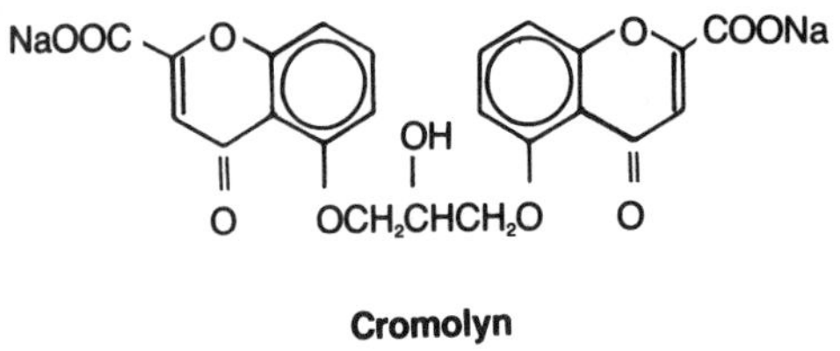

Cromolyn

Figure 13–3. Cromolyn.

Cromolyn

Cromolyn (Fig. 13–3) is also useful in the treatment of chronic asthma. This drug is believed to block the release of bronchoconstrictors from mast cells. It is used primarily as a prophylactic agent; it is not effective in terminating acute asthma attacks. Not all people respond to cromolyn; in particular, those individuals with acute inflammation may fail to respond. Thus, to determine if this agent is of value it may have to be administered for about 2 to 3 weeks. Cromolyn may be used chronically as a substitute for theophylline in moderate cases of asthma. However, it is used principally to prevent acute attacks of asthma and for this purpose must be administered prior to a known stimulus (e.g., exercise or exposure to an antigen). Cromolyn is not given orally, because it is very poorly absorbed from the GI tract. It is effective when deposited directly into the airways and is available in powder and aerosol forms for inhalational use. Toxicity is limited because the agent is poorly absorbed, but includes throat and trachea irritation, which can cause cough or bronchospasm. Allergic reactions may also be seen but are serious only rarely.

Glucocorticoids

When asthma is due to inflammation of the bronchial passages, glucocorticoid therapy is indicated. With chronic oral therapy, these agents should be administered every other day to minimize undesirable systemic effects (see Chapter 11, Endocrine Drugs). The marketing of glucocorticoids in forms for inhalational use has made glucocorticoid therapy far less risky. **Beclomethasone dipropionate** (Beclovent), when administered in aerosol form, is not appreciably absorbed; hence, its actions are limited primarily to the bronchial areas. Side effects with this form of therapy may be dysphonia and oral candidiasis.

In staticus asthmaticus daily intravenous infusions of a glucocorticoid may be necessary until the attack is controlled.

Anticholinergics

Recently an anticholinergic agent, **ipratropium bromide**, has been marketed in an inhalational form. Absorption is minimal and hence systemic effects are avoided. The bronchial dilating actions of this agent are additive with β_2-adrenoceptor stimulants. The addition of ipratropium to other agents is beneficial in some asthmatic patients.

Asthma Therapy

With the various drugs and forms of administration now available, symptoms of most patients with asthma can be relieved. With mild or occasional wheezing, the various drugs available in inhalational preparations may be sufficient. With more severe spasms, chronic treatment with theophylline or sympathomimetics or both may also be necessary. With severe, acute attacks, air flow may be so low that drugs given by inhalation may not reach airways in sufficient concentration; hence, injectable forms of sympathomimetics or theophylline may be necessary. In asthma associated with inflammation, steroids are indicated and may be combined with theophylline or sympathomimetics as necessary.

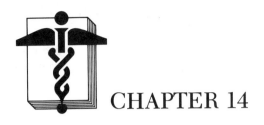

CHAPTER 14

Gastrointestinal Drugs

H. E. WILLIAMSON, Ph.D.

A variety of drugs are known to affect the gastrointestinal (GI) tract. In this chapter, those agents whose **primary** action is on the GI tract are discussed.

PEPTIC ULCER DISEASE THERAPY

Peptic ulcers, a major disease of the GI tract, can be of duodenal or gastric origin. Duodenal ulcers are associated with increased production of hydrochloric acid (HCl) in the stomach. To treat peptic ulcers, several different classes of drugs have been used. These have included anticholinergics, H_2-receptor antagonists, mucosal protectants, and antacids.

Anticholinergics

Although parasympathetic nerves are known to increase gastric acid secretion, the use of anticholinergics has not been very useful. To decrease HCl production, very large doses are necessary, and this results in numerous undesirable side effects related to anticholinergic activity. Furthermore, there is no evidence that these agents affect the course of the disease. Thus, these agents are no longer used.

H_2-Receptor Antagonists

The drugs most frequently used to treat peptic ulcers are the **H_2-receptor antagonists.** Whereas the H_1-histamine receptors are involved in contraction of smooth muscle, increased capillary permeability, the formation of wheal and flare, and immediate hypersensitivity, the H_2-histamine receptors are involved in gastric acid secretion. Older antihistaminic drugs affected only H_1 receptors. With the introduction of **cimetidine, ranitidine,** and recently **famotidine,** which are H_2-receptor antagonists, a major change occurred in the therapy of peptic ulcers. These agents are competitive inhibitors of histamine at H_2 receptors. They have little effect on H_1 receptors, β adrenoceptors, or muscarinic receptors. They have been found to be effective in decreasing HCl secretion induced by histamine, gastrin, food intake, and basal HCl secretion. These agents have become the drugs of choice in diseases in which a decrease in HCl secretion is desired. They are useful in the short-term treatment of duodenal and gastric peptic ulcers as well as prophylactically for duodenal ulcers. In the treatment of duodenal ulcers, H_2-receptor antagonists are reported to result in 85 to 90 percent cure within 8 weeks of therapy. They are also useful in Zollinger-Ellison syndrome, reflux esophagitis, stress ulcers, and systemic mastocytosis. Adverse reactions to cimetidine and ranitidine include headache, nausea, and skin rash. In addition, cimetidine exerts antiandrogenic activity such as gynecomastia and impotence, and rarely, has been reported to cause agranulocytosis and thrombocytopenia.

Mucosal Barrier Agents

Sucralfate (Carafate) is another agent that is useful in the treatment of duodenal peptic ulcers. This agent acts by binding to the necrotic tissue of ulcers. It serves as a barrier and hence protects the ulcer from acid or other potentially damaging substances. An acidic pH is necessary for activity. Thus, this compound cannot be administered with H_2-receptor antagonists or antacids. Results with this agent are comparable to those obtained with H_2-receptor antagonists or antacids. Another benefit of this agent is a low incidence of side effects. In a small percentage of patients, constipation may occur.

Antacids

Antacids (Table 14–1) are substances that are capable of neutralizing hydrochloric acid (HCl) secreted by the parietal cells of the stomach; they are used in treatment of a variety of hyperacidity conditions (e.g., peptic ulcer, gastritis, gastric hyperacidity, hiatal hernia, reflux esophagitis). The treatment of duodenal ulcers requires the use of large doses to accelerate healing, but

Table 14–1. ANTACIDS

Antacid	Onset	Duration	Side Effects/Precautions
Systemic			
Sodium bicarbonate	Rapid	Short	Short-term use only. Gas formation.
Sodium citrate	Rapid	Short	Short-term use only.
Nonsystemic Buffer			
Aluminum hydroxide ⎱ Aluminum phosphate ⎰ Dihydroxyaluminum aminoacetate ⎰	Slow	Long	May cause constipation. May cause nausea or vomiting. May affect drug absorption.
Magnesium trisilicate	Slow	Long	May cause diarrhea. Contraindicated in renal disease.
Nonbuffer			
Calcium carbonate	Rapid	Short	May stimulate HCl secretion. Gas formation. May cause constipation.
Magnesium hydroxide	Rapid	Short	May cause diarrhea. Contraindicated in renal disease.
Magnesium oxide ⎱ Magnesium carbonate ⎰	Slow	Long	May cause diarrhea. Contraindicated in renal disease.

the results are comparable to those seen with H_2-receptor antagonists. The large volumes and frequency of administration required of these antacids compared with only 1 tablet twice a day for the H_2-receptor antagonists has led to less frequent use of antacids. Antacids are available without prescription and are used extensively by individuals to self-treat **acid indigestion** (also referred to as heartburn or sour stomach). This condition is believed to be due to the regurgitation of stomach contents into the esophagus, where HCl can cause irritation of the esophageal lining. In susceptible individuals it occurs after eating—and usually after eating too large a meal.

The goal of treatment with antacids is to decrease the acidity of the stomach contents by increasing the pH from 1 or 2 to about 3.5 or 4. pH should not be increased to levels much above 4, as this inhibits the release of pepsin, a gastric enzyme involved in digestion of proteins. Furthermore, acid rebound will occur, since a high pH stimulates the release of HCl.

Antacids are usually classified as systemic or nonsystemic agents. A systemic antacid is absorbed and thus exerts effects internally as well as locally in the alimentary canal. Because of their systemic action, such agents are not recommended for chronic use. Nonsystemic antacids are not well absorbed and exert their action primarily in the alimentary canal. The nonsystemic agents may be further divided into buffer and nonbuffer agents. Buffer antacids increase the pH of stomach contents to about 4, whereas nonbuffer antacids can increase the pH to 7 or more.

Systemic Antacids

Sodium bicarbonate has a very fast onset of action, which is advantageous when quick relief is sought. Its disadvantages, in addition to being limited to short-term use, are its short duration of action and gas formation (release of carbon dioxide). Sodium bicarbonate may also increase the absorption of calcium ions from the intestines. With continual use, this could lead to the development of the milk alkali syndrome. Like sodium bicarbonate, **sodium citrate** has a fast onset and short duration of action. It does not form gas, however.

Both of the aforementioned systemic antacids are capable of increasing the pH of stomach contents to 7 or more. Thus, dosage of these agents must be regulated closely.

Nonsystemic-Buffer Antacids

Because agents of this type are not absorbed appreciably and increase stomach pH only to about 4, they are better suited for long-term usage.

Aluminum hydroxide has a slow onset of action but a long duration of action, and it does not form gas. Because of its astringent action, this agent can cause constipation. In addition, nausea and vomiting may also occur.

Since aluminum ions form an insoluble precipitate with phosphate ions, phosphate absorption is decreased. Upon long-term use this could lead to osteomalacia. Use may be made of this ability to increase phosphate loss in the prevention and treatment of renal calculi due to phosphate. Another use of this action is to treat hyperphosphatemia of chronic renal failure. The aluminum ion may also combine with other drugs and diminish their absorption. Tetracycline antibiotics are affected, as are drugs such as atropine.

Aluminum phosphate has only half the neutralizing capacity of aluminum hydroxide but may be useful in conditions in which plasma phosphate concentrations are decreased.

Dihydroxyaluminum aminoacetate is another aluminum antacid. It is similar in properties and usefulness to aluminum hydroxide.

Magnesium trisilicate, like aluminum hydroxide, has a slow onset and long duration of action and does not lead to gas formation. Its disadvantages include ability to cause diarrhea, especially at large doses. Because some magnesium ions are absorbed, this agent cannot be used in the presence of renal diseases in which Mg^{2+} excretion is depressed. Rarely, silica may be absorbed and this could lead to kidney stone formation.

Nonsystemic-Nonbuffer Antacids

With agents of this classification, dosage and schedule are very important, as these agents are capable of increasing stomach pH to 7 or more.

Calcium carbonate is a very fast-acting agent. It has numerous disadvantages, however, and probably should not be extensively used. Rebound secretion of acid can occur if too large a dose is given. This can happen for two reasons: (1) calcium ions in large quantities can stimulate the secretion of HCl, and (2) exessive neutralization can also stimulate HCl secretion. Gas formation occurs owing to the release of carbon dioxide, and the calcium ion is also capable of causing constipation.

Magnesium hydroxide (known as Milk of Magnesia as an 8 percent suspension) has a fast onset and short duration of action. Magnesium oxide and magnesium carbonate, other magnesium compounds in the nonsystemic-nonbuffer group of antacids, have a delayed onset and longer duration of action than magnesium hydroxide. Disadvantages of these three magnesium compounds include production of diarrhea when used in large doses. They are also contraindicated in patients with renal disease.

Preparations

Antacid products frequently contain two antacid compounds. Such products may combine an agent of fast onset (but short duration of action) such as $Mg(OH)_2$ with one that has a long duration (but delayed onset) such as aluminum hydroxide. Furthermore, undesirable effects may be offset by combining constipating agents (Al^{3+} or Ca^{2+} compounds) with diarrhea-producing agents (e.g., Mg^{2+} compounds). Antacid products are available in different forms (e.g., solutions, suspensions, tablets). Products with the smallest particle size are the most efficacious; thus, solutions are preferred, with suspensions next and tablets last. Most antacids useful for chronic use are too insoluble to be available as solutions but are available as suspensions. Tablet forms, although more convenient to use, have the largest particle size and should be chewed thoroughly to reduce particle size as much as possible.

OTC Monograph on Antacids

The Food and Drug Administration (FDA) has published a final monograph on antacids for over-the-counter (OTC) use. To be recognized as an efficacious product, the recommended dose of a given preparation must be capable of neutralizing 5 mEq of HCl in an *in vitro* test. Products meeting this test are considered efficacious in the treatment of acid indigestion or of upset stomach associated with acid indigestion. These are the only approved uses for antacids by laypersons.

ANTIFLATULENTS

Simethicone is an antiflatulent and is frequently used in combination with antacids to relieve symptoms of gas. It is recognized by the FDA as safe and effective for treatment of gas in the GI tract. Presumably, simethicone acts as a defrothicant to cause coalescence of bubbles of gas and thus to facilitate their expulsion from the GI tract.

LAXATIVES

Laxatives are agents that are used to promote evacuation of intestines (or bowels). Generally, the term "laxative" applies to agents that induce the production of a soft-formed stool. "Cathartic" is a term used to describe agents that induce a more fluid loss. However, cathartics are usually used in dosages that produce only a laxative-type response. Older terms such as "purgative" and "drastic" refer to agents that induce primarily fluid losses, and such agents are no longer employed. "Physic" is also an older term but is still used by the lay public, and is synonymous with "cathartic" or "laxative."

Laxatives have several uses. These include presurgical evacuation of the intestines, decreasing straining of defecation in cardiac patients or following GI tract surgery, hastening elimination of toxic substances from the intestines in poisonings, aiding in elimination of intestinal worms in anthelmintic therapy, aiding in visualizing organs in x-ray films of the abdomen, and treating constipation, which is the principal use of the drugs.

Constipation, defined as the infrequent or difficult evacuation of the feces, has many causes. One cause is an improper diet, i.e., one lacking in fiber (nonabsorbable polysaccharides). Fiber is needed to adsorb water and increase the solid volume of the feces, which in the large intestines helps to stimulate defecation. Inadequate fluid intake is another diet-related cause. Other causes include ignoring defecation impulses or changing habits when traveling. In addition, a number of drugs are known to cause constipation. Such agents include antispasmodics (e.g., atropine), other agents with anticholinergic activity such as antidepressants (e.g., imipramine), and major tranquilizers (e.g. chlorpromazine), as well as narcotic analgesics (e.g., morphine) and aluminum and calcium compounds.

Laxatives can themselves cause constipation. This can occur with the chronic use or misuse of cathartics. When an individual takes a laxative that is too strong, it is possible to empty the intestines completely. Because ingested food stuffs take as much as 4 to 7 days to move along the intestines, several days may be required to restore the volume of intestinal contents. After a few days, if unaware of this, one may believe oneself to be constipated again and take another large dose of a laxative; this could continue indefinitely. The chronic use of laxatives leads to a loss of defecation impulses and also to a decrease in smooth muscle of the colon. Such individuals become unable to defecate unless they take a laxative.

Laxatives are also frequently misused by individuals to treat conditions other than constipation. Older theories of medicine related many illnesses to the presence of toxic substances in the GI tract and relied heavily on purges for treatment. Although modern medicine has discarded these notions they are still held by many people, who take a laxative whenever they are ill. Another misuse of laxatives concerns the desire to be "normal" and the idea that this includes a daily bowel movement. There is a wide variation in intestinal elimination rates, and several studies indicate that three per week to three per day constitutes the "normal" range. Thus, much of laxative use is not necessary.

The agents described subsequently are classified according to the tentative final OTC monograph on laxatives. However, as indicated in the discussion of the various agents, some drugs may be acting by other mechanisms than that which classifies them. Agents are listed as cathartics or laxatives to indicate maximal activity. Table 14–2 summarizes the effects of these agents.

Irritant Cathartics

Irritant (or stimulant) agents are presumed to act by increasing motor activity of the intestines and are capable of producing a laxative or cathartic response, depending on the dose. Several different types of compounds are

Table 14–2. EFFECT AND LATENCY
OF REPRESENTATIVE LAXATIVES*

Effect/Latency	Laxative/Cathartic

Water evacuation
1 to 3 hours
	Irritant cathartic:
	  Castor oil
	Saline cathartics:
	  Dibasic sodium phosphate
	  Magnesium compounds
	  Rectal preparations

Soft or semifluid stool
6 to 12 hours
	Irritant cathartics:
	  Anthraquinone compounds (senna, cascara, aloe, danthron)
	  Diphenylmethane compounds (phenolphthalein, bisacodyl)

Softening of feces
1 to 3 days
	Bulk-forming laxatives:
	  Methylcellulose
	  Psyllium
	  Polycarbophil
	  Bran
	Emollient laxatives:
	  Sulfosuccinates (docusates)

*Usual clinical dosage.

classified as irritants, including anthraquinone compounds, diphenylmethane compounds, castor oil, and dehydrocholic acid.

Anthraquinone compounds include **cascara, senna, aloe,** and **danthron** (Dorbane). The first three substances are from plants and they contain the anthraquinone as a glycoside. As such it is inactive, but in the intestine, the glycoside is hydrolysed to release emodin, the anthraquinone compound. Danthron is a synthetic anthraquinone. Anthraquinones act on the large intestines (colon) to increase motor activity. They have a delayed onset of action of 6 to 10 hours and thus may be taken at bedtime. Since these are very potent agents, they can cause excessive loss of fluid and electrolytes, particularly with chronic use.

Anthraquinones are absorbed from the GI tract, and the excretion of a metabolic product, chrysophanic acid, causes urine to turn red when pH is alkaline and yellow when pH is acidic. Although harmless, patients unaware of this may be alarmed. A more serious problem could result from anthraquinone entering milk and affecting a nursing infant.

Agents classified as **diphenylmethane compounds** include **phenolphthalein** (found in Ex-Lax and Feen-A-mint) and **bisacodyl** (Dulcolax). Although classically believed to act by increasing motor activity of the large intestine, there is some evidence that indicates that phenolphthalein may inhibit Na^+, K^+-ATPase of the large intestine. This would decrease the absorption of sodium and water in this segment and thus induce defecation by increasing volume in the large intestines. The onset of these agents is 6 to 8 hours when taken orally. A suppository form of bisacodyl is available with an onset of action within an hour. Phenolphthalein is absorbed to some extent, and its excretion in urine can also cause a harmless discoloration (red in alkaline urine). The drug may also cause an allergic skin rash. A polychromatic rash (pink to deep purple) may occur in eruptions that range from pin-sized areas to areas as large as several inches, and the discoloration may persist for years. With both phenolphthalein and bisacodyl, chronic use can lead to excessive loss of electrolytes (sodium, potassium) and water. Excessive volume losses could result in hypotension or even circulatory collapse. Bisacodyl is a very irritating substance and thus is marketed in enteric-coated tablets.

The castor bean is the source of **castor oil,** a triglyceride. As such, it is a nonirritating oil. In the intestines, it is hydrolyzed by pancreatic lypase to ricinoleic acid, which is the active form. This substance acts on both the small and the large intestines to increase motor activity. The onset of action of castor oil is as short as from 1 to 3 hours. Because it acts throughout the intestines, it is a very potent agent, and the possibility of excessive volume and electrolyte loss is much greater with this agent; thus, its chronic use is not advisable.

Dehydrocholic acid is a bile salt and is a semisynthetic cholate. It acts on the large intestine and has a delayed onset of action (8 to 12 hours).

Saline Cathartics

Agents classified as saline cathartics are water soluble and are poorly absorbed from the GI tract. In the intestines, they exert an osmotic effect and retain fluid. The consequent distention of the intestines stimulates defecation. These substances are administered in hyperosmotic solutions and have an onset of action of a few hours. All of these agents are very potent and can result in excessive loss of fluid and electrolytes; thus, care must be exercised in their use.

One type of saline cathartic, **dibasic sodium phosphate,** may be given orally (Sal Hepatica) or rectally as an enema (Fleets Phospho-Soda). Because sodium absorption can occur, use of these agents by patients with congestive heart failure or hypertension is not recommended.

Magnesium compounds (magnesium hydroxide [**Milk of Magnesia**], **magnesium citrate,** and **magnesium sulfate**) are also employed as saline cathartics. In addition to their osmotic action, several reports indicate that magnesium ions also stimulate the release of cholecystokinin (CCK), which in turn stimulates motility of the GI tract. There is also evidence that magnesium ions may directly inhibit fluid absorption. Thus, several effects may be involved in the action of magnesium ions on the intestines. Some magnesium may be absorbed from the intestines. In patients with renal failure, plasma concentrations could increase to toxic levels.

Bulk-Forming Laxatives

Agents in this class add bulk or fiber to intestinal contents, causing a retention of water. This results in an increase in stool volume as well as a softening of stools. The action of the bulk-forming agents differs from that of the saline cathartics in that these osmotic agents retain water in the intestines outside of the stools, whereas the bulk-forming agents retain water within the stools. The onset of action of the bulk-forming agents is delayed (24 to 72 hours).

Compounds employed as bulk-forming agents include high molecular weight, nonmetabolizable carbohydrates such as **methylcellulose, psyllium, polycarbophil,** and **bran,** which are not absorbed from the GI tract. It is essential that these agents be taken with a full glass of water, as they may adhere to the esophagus or intestines and cause irritation, which could lead to obstruction. These agents may combine with other drugs such as salicylates, digitalis glycosides, or nitrofurantoins and deter their absorption. Thus, a time for administration must be selected when the agents will not interfere with the absorption of these other drugs.

Emollient Laxatives

The emollient laxatives are also referred to as stool-softener laxatives. These compounds are surface-acting agents. They soften stools by their wetting action, which allows water to enter. They have a delayed onset of action of 24 to 72 hours. Effective agents include various salts of **sulfosuccinates** (**docusates**). These agents markedly enhance the absorption of mineral oil, and so should not be used with this laxative. They are also capable of enhancing the absorption of other drugs from the GI tract, which could upset the schedules as well as increase the intensity of action of such drugs. Thus, it is not advisable to use these laxatives with other drugs.

Lubricant Laxatives

Lubricant laxatives include **mineral oil** or emulsions of mineral oil. These substances soften the feces and lubricate the GI tract. They are usually taken once daily at night. There are many disadvantages to these agents. They interfere with the absorption of fat-soluble vitamins. Thus, they are best given at bedtime on an empty stomach. It is not advisable to give them during pregnancy because they interfere with absorption of vitamin K, which could lead to hemorrhagic disease in the newborn. If mineral oil is aspirated into the lungs it causes lipid pneumonia. Hence, individuals who have difficulty in swallowing should not use these preparations. Mineral oil also retards healing of the GI tract. Since these preparations lubricate the entire GI tract including the anal sphincter, they can cause leakage. Such a problem is a sign of overdosage.

Rectal Preparations

Several agents are available that are capable of a laxative effect when given as a suppository. Glycerin and sorbitol are classified as hyperosmotic rectal preparations because they increase the osmotic concentration of the colon. They retain water, which expands the colon and then stimulates defecation.

A CO_2-releasing suppository is also available. This preparation contains sodium bicarbonate and sodium acid phosphate. The suppository is wetted just before insertion and the interaction of the two chemicals releases carbon dioxide. The released gas applies pressure to the large intestine to stimulate evacuation.

OTC Monograph on Laxatives

In the FDA's tentative final monograph on laxatives, there are many recommendations that would markedly change the formulations and recommendations for use of these agents. The types of action (e.g., stimulants, bulk-producing agents) must be indicated. It also states that if a laxative preparation contains two or more active ingredients, each agent must act by a different mechanism. Prior to this proposal, preparations have been marketed with up to eight different active ingredients. The monograph also recommends that when these preparations are used to treat constipation, they be used only for short-term relief. In addition, the monograph recommends that many substances be removed from the market because of potential toxicities. These include substances such as colcynth and jalap (too irritating), podophyllin (potential teratogen), and calomel (potential toxicity if absorbed). Finally, the monograph indicates that laxatives should not contain other drugs or substances, a statement that was directed at preparations containing vitamins and minerals; this does not seem to be the logical way to take such substances.

Laxative and Plasma Ammonia–Decreasing Agent

Lactulose is an agent used in hepatic encephalopathy to decrease plasma levels of ammonia. This agent is a synthetic disaccharide. It is not absorbed from the GI tract but is soluble in water and thus serves as an osmotic agent to retain water. It is not hydrolysed by the intestinal enzymes, but in the ileum and colon intestinal bacteria metabolize it to lactic acid and other organic acids. Because these are only partially absorbed, the hydrolysis increases the osmotic action of the agent. The laxative action of the agent increases the excretion of ammonia. The acidic compounds formed decrease the pH of the colon, in turn decreasing the rate of formation of ammonia by intestinal bacteria, decreasing absorption of ammonia from the GI tract, and trapping it as NH_4^+. As a result, plasma levels of ammonia may decrease by 25 to 50 percent. When used in chronic liver disease with hepatic encephalopathy, lactulose can lead to symptomatic improvement as well as some normalization of the EEG. Its undesirable effects include flatulence, cramps, and excessive diarrhea.

ANTIDIARRHEAL AGENTS

Useful agents in the treatment of diarrhea include **diphenoxylate** (an analog of meperidine), **loperamide,** and **paregoric** (camphorated tincture of opium). These agents act similarly to decrease intestinal motility and are discussed in more detail in Chapter 5.

Other agents used include adsorbents such as bismuth subsalicylate and kaolin. The usefulness of these agents is minimal; however, because they are available without a prescription they are widely used.

Hydrophilic colloids are another type of agent sometimes employed to treat diarrhea. Agents such as polycarbophil absorb water and form a synthetic stool. This may decrease the frequency of bowel movements.

EMETICS

Drugs that are capable of inducing vomiting are called emetics and are useful in treatment of some orally ingested poisons. Only two emetics are widely used. These are ipecac and apomorphine.

Ipecac is marketed as a syrup. At the request of the American Academy of Pediatrics, it is available without a prescription and thus is readily available for treatment of accidental poisonings. Because it acts on the chemoreceptor trigger zone (CTZ) in the fourth ventricle of the brain, it has a delayed onset of action.

Apomorphine is a morphine derivative but lacks analgesic activity. It also acts on the CTZ but since it is given by injection (subcutaneously) it has an onset of action of a few minutes. Overdosage of apomorphine will depress the emetic center.

ANTIEMETICS

Antiemetics are useful in the prevention and treatment of motion sickness. **Scopolamine**, an anticholinergic agent, has been used for many years. It has, however, many side effects because of its anticholinergic activity. The agents most frequently employed are the H_1-receptor antagonists **dimenhydrinate, meclizine,** and **cyclizine.** Their mechanism of action is not clear but may include central anticholinergic activity. Drowsiness is the most prominent side effect of these agents.

The phenothiazines, which inhibit dopamine receptors in the emetic center, are usually employed to treat postoperative nausea and vomiting, as well as that induced by radiation therapy (see Chapter 5).

MISCELLANEOUS GI AGENTS

Sulfasalazine is useful in the treatment of chronic inflammatory bowel disease (ulcerative colitis and Crohn's disease). The mechanism of action of this drug is not understood but may be related to the anti-inflammatory action of 5-aminosalicylic acid, which is formed as a result of bacterial breakdown of sulfasalazine in the intestines. There are numerous side effects associated with the use of this agent, including nausea and headache. Allergic responses may also be seen.

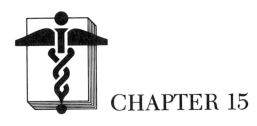

CHAPTER 15

Vitamins and Minerals

WILLIAM STEELE, Ph.D.

Vitamins are a group of 13 unique organic micronutrients that are required in trace amounts for the maintenance of health in humans. The nine water-soluble vitamins are **essential cofactors** in enzyme-mediated reactions. **Minerals** are a group of more than 16 inorganic micronutrients (elements) that are also required for maintenance of health. Nearly all trace elements are essential constituents of enzymes and other proteins. In spite of elaborate claims for the beneficial effects of supplements, food is the best source of vitamins and minerals. Additional vitamins and minerals are unnecessary in normal individuals who eat an adequate balanced diet and may in fact be harmful, as in the cases of vitamin A or D and of all minerals, particularly in children. Thus, vitamin and/or mineral supplementation is warranted only when there is evidence of a dietary deficiency or a valid physiological basis for therapy. In the United States, the Food and Nutrition Board of the National Academy of Sciences periodically issues recommended allowances of nutrients known as **Recommended Dietary Allowances** (RDA) that are intended to serve as a goal for good nutrition. These allowances are intentionally set at higher levels than necessary to prevent deficiency in order to compensate for individual variability. For labeling purposes, the Food and Drug Administration (FDA) has authorized a simplified and modified version of the RDA known as the **United States Recommended Daily Allowances** (USRDA), which enables the consumer to assess the suitability of a preparation in terms of percentages of the USRDA; amounts representing 50 to 150 percent of the USRDA are considered reasonable.

FAT-SOLUBLE VITAMINS

Vitamin A (Retinol)

Vitamin A is required for growth and development, reproduction, normal bone formation, vision in dim light, and maintenance of epithelial tissues. **Retinol** (vitamin A alcohol) is most abundant in meat, dairy products, and eggs. It can also be obtained from **provitamins,** β-carotene and other carotenoid pigments present in green and yellow vegetables and fruits. Most of the vitamin is stored in the liver in the form of retinol esters. A deficiency is usually slow to develop (due to body reserves and the vitamin's abundance in nature) and is generally a result of either impaired absorption, transport, or storage rather than inadequate intake. Night blindness (nyctalopia) is the earliest symptom. Prolonged deficiency in young children can lead to xerophthalmia and keratomalacia and ultimately to blindness and is a major cause of blindness worldwide. Chronic ingestion of large amounts of retinol, but not carotenoids, causes **hypervitaminosis A** (vitamin A toxicity) in children and adults; early manifestations include headache, bone pain, hyperostosis, fatigue, irritability, vomiting, loss of appetite, and skin changes (pruritus, desquamation, erythematous dermatitis, stomatitis). **Retinoic acid** (vitamin A acid) **isomers,** tretinoin (Retin-A) and isotretinoin (Accutane) in particular, are useful in the treatment of skin diseases (acne, Darier's disease, ichthyosis, psoriasis) because they are not stored in the liver and are rapidly excreted. They act by enhancing epidermal cell division and turnover. Tretinoin is used topically rather than orally to reduce the risk of hypervitaminosis. Side effects include erythema, desquamation, and sensitization of the skin to sunlight. Isotretinoin must be given orally and may cause hypervitaminosis-like side effects, including fetal abnormalities and spontaneous abortions. Retinoic acids are currently being studied for anticarcinogenic action (prevention of tumors of epithelial origin).

Vitamin D (Cholecalciferol)

1,25-Dihydroxyvitamin D is the hormone responsible for the regulation of intestinal absorption of calcium and phosphate; however, it is also capable of mobilizing calcium from bone by a permissive effect on parathyroid hormone action on bone. Vitamin D is available from two sources: the diet (natural vitamin D_3, vitamin D–supplemented milk and bread, and vitamin D_2 in plants) and photolytic conversion of the provitamin 7-dehydrocholesterol in the skin to vitamin D_3 by sunlight; hence, a deficiency is rare. Most of the vitamin is stored in the liver. The hormone, $1,25[OH]_2D$, is formed by hydroxylation of vitamin D in the liver to 25-hydroxyvitamin D, followed by hydroxylation of the latter metabolite in the kidney to $1,25[OH]_2D$ by 1-α-hydroxylase. $1,25[OH]_2D$ production is controlled by regulation of 1-α-hydroxylase synthesis; an increase in parathyroid hormone or a decrease in serum phosphate stimulates renal synthesis of the hydroxylase, thereby increasing hormone production. Deficiency may occur as a result of hypoparathyroidism, genetic defects, malabsorption syndromes, or prolonged anticonvulsant therapy (barbiturates or phenytoin [Dilantin]). Chronic deficiency causes rickets in the young and osteomalacia in adults as a result of parathyroid hormone–mediated increases in calcium mobilization from bone. Vitamin D in large doses is toxic in both children and adults, causing hypercalcemia manifested by weakness, loss of appetite, vomiting, diarrhea, polyuria, EKG changes, and mental changes. Chronic intoxication can lead to soft tissue calcification, renal failure, and death.

Vitamin E (Tocopherol)

The role of vitamin E in nutrition is poorly understood; however, it is thought to act as an **antioxidant,** either preventing the oxidation of cell constituents or preventing the formation of toxic lipid peroxides from polyunsaturated fatty acids. Vitamin E is widely distributed in nature. Recently, a deficiency manifested by ataxia, areflexia, and decreased proprioception has been documented in children with chronic cholestasis. Deficiency may also occur as a result of prolonged therapy with iron or thyroid hormones. There is no compelling evidence at present to support the notion that vitamin E has any therapeutic value other than in the treatment of deficiency states.

Vitamin K (Phytonadione, Vitamin K₁)

This vitamin is required for a terminal step in the synthesis of the **vitamin K–dependent clotting factor proteins** II, VII, IX, and X in the liver (post-translational carboxylation of glutamyl residues to form γ-carboxyglutamyl residues, which confer biological activity on these proteins by allowing them to bind calcium ions and attach to phospholipid micelles). It is available from two sources: the diet and intestinal bacteria. Most of the vitamin is stored in the liver, but it is not retained for long periods. A deficiency is uncommon but may occur as a result of malabsorption of fats, liver disease, hyperthyroidism, or prolonged therapy with antibiotics or supplementation with large doses of other fat-soluble vitamins; the principal manifestation is bleeding (ecchymoses, epistaxis, hematuria, GI bleeding). Vitamin K is used routinely in the treatment of decreased clotting factor synthesis in newborn infants and in accidental overdosage with **coumarin anticoagulants** (warfarin [Anthrombin-K, Coumadin, Panwarfin] and dicumarol). Single large doses of vitamin K may cause hemolytic anemia in neonates by increasing plasma levels of unbound bilirubin and severe hypersensitivity reactions in adults receiving the vitamin intravenously. Menadione (vitamin K₃), a synthetic water-insoluble analog of natural vitamin K, and menadiol sodium phosphate [Kappadione, Synkayvite] and menadione sodium bisulfite, synthetic water-soluble derivatives of vitamin K₃, cause hemolysis in patients with glucose-6-phosphate dehydrogenase (G-6-PD) deficiency. Further, they are not recommended for use in the newborn infant or in the treatment of oral anticoagulant overdosage.

WATER-SOLUBLE VITAMINS

Thiamine (Vitamin B₁)

Thiamine pyrophosphate, the biologically active form of this vitamin, is a **coenzyme** for several important processes in carbohydrate metabolism (decarboxylation of pyruvate and α-ketoglutarate and metabolism of pentose *via* the hexose monophosphate shunt). Thiamine is widely distributed in nature, but thiamine-rich foods, such as grains, are rare and their thiamine content is depleted by milling. Mild deficiency may occur in association with increased energy demands (pregnancy, lactation, hyperthyroidism, and heavy manual labor), as requirement is determined by caloric intake and carbohydrate intake in particular. Severe deficiency (beriberi) is rare except in individuals with impaired absorption (prolonged diarrhea or other malabsorption syndromes), impaired utilization (liver disease), or malnutrition (alcoholism, polished rice diet). Manifestations of deficiency in **dry beriberi** are neurological (e.g., peripheral neuropathy and, in chronic alcoholism, Wernicke's encephalopathy and Korsakoff's syndrome). In **wet beriberi,** they are cardiovascular (e.g., edema and high-output heart failure in deficiency produced by a polished rice diet). Thiamine is safe when given orally or intravenously and has no therapeutic use apart from the treatment of deficiency.

Riboflavin (Vitamin B$_2$)

The biologically active forms of this vitamin, **flavin mononucleotide** (FMN) and **flavin adenine dinucleotide** (FAD), are coenzymes in various oxidative systems. Riboflavin is widely distributed in nature and particularly rich in organ meats. Deficiency is rare but may occur in association with deficiencies of other B-complex vitamins, niacin in particular, in malabsorption syndromes and in alcoholism. Deficiency is characterized by lesions of the mucous membranes and skin (sore throat, angular stomatitis, glossitis, cheilosis, dermatitis). Riboflavin is safe when given orally or parenterally and has no therapeutic use other than the treatment of deficiency.

Pyridoxine (Vitamin B$_6$)

The biologically active form of this vitamin, **pyridoxal phosphate,** is a coenzyme for various steps in amino acid metabolism, that is, transamination and decarboxylation (e.g., in neurotransmitter biosynthesis: glutamate to GABA, levodopa to dopamine, and 5-OH-tryptophan to serotonin). Pyridoxal phosphate is also required for the first step in heme biosynthesis. The vitamin is widely distributed in nature, and dietary deficiency is rare. However, deficiency may occur as a result of deficiencies of other B-complex vitamins (e.g., alcoholism), genetic defects in utilization, or treatment with antagonists (cycloserine [Seromycin], hydralazine [Apresoline], isoniazid [Nydrazid], or penicillamine [Cuprimine, Depen]). Deficiency is characterized by skin lesions around the eyes, nose, and throat; hyperexcitability and seizures (possible due to a fall in GABA levels); and peripheral neuritis associated with synovial swelling. Pyridoxine is safe when given orally or intravenously in therapeutic amounts (prolonged intake of large doses may cause peripheral sensory neuropathy with ataxia) and has no therapeutic use other than the treatment of deficiency. It can, however, anatagonize levodopa's (Dopar, Larodopa) action in the treatment of Parkinson's disease by increasing the conversion of levodopa to dopamine, which does not cross the blood-brain barrier.

Niacin (Vitamin B₃, Nicotinic Acid)

The biologically active forms of this vitamin, **nicotinamide adenine dinucleotide** (NAD) and **nicotinamide adenine dinucleotide phosphate** (NADP), are coenzymes in various oxidative systems. Niacin is widely distributed in nature and can also be obtained from tryptophan by a series of conversions requiring riboflavin, pyridoxine, and thiamine. Deficiency is rare, but may occur as a result of malabsorption syndromes, prolonged isoniazid (Nydrazid) therapy, cirrhosis, or use of corn (which is deficient in tryptophan) as the sole source of dietary protein. Severe deficiency (pellagra) is characterized by erythematous lesions on areas of the skin exposed to sunlight, diarrhea, and psychoses (hallucinations and dementia), that is, the three D's: diarrhea, dermatitis, and dementia. Therapeutic doses of niacin may cause flushing, headache, pruritus, and gastrointestinal distress, whereas large doses may activate peptic ulcer disease or cause hepatotoxicity. Niacin in combination with a bile acid-binding resin has been found to lower LDL levels in patients with heterozygous familial hypercholesterolemia.

Pantothenic Acid

The biologically active form of this vitamin, **coenzyme A,** is an essential cofactor in fat, carbohydrate, and protein metabolism and in the synthesis of acetylcholine, porphyrins, and steroids; its main biological role is the transfer of acetyl units. Pantothenic acid is widely distributed in nature and a dietary deficiency is unlikely, except in severe malnutrition. It is safe when given orally and has no therapeutic use other than the treatment of deficiency.

Biotin

Biotin is a coenzyme for carboxylation reactions in both carbohydrate and fat metabolism. It is available from two sources: the diet and intestinal bacteria. Deficiency can result from ingestion of raw egg white (which contains **avidin,** a high-affinity, biotin-binding protein), long-term parenteral nutrition, severe malnutrition, or genetic defects in biotin-dependent enzymes. Deficiency is characterized by dermatitis, anorexia, muscle pain, and mental depression. Biotin is safe when given orally and has no therapeutic use other than the treatment of deficiency.

Cyanocobalamin (Vitamin B$_{12}$)

This vitamin is a coenzyme in fat and carbohydrate metabolism (**deoxy-adenosylcobalamin**) and in methionine synthesis (**methylcobalamin**), which is essential for normal folate metabolism. It is available only from animal tissues. Absorption depends on **intrinsic factor,** a glycoprotein synthesized by gastric parietal cells, and on receptor-mediated absorption of the intrinsic factor–vitamin B$_{12}$ complex in the ileum. After absorption, it binds to transcobalamin II in plasma. Vitamin B$_{12}$ is stored in the liver, secreted into bile, and avidly reabsorbed in the intestine. A deficiency inhibits methionine synthesis and leads to the accumulation of **methyltetrahydrofolate** (the source of the methionine methyl group and the principal form of folate supplied to the cell), which in turn causes a deficiency of **tetrahydrofolate.** This inhibits thymidylate synthesis, a rate-limiting step for DNA synthesis in rapidly proliferating cells such as the erythroblast and produces megaloblastic anemia and neurological damage (degeneration of posterior and lateral columns of the spinal cord and cerebral degeneration), which is irreversible. Deficiency is rare and develops slowly owing to extensive vitamin B$_{12}$ storage in the liver and to low daily requirement but may occur as a result of **pernicious anemia,** gastric atrophy or resection (blocks the formation of intrinsic factor required for intestinal absorption of the vitamin, causing vitamin malabsorption like that in pernicious anemia), ileal disease, impaired utilization, intestinal parasites, chronic disease, or strict vegetarian diet. Vitamin B$_{12}$ is safe when given orally or parenterally; the latter route must be used following total gastrectomy and resection of the distal ileum, in pernicious anemia for life, and in malabsorption syndromes. It has no therapeutic use other than the treatment of deficiency.

Folic Acid

The biologically active forms of this vitamin, **dihydrofolate** and **tetrahydrofolate,** are coenzymes in a variety of conversions involving one-carbon units (e.g., amino acid, purine, and thymidylate synthesis). Folate is widely distributed in nature. It is stored in cells as polyglutamates, but body stores are more rapidly depleted than are those of vitamin B$_{12}$. A deficiency is rare but may occur as a result of malabsorption syndromes, acute or chronic alcoholism, hemolytic anemia, therapy with **inhibitors of dihydrofolate reductase,** such as **methotrexate** (Mexate) or **trimethoprim** (as in Bactrim, Septra) or with inhibitors of folate absorption, such as phenytoin (Dilantin), or increased requirement (pregnancy). Deficiency causes megaloblastic anemia (due to inhibition of thymidylate synthesis, the rate-limiting step in DNA synthesis in erythroblasts) identical to that seen in vitamin B$_{12}$ deficiency; however, it is rarely associated with neurological abnormalities. Folate (Folvite) is safe when given orally or intravenously; the oral route is used to treat all deficiencies except those induced by dihydrofolate reductase inhibitors (methotrexate, in particular), which require parenteral administration of **leucovorin** (formyltetrahydrofolate), a reduced form of folate. Large doses of folate can produce hematological improvement in megaloblastic anemia caused by vitamin B_{12} deficiency but do not prevent the progression of neurological damage associated with vitamin B_{12} deficiency and therefore should not be used indiscriminately in the treatment of megaloblastic anemias.

Ascorbic Acid (Vitamin C)

This vitamin is involved in the synthesis of collagen, bone matrix, ground substance, and steroids. It is available from citrus and vegetables and is readily destroyed by cooking. A deficiency is rare but may occur in alcoholics or others with low vitamin intake or in those who have rapidly withdrawn from chronic high-dose therapy, including newborn infants of women who have taken high doses of vitamin C during pregnancy. Deficiency causes **scurvy,** which is characterized initially by nosebleeds and petechial hemorrhages and ultimately by defective ground substance formation, capillary fragility, defective development of teeth, and hemorrhages into muscle and joints. Ascorbate is safe when given orally in moderate amounts; however, doses greater than 1 g per day may cause diarrhea, renal calculi, urethritis, excessive iron absorption, and sickle cell crisis. The claims that massive doses are effective in the prevention of the common cold or rectal cancer have not yet been satisfactorily validated.

MINERALS

Mineral elements can be divided into two classes based on their abundance in the body: **abundant elements** (calcium, magnesium, potassium, sodium, chloride, phosphorus, and sulfur) and **trace elements** (chromium, cobalt, copper, fluorine, iodine, iron, maganese, molybdenum, selenium, and zinc). As excessive amounts of minerals can cause tissue damage, supplementation should be restricted to the treatment or prevention of deficiency.

Abundant Elements

Calcium

Calcium, the most abundant mineral in the body, is a major structural component of bone. Apart from its structural function, calcium plays an important role in blood coagulation, cardiac function, muscle contraction, neuromuscular transmission, and membrane integrity. The concentration of calcium in the plasma is controlled by parathyroid hormone and vitamin D. Calcium is widely distributed in nature, but the principal source in the diet is dairy products. Requirement is increased by rapid growth, pregnancy, and lactation. Supplementation is required in infants maintained on skim milk or formulas; however, the efficacy of routine calcium supplementation in postmenopausal women for preventing osteoporosis is controversial. Supplementation in excess of requirements is inappropriate and unnecessary. Calcium salts are the drug of choice in the treatment of low-calcium tetany (hypocalcemia) due to deprivation of calcium and vitamin D, hypoparathyroidism, renal insufficiency accompanied by hyperphosphatemia, or massive transfusions with citrated blood.

Magnesium

Magnesium is a minor constituent of bone and a cofactor for many enzymes. It plays an important role in protein synthesis, oxidative phosphorylation, nerve excitability, and muscular contractility. It is widely distributed in nature, and dietary deficiency is rare. Hypomagnesemia may occur as a result of chronic alcoholism, malabsorption syndromes, diabetes, diuretic therapy, or renal damage. Severe hypomagnesemia may lead to tetany and convulsions. High plasma levels of magnesium are generally associated with renal insufficiency; ingestion of large amounts of magnesium (in the form of antacids or cathartics) in the presence of renal insufficiency may lead to respiratory failure and cardiac arrest.

Potassium

Potassium, the most abundant **intracellular cation,** plays an essential role in neuronal and muscular excitability and in protein synthesis. It is widely distributed in nature and dietary deficiency is rare, but hypokalemia may occur as a result of diarrhea, vomiting, metabolic alkalosis, prolonged use of corticosteroids, or diuretic therapy with furosemide (Lasix) or thiazides. Neuromuscular disorders are the most common adverse effect of hypokalemia. Hyperkalemia can be caused by renal failure, metabolic acidosis, potassium-sparing diuretics, or adrenal insufficiency; the main clinical manifestation is cardiac arrhythmias.

Sodium

Sodium, the most abundant **extracellular cation,** plays an essential role in fluid balance and volume. Sodium intake *via* processed foods and salt usage is generally far in excess of normal requirements and may lead to hypertension. Serum sodium is regulated by the kidney, aldosterone, atrial natriuretic factor, and antidiuretic hormone (ADH) (indirectly by regulating H_2O excretion). Hyponatremia is rare, since the kidney will excrete essentially salt-free urine following dietary restriction. However, it may occur as a result of prolonged diarrhea or vomiting, excessive sweating, renal disorders, adrenocortical insufficiency, cystic fibrosis, or diuretic therapy; the dominant symptoms are confusion and weakness.

Chloride

Chloride is the most abundant extracellular **anion** and is essential for maintenance of electrolyte balance. Chloride loss may occur as a result of prolonged vomiting, diuretic therapy, or other conditions that lead to excessive loss of sodium.

Phosphorus

Phosphorus in the form of various phosphorylated compounds plays an essential role in intermediary and energy metabolism, and phosphate is a major structural component of bone. Phosphorus is widely distributed in nature and deficiency is rare. Serum phosphate is regulated by parathyroid hormone and vitamin D. However, hypophosphatemia may occur as a result of chronic alcoholism, excessive use of calcium- or aluminum-containing antacids, liver disease, prolonged vomiting, or hyperparathyroidism.

Sulfur

Sulfur is a constituent of several amino acids and vitamins. It is widely distributed in nature, and deficiency is unknown. No daily requirement has been set for sulfur.

Trace Elements

Chromium

Chromium is a constituent of the glucose tolerance factor, which facilitates the binding of insulin to its receptor. Dietary deficiency is unknown, but has been suspected in individuals maintained for months or years by parenteral nutrition whose symptoms of glucose intolerance were corrected by supplementation.

Cobalt

Cobalt is a constituent of cyanocobalamin. It is present in adequate amounts in a balanced diet. The claims that cobalt has a beneficial effect in refractory anemias are questionable.

Copper

Copper is a constituent of several enzymes and other proteins. It is widely distributed in nature and deficiency is rare. However, deficiency may occur as a result of defects in transport (Menkes' syndrome, genetic disorders, and premature infants) or malabsorption syndromes. Large doses of copper salts cause gastrointestinal distress, renal damage, and hemolysis. Copper retention (Wilson's disease) and intoxication is best treated with the copper **chelators** dimercaprol and penicillamine (Cuprimine, Depen).

Fluoride

Fluoride is a constituent of bone and teeth and when present in optimal amounts reduces the incidence of vertebral fractures and dental caries. The principal source of fluoride in the diet is water in those areas where it occurs naturally or where fluoridation is practiced. Fluoride supplements are required only in areas where the water supply contains less than 0.3 ppm. Excess fluoride in the drinking water or air (insecticides or industrial pollutants) causes mottling of dental enamel (dental fluorosis), an irreversible condition.

Iodine

Iodine is a constituent of the **thyroid hormones**. The principal source of iodine in the diet is iodized salt and seafood. Nutritional deficiency is generally attended by thyroid gland enlargement (endemic goiter). The prevalence of this disorder has been sharply reduced following the addition of iodate to table salt and bread. Chronic ingestion of large amounts of iodide can inhibit thyroid hormone synthesis and lead to hypothyroidism (iodine goiter).

Iron

Iron is a constituent of both **functional forms** (hemoglobin, myoglobin, cytochromes, transferrin) and **storage forms** (ferritin and hemosiderin) **of iron**. It is widely distributed in nature, but meat is the principal source of readily available iron (**heme iron**). Deficiency occurs more frequently than thought, as a result of increased requirement (infants, children, pregnancy) or increased loss (menstruation, lactation, bleeding); supplementation with ferrous salts should be continued in such individuals until iron stores are replenished. Deficiency can also result from malabsorption syndromes, gastrectomy, achlorhydria, copper deficiency, or excessive use of antacids that convert iron to insoluble compounds. Microcytic, hypochromic anemia develops when iron stores are depleted. Acute iron poisoning is rare in adults but common and generally fatal in young children following ingestion of 2 to 10 g of iron. Chronic iron toxicity can result from increased intestinal iron absorption in patients with hemochromatosis owing to deposition of iron in the heart, liver, pancreas, and other organs or from multiple red cell transfusions over a long time period.

Manganese

Manganese is a constituent of many enzymes. It is widely distributed in nature, and deficiency is unknown. Chronic exposure to high levels of manganese compounds (mining and processing) leads to parkinsonian symptoms.

Molybdenum

Molybdenum is a constituent of several enzymes. Although it is unevenly distributed in nature, deficiency is rare. Chronic molybdenum supplementation may cause increased excretion of copper.

Selenium

Selenium is a constituent of several enzymes including **glutathione peroxidase,** which protects cells against free radical damage by destroying hydroperoxides and lipoperoxides. It is unevenly distributed in nature, but deficiency is rare. However, chronic deficiency has been associated with fatal cardiomyopathy in children and young women in China. In certain areas selenium toxicity (selenosis) is a serious concern of animal producers.

Zinc

Zinc is a constituent of many enzymes. It plays an important role in growth and tissue repair as a consequence of its presence in nucleic acid **polymerases.** Zinc is widely distributed in nature, but the principal source in the diet is meat, because the forms of zinc in plants are unavailable. Deficiency is rare but can result from inadequate intake (poor diet, total parenteral nutrition) or increased requirement (children, pregnancy, lactation). Manifestations of deficiency include anorexia, slow wound healing, dermatitis, decreased taste sensation, and suboptimal growth. Chronic zinc supplementation may interfere with the absorption or utilization of other minerals (iron and copper) and cause nausea, vomiting, and abdominal pain.

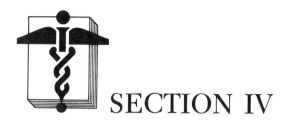

SECTION IV

Chemotherapy for Infection and Neoplasm

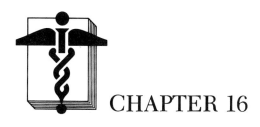

CHAPTER 16

Antimicrobial Drugs

JAMES L. SPRATT, M.D., Ph.D.

363

Paul Ehrlich first defined **chemotherapy** in 1913 as the treatment of a systemic infection by a specific drug. The term is very much used in the same fashion today in relation to the use of systemic antibiotics, synthetic antimicrobial drugs, and certain cancer chemotherapy drugs. The term **local anti-infectives** is used to refer to **antiseptics** and **disinfectants** that are used topically (antiseptics) or on inanimate objects (disinfectants).

Ehrlich is also responsible for the concept of **chemotherapeutic index,** relating the drug effect on the microorganism to the drug effect on the host. It is often expressed as the maximum dose tolerated by the host divided by the minimum curative dose. In quantitative laboratory terms, it is sometimes expressed as LD_{50} (lethal dose$_{50}$) $\div CD_{50}$ (curative dose$_{50}$).

The Darwinian concept of **antibiosis** (literally "antilife") was used by Sellman Waksman in defining the term **antibiotic**. He was referring to substances produced by living organisms which are antagonistic to the life of other microorganisms. The generic term **antimicrobial** includes various synthetic agents such as the sulfonamides, nitrofurans, and so forth.

Chemotherapeutic **spectrum** refers to the range of organisms against which the drug is effective. Agents effective against a wide variety of organisms are called broad-spectrum (as opposed to narrow- or medium-spectrum) agents. These terms are quite relative, and thorough diagnostic procedures should be followed before specific therapy is initiated. Additionally, the features of a given drug and the availability of other drugs may cause its clinically useful spectrum to differ from its microbiological spectrum.

Antimicrobial **potency** is usually expressed as activity per milligram and refers to the toxic effects of the compound on a specific microorganism, not the host. Although antimicrobial agents can have toxic effects on both the host and the invading microorganism, the term **toxicity** in this area usually refers to toxic effects on the host.

Antimicrobial drugs may have either **bactericidal activity** (killing microorganisms) or **bacteriostatic activity** (inhibiting multiplication of organisms), and the nature of the activity may depend on drug concentration. Bactericidal drugs generally include the penicillins, cephalosporins, and aminoglycosides. Bacteriostatic drugs generally include erythromycin, clindamycin, chloramphenicol, tetracyclines, and the sulfonamides.

Synergism and **antagonism** of antimicrobial drugs refer to the actions of the drugs on the microorganism, not the host. These terms are further discussed in this chapter.

Each component of the host-drug-microorganism triad is interactive with each of the other two components. The drug response in the *in vivo* situation therefore may or may not be equivalent to that noted in the *in vitro* situation. For example, the host may metabolize an active compound to an inactive compound or, conversely, metabolize an inactive compound to an active compound. Prominent effects on normal flora (particularly of the respiratory, GI, and genitourinary tracts) can influence the therapeutic response and the general health of the patient. Likewise, **suprainfections** can develop. Such suprainfections are infections that are superimposed on a pre-existing infection that is being treated. Unfortunately common suprainfections include vaginal moniliasis (*Candida albicans* infection) with tetracycline therapy and penicillinase-producing staphylococcal infections with penicillin G therapy.

MECHANISMS OF ACTION OF ANTIMICROBIAL DRUGS

The mechanisms by which antimicrobial drugs act on bacteria are categorized in Figure 16–1.

Inhibition of Cell Wall Synthesis

Bacteria, as opposed to animal cells, have a cell wall that maintains the cell shape and an internal osmotic pressure of 5 to 20 atmospheres. The inter-

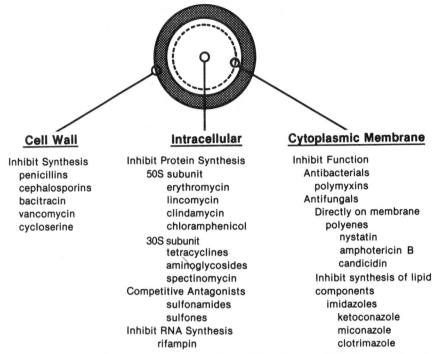

Cell Wall	Intracellular	Cytoplasmic Membrane
Inhibit Synthesis	Inhibit Protein Synthesis	Inhibit Function
penicillins	50S subunit	Antibacterials
cephalosporins	erythromycin	polymyxins
bacitracin	lincomycin	Antifungals
vancomycin	clindamycin	Directly on membrane
cycloserine	chloramphenicol	polyenes
	30S subunit	nystatin
	tetracyclines	amphotericin B
	aminoglycosides	candicidin
	spectinomycin	Inhibit synthesis of lipid
	Competitive Antagonists	components
	sulfonamides	imidazoles
	sulfones	ketoconazole
	Inhibit RNA Synthesis	miconazole
	rifampin	clotrimazole

Figure 16–1. Sites of antibiotic action. (Adapted from Cowan, FW: Pharmacology for the Dental Hygienist. Lea & Febiger, Philadelphia, 1978, p 238.)

nal osmotic pressure is threefold to fivefold greater in Gram-positive than in Gram-negative bacteria owing to differences in the structural rigidity of their cell walls. Inhibition of cell wall synthesis impairs the cell wall rigidity, the cell imbibes water, and it will literally explode in an isotonic environment.

The bacterial cell wall formation occurs (1) by synthesis of precursors, (2) by formation of peptidoglycans, which are the basic cell wall components, and finally (3) by cross-linking of the polymeric forms of the peptidoglycans *via* transpeptidation.

Cycloserine, a secondary antitubercular drug, is an analog of D-alanine which blocks alanine racemase, therefore blocking synthesis of the precursor pentapeptide component of the peptidoglycan.

Bacitracin and **vancomycin** are examples of the formation of peptidoglycans, acting early in the synthetic processes before the cross-linking step. These synthetic steps are in the cell membrane, and the drugs must get into the cell to be effective. These drugs, therefore, only affect certain kinds of bacteria.

The **penicillins** and **cephalosporins,** the most commonly used of all antibiotics, act at the cross-linking step. Penicillin binds to a penicillin-binding protein receptor, causing a defect in the integrity of the cell wall by supplanting the structurally similar acyl-D-alanyl-D-alanine, resulting in inhibition of the transpeptidation reaction. The drug may also cause inhibition of an inhibitor of autolysis, thereby promoting autolytic activity.

All of the penicillins and cephalosporins (the **beta-lactams**) appear to work in similar fashion.

Inhibition of Protein Synthesis

A number of antimicrobial drug groups act by inhibiting protein synthesis.

Streptomycin, an aminoglycoside, attaches to a specific receptor protein on the 30S subunit of the bacterial microsomal ribosome and blocks the initiation complex for peptide formation, thereby causing RNA to be misread. The wrong amino acid is put into the peptide chain, leading to a nonfunctional protein. All aminoglycosides are believed to work in a similar fashion.

The **tetracyclines** attach to a specific receptor protein on the 30S subunit to block the attachment of an aminoacyl-tRNA. This blocks the introduction of a new amino acid into the peptide chain, thus terminating it.

Chloramphenicol works at the 50S subunit. It prevents the binding of a new amino acid by inhibiting peptidyl transferase.

The **macrolides** (e.g., erythromycin) and **lincosamides** (lincomycin and clindamycin) act at the 50S subunit, interfering with initiation complex formation or aminoacyl translocation.

Inhibition of Cytoplasmic Membrane Function

The cytoplasmic membrane of bacteria regulates cell permeability and the composition of its internal environment. Certain drugs affect the integrity of the cytoplasmic membrane of microorganisms more than the cytoplasmic membrane of animal cells. The **polymyxins** act on the cell membrane of bacteria, but not on that of fungi. They interact with phosphatidylethanolamine, which is abundant in bacterial cell membranes, but not in that of fungi. **Polyenes** such as **amphotericin B** act on fungal cell membranes but not on those of bacteria. They interact with ergosterol as the receptor substance. It should be noted that the **imidazoles,** such as **ketoconazole,** act on fungi by inhibiting the synthesis of the fungal membrane lipids. Although the end result is somewhat similar, their mechanisms are different from those of the polyenes.

Competitive Antagonism

The **sulfonamides** are structural analogs of para-aminobenzoic acid (PABA), which will substitute for it in the production of folic acid. The resultant nonfunctional analog of folic acid prevents the growth of bacteria, as folic acid is essential for their growth. This drug effect is not apparent in the patient, since humans need preformed folic acid. The effect is apparent in bacteria because they cannot use preformed folic acid.

Inhibition of Nucleic Acid Synthesis

The **rifamycins** such as **rifampin** bind to DNA-dependent RNA polymerase of bacteria to inhibit RNA synthesis.

RESISTANCE DEVELOPMENT

Mechanisms

The development of drug-resistant strains of bacteria can occur through a variety of mechanisms. The utilization of antimicrobial drugs exerts a selection pressure encouraging the development of resistant strains.

1. Organisms may produce an **enzyme that destroys the active drug.** Staphylococci may produce beta-lactamases (penicillinases/cephalosporinases). Acetylating and phosphorylating enzymes may be produced by bacteria, thereby rendering certain antimicrobial drugs ineffective.
2. Organisms may **alter their permeability** to a given drug. For example, tetracycline accumulation in certain susceptible organisms can be controlled by active transport through the cell membrane. These organisms may change their permeabilty to tetracyclines, leading to resistance.
3. By **altering drug receptors** in the microorganism, resistance to aminoglycosides can occur by loss of a binding protein on the 30S subunit of the bacterial ribosome.
4. Resistance may occur by **altering a metabolic pathway,** as in developing the ability to use preformed folic acid and thereby becoming resistant to sulfonamides.
5. **Alteration of target enzymes** may explain other instances of resistance. If a given target enzyme of the microorganism is ordinarily inhibited by specific antibiotics, its newly altered enzyme may be less affected and therefore allow the microorganism to survive.

Propagation

The propagation of antimicrobial resistance in bacterial populations can be conveniently classified into **chromosomal** and **extrachromosomal.** In this context, chromosomal refers to the random process of mutation. This is an unlikely explanation for resistance occurring in a given patient because mutation is infrequent in comparison to the time course of therapy for an individual patient. Plasmids or extrachromosomal pieces of genetic material free in the cytosol are the basis of extrachromosomal resistance transfer. **Transduction** occurs when bacteriophages transport plasmids from bacteria to bacteria. **Transformation** occurs when a bacterium picks up naked DNA from the environment. **Conjugation** is a mechanism whereby genetic material is passed directly from one bacterium to another.

The transfer of resistance factors *via* conjugation has also been termed **infectious drug resistance** because of its implications. Cell-to-cell contact is required. It occurs most often in the GI tract. Conjugation can occur between two different strains or species of bacteria, including nonpathogenic-to-pathogenic transfer. The transference of resistance to as many as six drugs can occur simultaneously.

The term **cross-resistance** is used in reference to the situation in which an organism is resistant to a drug to which it has never been exposed. When this occurs, it usually occurs among structurally related drugs.

The term **persisters** describes bacteria that are metabolically inactive during therapy. If they do become metabolically active, they are totally susceptible to the action of the antibiotic. In a sense, it is a temporal (nongenetic) resistance, but not a true resistance to the drug. Persisters can be a problem if the antibiotic is not prescribed for an adequate length of time or if patient compliance is a problem before the prescribed duration has been completed.

Drug Choice

Certain steps can be followed to minimize development of resistance problems in both the individual patient and the population at large. As a rule, the best antimicrobial to use is the one that has the most narrow spectrum and yet is effective. This will cause the least problems to the individual's microflora and minimize the hazards of resistance development for the patient population in general. A **sufficient amount of the right drug** should be used for an **adequate amount of time**. On rare occasions, simultaneous use of more than one drug is warranted (e.g., as in tuberculosis). One should also avoid the use of quite valuable drugs when their use is not warranted.

The host-drug relationship for antimicrobial agents is often minimal and no real pharmacological actions of these drugs are usually apparent at therapeutic doses. However, **adverse effects** do occur and consist of (a) direct **toxic effects** which **often are dose-related** and **predictable** and (b) **allergic reactions** which **often are not dose-related** and **not predictable**. Although not a host-drug direct interaction, suprainfections certainly have their adverse consequences for the host.

Because of the potential for these adverse effects, drug choice is always based on the severity of the illness and its potential for morbidity, mortality, or both. Any kind of allergic response (e.g., rashes, fever, urticaria, jaundice, depression of the hematopoietic system, anaphylactic shock) may occur.

ANTIBACTERIAL AGENTS

Inhibitors of Cell Wall Synthesis

The Penicillins

The generic chemical term **beta-lactams** refers to both the penicillins and the cephalosporins. The penicillins (Table 16–1) are still the most often used and are still considered to be the most important of the currently used antibiotics. The penicillins interfere with the cross-linking step in bacterial cell wall synthesis, thereby leading to bacterial destruction *via* osmotic forces or normal defense mechanisms or both.

Structure. The mold *Penicillium chrysogenum* has supplanted Alexander Fleming's original *P. notatum* as the world's supplier of the natural penicillins F, K, X, G, and O. All of these naturally occurring penicillins have the **6-amino-penicillanic acid** portion and each has its own side chain (Fig. 16–2). The 6-amino-penicillanic acid portion must be present to get antibacterial activity.

Penicillin G, first discovered by Fleming in 1929, is the only naturally occurring penicillin still used. Other than penicillin G, currently used penicillins are manufactured by adding **amidase** to the naturally occurring penicillins to split off the side chains. Subsequently, semisynthetic penicillins are produced by adding back specific side chains to give particular characteristics to that individual new penicillin molecule. The nature of the side chain determines the drug's spectrum, chemical stability, and degree of plasma protein binding. Whereas penicillin G is very water soluble and labile in solution—particularly in acid—the newer semisynthetic penicillins are designed to be less susceptible to gastric acid, to have a broader spectrum, or to be penicillinase-resistant.

Penicillin G. A narrow-spectrum antibiotic, penicillin G is primarily effective against Gram-positive cocci. It is also useful against gonococci, spirochetes, *Actinomyces*, and some anaerobes. It is most effective against rapidly growing bacteria and can be both bacteriostatic and bactericidal. If the organism is susceptible to the drug, it will be bactericidal if the dose is high enough.

Penicillin G is extremely potent against susceptible bacteria, but development of resistance has limited its usefulness. Resistance often occurs by organisms producing a beta-lactamase (penicillinase), which destroys the activity of the drug by scission of the beta-lactam ring.

Table 16–1. PENICILLINS AND RELATED DRUGS

Generic Name	Trade Names	Comments

1. **Penicillinase-susceptible, narrow-spectrum:** Clinically useful spectrum includes *Streptococci, Neisseria,* spirochetes, many anaerobes (not *Bacteroides*)
   A. *Penicillin G*

potassium penicillin G		All dosage routes and prompt action
sodium penicillin G		IM or IV and prompt acting

   B. *Depot Penicillin G*

procaine penicillin G	Duracillin	IM for long action
benzathine penicillin G	Bicillin	IM for long action
	Permapen	

2. Same as 1 but **acid-resistant**
   A. *Phenoxymethyl Penicillins*

hydrabamine penicillin-V	Compocillin-V	Oral use
penicillin-V	Penicillin V	Oral use
	Pen-Vee	
	V-Cillin	
potassium penicillin-V	Compocillin-Vk	Oral use
	Pen-Vee-K	
	V-Cillin	

   B. *Potassium Phenethicillin*

	Maxipen	Oral use
	Syncillin	

3. **Broader-spectrum:** More active than penicillin G against some Gram-negatives, but not penicillinase resistant
   A. *Broader-Spectrum*
   Clinically useful spectrum includes *Haemophilis influenzae, Escherichia coli, Proteus mirabilis,* enterococci, *Neisseria gonorrhoeae*

ampicillin	Penbritin	
amoxicillin	Amoxil	Like ampicillin
	Larocin	
proampicillins		To ampicillin *in vivo*
hetacillin	Versapen	
bacampicillin	Spectrobid	
cyclacillin	Cyclapen	

   B. *Antipseudomonal*
   Clinically useful spectrum as for 3A above and *Pseudomonas aeruginosa, Enterobacter,* indole-positive *Proteus*

carbenicillin	Pyopen	Parenteral use
	Geopen	
carbenicillin indanyl (ester)	Geocillin	Oral ($\rightarrow$ split)
ticarcillin	Ticar	Parenteral
azlocillin	Azlin	Parenteral

Table 16–1. (Continued)

Generic Name	Trade Names	Comments

C. *Extended-Spectrum*
Clinically useful spectrum as for 3B with increased activity for *Enterobacteria-ceae* such as *Klebsiella*, with some anaerobes including *Bacteroides fragilis*

mezlocillin	Mezlin	Parenteral
piperacillin	Pipracil	Parenteral

4. **Penicillinase resistant** with spectrum similar to that of penicillin G, but clinically useful spectrum is penicillinase-producing *Staphylococcus aureus*

methicillin	Staphcillin	For IM or IV use, *not oral*
	Dimocillin	
oxacillin	Prostaphlin	Oral or parenterally
	Resistopen	
cloxacillin	Orbenin	Oral use
	Tegopen	
dicloxacillin	Veracillin	Oral use
	Dynapen	
	Pathocil	
nafcillin	Unipen	Oral or parenterally

5. **Amidinopenicillins:** More active against G −, including *E. coli* and many *Shigella*, *Klebsiella*, and *Enterobacter* strains

amdinocillin (mecillinam)	Coactin

6. **Monobactams:** Beta-lactamase resistant with G − spectrum. Clinically useful spectrum includes *Pseudomonas, Serratia,* and *E. coli;* inactive against G +

aztreonam	Azactam

7. **Carbapenems:** Both G + and G −, as well as beta-lactamase resistant; renal metabolism inhibited by cilastatin

imipenem	Primaxin	Primaxin includes cilastatin

G − = Gram-negative.
G + = Gram-positive.

Disposition. Penicillins are used both orally and parenterally. They should not be used topically, because of the potential for allergic sensitization and increasing drug-resistant organisms. It is estimated that only 5 to 35 percent of an oral dose of penicillin G is absorbed, whereas a parenteral dose of a penicillin preparation is totally absorbed. This explains why the oral dose of penicillin G is five or more times the parenteral dose. The benzocaine and procaine salts of penicillin G are quite long lasting, with antimicrobial activity still present up to 3 weeks after a dose of benzocaine penicillin G.

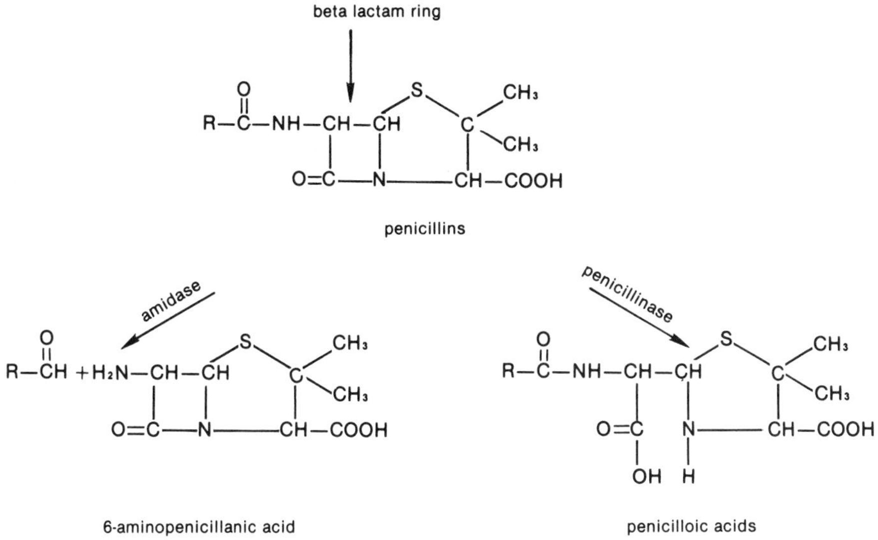

beta lactam ring

penicillins

amidase

penicillinase

6-aminopenicillanic acid

penicilloic acids

Figure 16–2. Structure of penicillins.

Penicillins are used orally (1) in less serious infections; (2) after an infection has been brought under control by parenteral use; (3) prophylactically for the prevention of endocarditis, such as prior to tonsillectomy, tooth extractions, or teeth cleaning; and (4) prophylactically for some prosthetic cases.

Parenteral penicillins are used in patients with serious infections and in patients who probably cannot or will not comply with an oral dosage regimen. The latter may include the very young and the very old.

Penicillins are distributed to all tissues, including the fetus. For penicillin G, tissue levels are about 20 percent that found in blood. Penetration into the central nervous system is usually inadequate unless large parenteral doses are given or functioning of the blood-brain barrier is significantly damaged, or both.

Plasma protein binding can be prominent and varies from one penicillin to another. This protein binding has been taken into consideration when dosage regimens are recommended for individual disease entities. The blood level is maximal at one-half to 1 hour after an oral dose. To minimize problems with gastric acid and binding to food protein, penicillins should be taken one-half hour before or 3 hours after a meal when possible.

Approximately 90 percent of penicillin G is excreted unchanged, with the other 10 percent being metabolized. The urinary excretion is approximately 10 percent by glomerular filtration and 90 percent by tubular secretion, with a maximum of 2 grams per hour excreted in a normal adult. This prominent urinary excretion is one of the features that make the penicillins useful in the treatment of certain urinary tract infections. Decreased renal function in the newborn, elderly, or patients with renal disease will tend to maintain blood levels.

Toxicity and Allergic Reactions. The adverse effects of the penicillins include toxicity, allergic reactions, and the inhibition of normal flora. The latter may promote suprainfections.

The penicillins are among the least toxic of available drugs. Allergic reactions are the important concern. Large oral doses can produce gastrointestinal upset, intramuscular administration can cause local pain, and intravenous use can cause sclerosing phlebitis. In other words, it is a chemical irritant to tissues.

It is now evident that all penicillins are cross-sensitizing, so that patients who are truly allergic to one penicillin are allergic to all penicillins. Penicillin metabolism in the patient produces penicillanic acid and penicilloic acid which can form dimers and trimers with one another and can subsequently conjugate to proteins to become immunogens. Noncontaminated penicillin, therefore, may be the original source of true allergy to penicillins.

However, prior to the early 1970s, batches of penicillin contained trace amounts of penicillin conjugated to proteinaceous material.[28] The protein could have come from the mycelium of the mold used to make the natural penicillins or could have come from the amidase that is added to the brew to hydrolyze the natural penicillins. If someone became allergic to the mycelial protein that did not have penicillin conjugated thereto, that person would be allergic to the protein but not to penicillin. Such an individual could have a reported history of allergy to penicillin but could "lose" this penicillin allergy if uncontaminated penicillin were subsequently used.

Another source of original exposure can be from dermatophytes that live on human skin surfaces. These dermatophytes can produce penicillin-like molecules that can be cross-sensitizing with the penicillins. Environmental molds also may produce penicillin-like molecules that can be cross-sensitizing. The drinking of penicillin-contaminated milk is yet another source of an unrecognized exposure to penicillin.

Of the skin eruptions with ampicillin, it is estimated that about one third are actually due to an allergic response. Those with an urticarial response are probably due to allergy, whereas other skin reactions may be questionable. This does not imply that one should be casual concerning the interpretation of an eczematous response to ampicillin. Individuals with infectious mononucleosis and individuals taking drugs that affect uric acid metabolism have a high incidence of rashes with ampicillin.

Allergic responses to penicillin occur most often with topical use and least often with oral use. It is estimated that up to 5 to 10 percent of adults and an extremely low percentage of children are allergic to the penicillins. About 10 percent of allergic reactions are of reasonably serious consequence.

Allergic reactions to penicillin can be approximately categorized in reference to time as (1) immediate (less than 20 minutes), (2) intermediate (2 hours to 2 days), and (3) delayed or late (greater than 2 days). The initial symptoms of an immediate reaction is often nasal and labial pruritus and/or cutaneous urticaria (hives), asthma, rhinitis, anaphylaxis, or laryngeal edema progressing to vascular collapse. Both anaphylaxis (estimated at 0.05 percent of recipients) and laryngeal edema are, of course, life-threatening reactions. The intermediate reactions are often urticarial, but may also consist of fever, abdominal crises, and so forth. Late reactions may occur even after the antibiotic has been stopped and can consist of serum sickness, rashes, thrombocytopenia, anemias, and so forth.

A history of penicillin allergy dictates use of another antibiotic. If a penicillin is deemed absolutely essential, skin testing with penicilloyl-polylysine and other determinants must be carefully performed by an individual well versed in the hazards of such procedures.

Resistance. Resistance to penicillins is a significant problem. Organisms may (1) be naturally resistant, (2) produce penicillinase, (3) produce amidase, or (4) lack penicillin receptors. Penicillinase-producing staphylococci have always been a significant problem. The penicillinase-resistant penicillins are specifically designed for such situations. The combination of clavulanic acid and amoxicillin is now available. The clavulanic acid serves as an inhibitor of penicillinase so that the amoxicillin is available to have its effect on cell wall synthesis. Although pneumococcus had been sensitive to penicillin G for many years, some resistance to penicillin G is now known to occur. Penicillin-resistant organisms are particularly a problem in hospitals. Besides being well demonstrated epidemiologically, it has been noted that sewage from residential areas containing hospitals has many more resistant strains than that from other residential and industrial areas.

Penicillin Groups. The various **penicillin groups** are shown in Table 16–1. The **penicillin G group** is primarily useful in Gram-positive infections and actinomycosis. Parenteral use is recommended in serious infections. The **penicillin V group,** which was designed to give protection in gastric acid, provides a blood level that is three to five times that of penicillin G for a comparable oral dose. This currently is the most widely used penicillin group.

The **broader-spectrum penicillins** can be useful against *Haemophilus influenzae, Escherichia coli, Proteus,* and a number of other organisms. Ampicillin is the prototype of this group and the oldest member thereof. Hetacillin and bacampicillin produce ampicillin *in vivo* and it is purported that bacampicillin and amoxicillin reach higher blood levels that ampicillin. Cyclacillin can give higher blood levels that ampicillin, but it is also excreted faster.

The carbenicillin/ticarcillin subgroup is particularly active and useful against *Pseudomonas,* as well as *Enterobacter* and *Proteus.* Hypokalemia and altered platelet function with bleeding have been noted with the drugs of this subgroup.

The azlocillin/piperacillin subgroup is additionally useful against *Klebsiella* as well as *Pseudomonas.*

The penicillins used against *Pseudomonas* are sometimes combined with an aminoglycoside, as this combination can be synergistic against *Pseudomonas*. Although this occurs *in vivo*, it must be recalled that the penicillin drug and the aminoglycoside must not be given in the same intravenous solution or syringe; in the same solution, they can physically interact to negate their effectiveness.

The **penicillinase-resistant penicillins** should be used only against penicillinase-producing organisms. Bone marrow depression with granulocytopenia may occur with the use of these agents. Interstitial nephritis, particularly with the use of methicillin, can also occur.

The **amidinopenicillins** are a new group with amdinocillin (mecillinam) as the initial prototype. It binds to the penicillin binding protein 2 only, thereby presumably explaining how it may be synergistic with penicillins that bind to other bacterial receptor proteins. It is more active against Gram-negative than Gram-positive bacteria.

Combined **penicillin/beta-lactamase inhibitors** are available as amoxicillin/clavulanic acid (Augmentin), ticarcillin/clavulanic acid (Timentin), and ampicillin/sulbactam (Unasyn). The rationale of the combination is that the clavulanic acid or sulbactam (a penicillanic acid sulfone) will increase the effectiveness of the given penicillin by inhibiting bacterial beta-lactamase.

The Cephalosporins

The **cephalosporins**, like the penicillins, are beta-lactams. They have a **7-aminocephalosporanic acid** portion of the molecule that is comparable to that of the 6-aminopenicillanic acid portion of the penicillins (Fig. 16–3). These cephalosporins likewise have different side chains that confer the various properties of the individual drugs. Like the penicillins, the cephalosporins are bactericidal and inhibit cell wall synthesis in a comparable fashion. They may or may not be effective against a specific strain of penicillin-resistant organisms.

Classification. The cephalosporins are often classified as first, second, and third generations. This terminology is that of marketing rather than of scientific origin, but for some time did follow the chronological development of the cephalosporins. However, some of the most recently released cephalosporins do not necessarily resemble those of the usual third-generation cephalosporins.

Rather than its original chronology and marketing context, the cephalosporin generation terminology is now more applicable to the concept of spectrum. First-generation drugs have good activity against a number of Gram-positive organisms and limited selective activity against Gram-negative organisms such as *E. coli*, *Klebsiella*, and *Proteus*. Second-generation drugs have a still broader spectrum, particularly against Gram-negative organisms; however, there may also be decreased effectiveness against some Gram-posi-

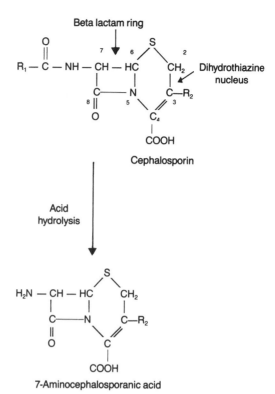

Figure 16–3. Structure of cephalosporins. R_1 and R_2 are sites for substitution. (Adapted from Snyder, IS and Finch, FG: β-Lactam Antibiotics [Penicillins and Cephalosporins]. In Craig, CR and Stitzel, RE [eds]: Modern Pharmacology, ed 2. Little, Brown & Co., Boston, 1986, p 673.)

tive cocci. The third-generation drugs add on even newer and more specific spectrum characteristics but lose effectiveness against many of those organisms that are affected by the earlier cephalosporins. As one progresses from first- to third-generation drugs, effectiveness against Gram-negative organisms increases while effectiveness against Gram-positive organisms decreases.

Resistance. The sometimes confusing question of **cross-resistance** or lack thereof may be based on the presence of beta-lactamases. Historically, there were vigorous discussions on whether or not cephalosporinase (which degrades cephalosporins) and penicillinase (which degrades penicillins) were the same enzyme. In time it was found that there are at least 50 different isozymes of these beta-lactamases and the substrate specificity can be quite different among the different isozymes. The potential for induction by various substrates can also differ among the various beta-lactamases.

Disposition. Many of the cephalosporins are poorly absorbed from the gastrointestinal tract and therefore are administered parenterally. Like the penicillins, most cephalosporins are excreted primarily by secretion in the kidney.

Toxicity and Allergic Reactions. As with the penicillins, adverse reactions to the cephalosporins include tissue irritation at the site of injection and irritation of the gastrointestinal mucosa when taken orally. Again, suprainfections consequent to influences on normal flora are always a possibility, particularly with the broader-spectrum drugs.

Renal toxicity was of particular concern with the earliest cephalosporins. An increase in BUN or creatinine, especially with a history of prior renal damage, can still be of concern, particularly when cephalosporins are used with aminoglycosides.

The likelihood and types of allergic reactions are comparable to those with penicillins. Because the cephalosporins historically appeared much later than the penicillins, allergic sensitization due to contamination (as occurred with penicillins) should not be a comparable problem with cephalosporins. Likewise, freshly prepared parenteral solutions of both penicillins and cephalosporins are less likely to contain degradation products that could conjugate with proteins to form immunogens.

Cross-sensitivity with penicillins has been reported but is not necessarily a constant. Since half of patients whose skin tests positive for penicillin also test positive for cephalothin,[29] prudence would dictate the use of an alternate to beta-lactams when feasible in penicillin-sensitive individuals, particularly if documented with a recent skin test. If a beta-lactam is deemed essential, such as penicillin in endocarditis, cautious desensitization with the specific drug may be warranted.[30]

Choice of Cephalosporins. Newer cephalosporins are constantly being added to those listed in Table 16–2. Full particulars on individual drugs cannot be given in this limited presentation. For example, among the first-generation drugs, many consider cefazolin to be much less painful on intramuscular injection than others in the group. Among second-generation drugs, cefamandole and cefaclor are purported to be much more active against *H. influenzae*. Cefoxitin is active against *Bacteroides fragilis* and some other anaerobes. Cefuroxine and cefonicid have similarities to cefamandole, but cefonicid has a long half-life with once-per-day dosage.

The third-generation cephalosporins are not first-choice agents for Gram-positive infections; on the contrary, they are often specialty drugs for life-threatening situations with Gram-negative organisms. A recent exception is the use of ceftriaxone in penicillinase-resistant gonorrhea. They all have longer elimination half-lives than the early cephalosporins and are comparatively very expensive. In addition to adverse reactions that can occur with any cephalosporin (local pain, transient liver enzyme abnormalities, gastrointestinal disturbances, leukopenia, and thrombocytopenia) moxalactam and cefoperazone have been associated with hypoprothrombinemia and bleeding. Additionally, moxalactam, cefoperazone, and the second-generation cefamandole have been associated with disulfiram-type reactions due to inhibition of acetaldehyde dehydrogenase. Alcohol consumption should therefore be avoided during and for several days following treatment with these agents.

Table 16–2. CEPHALOSPORINS

Drug	Trade Name(s)	Route

"First Generation"
Active against G+ *Staph. aureus* (not methicillin resistant), *Staph. epidermidis*, and streptococci (not enterococci). Moderately active against community-acquired G− strains of *E. coli*, *Klebsiella pneumoniae*, and *Proteus mirabilis*. Anaerobes (not *Bacteroides fragilis*) usually susceptible *in vitro*.

Drug	Trade Name(s)	Route
cephalothin	Keflin	Parenteral
cefazolin	Ancef	Parenteral
	Kefzol	
cephapirin	Cefadyl	Parenteral
cephradine	Velosef	Oral, parenteral
	Anspor	Oral
cephalexin	Keflex	Oral
cefadroxil	Duricef	Oral
	Ultracef	

"Second Generation"
Less effective than "first-generation" against G+, but more effective against G− species noted above.

Drug	Trade Name(s)	Route
cefamandole	Mandol	Parenteral; useful for *Enterobacter*, indole-positive *Proteus*, and anaerobes.
cefuroxime	Zinacef	Parenteral. Axetil ester for oral use.
cefonicid	Monocid	Parenteral; once per day may be sufficient.
cefoxitin	Mefoxin	Parenteral; useful for *Bacteroides fragilis* and *Serratia marcescens*.
cefaclor	Ceclor	Oral; useful for *H. influenzae*.
cefotetan	Cefotan	Parenteral

"Third Generation"
Greater activity against G− named above plus *Providentia*, *Pseudomonas*, and *Bacteroides fragilis*.

Drug	Trade Name(s)	Route
cefotaxime	Claforan	Parenteral
ceftriaxone	Rocephin	Parenteral once per day
moxalactam	Moxam	Parenteral
cefoperazone	Cefobid	Parenteral
ceftizoxime	Cefizox	Parenteral
ceforamide	Precef	Parenteral
ceftazidime	Fortaz	Parenteral

G+ = Gram-positive.
G− = Gram-negative.

Other Inhibitors of Cell Wall Synthesis

The **monobactam**, aztreonam, is a monocyclic beta-lactam, which is resistant to beta-lactamases and active against a number of aerobic Gram-negative organisms. It does not appear to be cross-allergenic with penicillins.

Another group of beta-lactam drugs (having different stereochemical configuration) are the **carbapenems**, exemplified by imipenem. It too is beta-lactamase resistant. Its spectrum includes a number of both Gram-positive and Gram-negative organisms. Because it is readily metabolized in the kidney, it is coadministered with cilastatin, which inhibits this renal metabolism of imipenem. Imipenem can be cross-allergenic with penicillins.

Cycloserine, a secondary drug used to treat tuberculosis, acts on susceptible bacteria at the first phase of cell wall synthesis (i.e., synthesis of the nucleotide intermediates). It does not have a prominent place in therapy other than the aforementioned use.

Bacitracin, a useful **topical** agent against **Gram-positive infections,** has a **bactericidal** spectrum similar to that of penicillin G. It interferes with cell wall synthesis *via* the interference with the phospholipid carrier for the mucopeptide used in cell wall synthesis. Its potential for nephrotoxicity when used parenterally negates such usage. Sensitivity reactions do occur, but not commonly. No cross-resistance occurs with other antimicrobial drugs.

Like bacitracin, **vancomycin** also acts on phase two of cell wall synthesis in bacteria. Vancomycin is bactericidal against a number of Gram-positive organisms. It is poorly absorbed orally and therefore is used intravenously in severely ill hospitalized patients, particularly in cases of rampant staphylococcal infection or enterococcal endocarditis not responding to other therapy. Rapid infusion may cause a flush on the upper body. Toxic manifestations such as fever, chills, colitis, rashes, and auditory and renal impairment argue for the use of less toxic antibiotics if possible. These toxic effects were even more prominent in earlier years when less purified drug preparations were being used.

Vancomycin may also be used orally for enterocolitis due to either staphylococci or *Clostridium difficile,* and can be life saving in such conditions.

Inhibitors of Protein Synthesis

Erythromycin

The only currently used **macrolide** in this country is **erythromycin** in its various forms. Erythromycin inhibits aminoacyl translocation by reacting with a receptor on the 50S subunit. This inhibition of protein synthesis is bacteriostatic, but may be bactericidal at high concentrations. The drug contains large lactone rings glycosidically linked to sugars. The nature of the molecule may explain why many Gram-negative bacteria are impermeable to the molecule.

It is therefore most useful in a variety of Gram-positive infections such as those of the pneumococcus, *Streptococcus pyogenes,* and *S. viridans.* It is also of use in treating diphtheria, mycoplasma pneumonia, and infections with legionella. It is a useful substitute for penicillin in individuals who are allergic to penicillin. It can likewise be useful against some penicillin-resistant strains of organisms.

Staphylococci can methylate the rRNA receptor site so that the drug will not bind and the organism therefore becomes resistant. This resistance can be plasmid transferred. When resistance occurs, there may be cross-resistance with lincomycin.

Preparations of erythromycin include

1. Free base—oral and topical use (unstable in acid or alkali and therefore able to be destroyed by gastric juice)
2. Estolate (i.e., lauryl sulfate salt of erythromycin propionic acid ester)—oral use (more palatable and somewhat acid stable)
3. Flavored suspension of stearate (and ethylsuccinate)—oral use
4. Intravenous powders (lactobionate and gluceptate)

Erythromycin is concentrated in the liver and excreted *via* the bile (up to 50 times blood level) and feces. A smaller amount (5 percent) is excreted in the urine.

Impaired liver function and jaundice have been reported following the estolate, but this is reversible. It appears to be an unpredictable hypersensitivity phenomenon producing intrahepatic cholestasis.

If fever, eosinophilia, or rash occurs, they too will subside after stopping the drug. Reversible hearing loss may occur with high dosage.

Erythromycin can be irritating to tissue and the symptoms will be dependent on the route of administration (e.g., oral use may produce nausea, vomiting, and diarrhea).

The Lincosamides

The **lincosamides,** lincomycin and clindamycin, also inhibit protein synthesis at the 50S subunit.

Lincomycin is the earlier of the pair and often substituted for erythromycin in the past. It resembles erythromycin in spectrum, and cross-resistance with erythromycin can occur. It continued to be used less with the advent of clindamycin, which is more potent and has fewer adverse effects.

Clindamycin is a chemical derivative of lincomycin which can be used orally or parenterally. It can be effective against a number of Gram-positive cocci and some anaerobes. It should not be used against Gram-positive cocci if a penicillin or erythromycin can be used.

Although mild GI symptoms are common, the occurrence of pseudomembranous colitis is potentially fatal. Although other organisms may be involved, the exotoxin of *Clostridium difficile* is often the problem. Although initially described as clindamycin colitis, this condition has now been associated with a wide variety of antibiotics including the penicillins, cephalosporins, erythromycin, chloramphenicol, tetracyclines, streptomycin, and cotrimoxazole. As mentioned earlier, discontinuation of the involved antibiotic and the utilization of oral vancomycin can be life saving in this situation.

In addition to common mild GI symptoms, rashes occur in about 10 percent of patients.

The drug is especially useful for non-CNS *Bacteroides fragilis* infection. Clindamycin does not usually cross the blood-brain barrier and therefore is not useful in *B. fragilis* infections of the central nervous system.

Chloramphenicol

Chloramphenicol, along with the tetracyclines, is a true broad-spectrum antibiotic. Chloramphenicol is a small synthetic molecule that is effective against a number of Gram-positive and Gram-negative bacteria, as well as certain rickettsiae. It is particularly useful in (1) significant *Salmonella* infection (e.g., typhoid or paratyphoid fever), (2) *H. influenzae* meningitis or laryngotracheitis (with ampicillin or a third-generation cephalosporin as an alternative choice of drug), and (3) rarely, Gram-negative bacteremia.

Chloramphenicol is bacteriostatic, inhibiting protein synthesis at the 50S subunit by preventing the binding of new amino acids *via* inhibition of peptidyl transferase. The drug can also inhibit mitochondrial protein synthesis in mammalian cells, particularly in erythropoietic cells in debilitated patients.

Resistant mutants do not emerge rapidly, and cross-resistance does not occur between chloramphenicol and other drugs. When resistance does develop, it may be due to a plasmid-controlled acetylating enzyme.

Chloramphenicol is quite rapidly and essentially completely absorbed from the gastrointestinal tract and widely distributed to all tissues and body fluids. About 10 percent is excreted unchanged in the urine and 90 percent is excreted *via* the same route as inactive metabolic products (glucuronic acid conjugate and reduced derivatives).

Local irritation from the drug can produce nausea, vomiting, or diarrhea in the first few days of therapy. If such symptoms occur a number of days after the initiation of therapy, the possibility of suprainfection from inhibition of gut flora must be considered.

Because the drug is toxic to the erythropoietic system at high levels, high dosage can produce a maturation arrest of red cells, which will subside upon discontinuance of the drug.

The so-called gray baby syndrome, with vomiting, diarrhea, flaccidity, and shock, is due to toxic levels of chloramphenicol accumulating secondary to the relative absence of effective glucuronyltransferase activity in the newborn. This decreased enzyme activity and decreased renal function contraindicates the use of chloramphenicol in the newborn.

The rare aplastic anemia (estimated at 1 in 30,000) that can occur with chloramphenicol is not necessarily related to doses or the duration of therapy. This can be fatal. If the patient survives, he or she may later get leukemia.

Although not common, rashes and fever may occur with the drug.

Since there are now other drugs available and there is the possibility of aplastic anemia, chloramphenicol should be used only if other effective drugs cannot be used in the particular circumstances.

Tetracyclines

The **tetracyclines,** like chloramphenicol, are broad-spectrum drugs that are bacteriostatic *via* inhibition of protein synthesis. Other than some differences in regard to persistence in the body, all drugs of this group are chemically similar and have similar spectra and toxicity. They are effective against a number of Gram-positive bacteria, Gram-negative bacteria, spirochetes, leptospira, chlamydiae, mycoplasmae, amebae, and some rickettsiae.

The tetracyclines act on bacteria by preventing access of aminoacyl tRNA to the acceptor site on the mRNA-ribosome complex, thereby preventing adding of amino acids to the growing peptide chain. This effect can also occur in mammalian cells at high concentrations, particularly in debilitated individuals.

The oral route of administration is usual, but absorption is variable. Intramuscular absorption is often poor and the site can be painful. Intravenously, the drug should be given slowly over several minutes or by drip because of its irritating properties. It should be noted that the intravenous route can cause severe hepatic injury, with a greater frequency of complications in pregnant patients and those with renal disease.

From one fifth to one half of the absorbed drug is bound to serum proteins. It distributes to all tissues of the body, being somewhat higher in bone and liver and quite low in the cerebrospinal and synovial fluids.

The drug can chelate a number of metallic ions; therefore, calcium and aluminum salts tend to impair gastrointestinal absorption.

The four-ring tetracycline skeleton is not metabolized by mammals, but one does see metabolic changes in the substituent groups.

Excretion is primarily in the urine (glomerular filtration) and secondarily in bile. The bile level may be 10 times that of the serum. Kidney damage and oliguria shift the excretory load to the liver, thereby increasing the possibility of hepatotoxicity.

Toxicity and Allergic Reactions. Toxic effects of tetracyclines can include early gastrointestinal upset and diarrhea due to simple chemical irritation. More severe symptoms may be due to changed gut flora with fungal overgrowth, which may respond to buttermilk or sour cream therapy. However, resistant staphylococcal enterocolitis can also occur and it carries a 50 percent mortality. Pseudomembranous colitis with a bloody, white-cell–containing diarrhea may be due to *C. difficile*. The latter two life-threatening conditions may require vancomycin and the care of therapists who are comfortable with the treatment of such conditions.

The possibility of severe liver and pancreatic damage from large doses, particularly intravenously, has been noted earlier. With current knowledge, the previously reported renal toxicity from the use of outdated tetracyclines should no longer occur.

The deposition in teeth and bones of the fetus and premature with brownish discoloration of enamel, tooth defects, and slowing of bone growth is well known. Tetracyclines should therefore be avoided in women throughout the last half of pregnancy and in children until age 7.

Blood dyscrasias may occur from long-term use of tetracyclines, and an antianabolic effect with negative nitrogen balance can occur in the undernourished owing to inhibition of protein synthesis. Photosensitivity has been known to occur, particularly with demeclocycline (demethylchlortetracycline).

A variety of allergic/hypersensitivity reactions such as glossitis, skin eruptions, angioedema, fever, and a burning sensation of the eyes are known to occur. Anaphylaxis has occurred. All of the tetracyclines are cross-sensitizing.

Resistance. Resistance has occurred to the extent that the tetracyclines are no longer effective in the majority of staphylococcal infections. They are no longer effective in treating streptococcal infections of the heart. Tetracycline resistance can sometimes be explained by organisms that lack permeability to tetracyclines and also by mutants that lose a normally present active transport mechanism for tetracyclines and therefore no longer concentrate the drug within the cell. The latter type of tetracycline resistance is plasmid controlled.

For many years it was dogma that there is complete cross-resistance among the various tetracyclines. This is generally true, but some staphylococcal strains have been reported to be still sensitive to minocycline.

Use in Treatment of Acne. The use of tetracyclines in treating acne is a source of continuing discussion. *Corynebacterium acnes* or *Propionibacterium acnes*, an anaerobic organism, grows in the sebaceous follicles and produces a lipase that hydrolyzes the triglycerides in sebum to fatty acids. The sebum and particularly the fatty acids are irritating. Tetracyclines can inhibit both the growth of the organism and the lipase enzyme itself. The risk side of the equation is the fostering of antibiotic resistance by bacteria. The scarring sequelae of severe pustular acne is the prevailing argument in favor of tetracycline use in such cases. Rigorous attention to hygiene and diet, as well as judicious use of nonantibiotic topical preparations, are the measures of choice in less severe situations.

Choice of Tetracyclines. From their structure and this discussion, it can be seen that any given practitioner need be familiar with only one or possibly two of the tetracyclines. As shown in Table 16–3, some of the tetracyclines

Table 16–3. TETRACYCLINES

Generic Name	Trade Name(s)	Comments

Clinically useful spectrum includes G + cocci (but resistance often a problem and better drugs available); G − non-resistant strains of *Neisseria gonorrhoeae* and *N. meningitidis, H. influenzae, Brucella, Vibrio cholerae;* spirochaetes, rickettsiae, mycoplasma, and chlamydia.

A. Short Duration. Avoid in renal failure

tetracycline	Achromycin	$t_{1/2} = 8$ hr
	Panmycin	
	Polycycline	
	Tetracyn	
chlortetracycline	Aureomycin	$t_{1/2} = 6$ hr
oxytetracycline	Terramycin	$t_{1/2} = 9$ hr

B. Intermediate Duration: Two doses per day; avoid in renal failure

demeclocycline	Declomycin	$t_{1/2} = 12$–14 hr
methacycline	Rondomycin	$t_{1/2} = 12$–14 hr

C. Longer duration: Two doses per day

doxycycline	Vibramycin	$t_{1/2} = 15$–21 hr (15–36 in anuric); safest for extrarenal infection in renal failure
minocycline	Minocin	$t_{1/2} = 12$–13 hr (17–30 in anuric)

G + = Gram-positive.
G − = Gram-negative.

have a longer persistence in the body and require fewer doses per day. Demeclocycline persists in the body for a slightly longer time and has only slightly greater potency than the original three tetracyclines, but has the potential for photosensitivity. Doxycycline does not accumulate in the blood in patients with renal failure and is therefore recommended for extrarenal infections in such individuals. Vestibular toxicity has been reported with minocycline.

Because of their high-lipid solubility, doxycycline and minocycline have the best oral absorption (95 to 100 percent) among the tetracyclines. A potentially important drug interaction is that the $T_{1/2}$ of doxycycline can be shortened from 20 hours to 7 hours with concurrent chronic therapy using phenobarbital or phenytoin.

Spectinomycin

Spectinomycin (Trobicin) is an aminocyclitol that inhibits protein synthesis at the 30S ribosomal subunit by inhibiting translocation. It is not a tetracycline but is included at this juncture based on its mechanism. It is clinically useful only against gonorrhea, particularly when penicillin is not effective or when the patient is allergic to penicillin. It is given in a single intramuscular dose.

Mupirocin

Mupirocin (pseudomonic acid, Bactroban) is now available for topical therapy of impetigo. It prevents incorporation of isoleucine into bacterial protein by binding to bacterial isoleucyl transfer-RNA synthetase. Local itching, stinging, and rash have been reported.

The Aminoglycosides

The **aminoglycosides** (Table 16–4) are very important drugs in the treatment of Gram-negative infections. They inhibit protein synthesis by causing abnormal initiation complex formation and misreading of mRNA with consequent nonfunctional proteins being formed. Unlike other inhibitors of bacterial protein synthesis, they are bactericidal.

Although the microbiological spectrum of a given aminoglycoside may include Gram-positive bacteria, Gram-negative bacteria, and even mycobacteria, the clinically useful spectrum and useful modes of administration are dictated by their toxicity and the presence or absence of more appropriate drugs for a given infection. Their important systemic use against bacteremia with Gram-negative enteric bacteria is noted with the gentamicin discussion.

Toxicity. The aminoglycosides are both ototoxic and nephrotoxic when

Table 16–4. AMINOGLYCOSIDES

Drug	Trade Name(s)	Comments
Clinically useful spectrum as below, but use limited by toxicity and/or resistant organisms.		
streptomycin		Tuberculosis use
neomycin		Topical use and bowel "sterilization"
kanamycin	Kantrex	Topical use and bowel "sterilization"
Clinically useful spectrum primarily aerobic G − including *E. coli, Proteus, Pseudomonas, Klebsiella, Enterobacter,* and *Serratia.*		
gentamicin	Garamycin	
tobramycin	Nebcin	
amikacin	Amikin	
netilmicin	Netromycin	

G − = Gram-negative.

given parenterally. The ototoxicity can cause both hearing and equilibrium disturbances and is worse when the patient is hearing impaired or elderly, and when given concurrently with potent diuretics such as ethacrynic acid or furosemide. The nephrotoxicity is worse when patients are elderly, in shock, or dehydrated, and in those with a history of prior renal disease, with oliguria, or receiving concurrent therapy with a cephalosporin. The effect is an acute tubular necrosis that is usually reversible.

The curare-like neuromuscular blockade from the use of high-dose aminoglycosides in abdominal surgery years ago should no longer occur, as this high-dose toxicity is well documented. It also recommends caution whenever aminoglycosides and neuromuscular blockers are being used concurrently.

The potential for toxicity with systemic use of aminoglycosides prompts the use of drug blood level determination at the peak (one half to 1 hour after infusion) and at the trough (prior to infusion) in an attempt to maintain a nontoxic but therapeutically effective blood concentration. Likewise, as these drugs are excreted by glomerular filtration and the $t_{1/2}$ can increase from 2.5 hours to 2.5 days in renal failure, the correction of either the dose level or the dose interval will depend on the creatinine clearance (not the creatinine concentration). Nomograms for the specific drug need to be consulted while also recognizing that changes in other factors such as volume of distribution may also occur in disease states.

Resistance. Resistance to aminoglycosides can occur by (1) altered ribosomal receptors, (2) changes in cell permeability to the drug or drugs, and (3) development of enzymes responsible for metabolism of a given drug or drugs. The latter is probably the most important among the mechanisms and is plasmid mediated.

Choice of Aminoglycosides. Streptomycin is classified as an aminoglycoside and has many of the general features of aminoglycosides just noted. Although sometimes used for other purposes, it will be discussed with antitubercular drugs.

Neomycin is a rather wide-spectrum aminoglycoside, affecting a number of Gram-positive and Gram-negative organisms. It is not readily inactivated by exudates, enzymes, gastrointestinal secretions, or bacterial by-products. It is also the most nephrotoxic of the aminoglycosides. For these reasons it is useful topically but its marked parenteral toxicity prevents its use for systemic infections. Its oral use to preoperatively reduce gut flora and also to inhibit ammonia-producing gut flora in hepatic coma can be considered topical uses, as it is not absorbed from the gut. It is not to be confused with nystatin (an antifungal agent).

Kanamycin (Fig. 16–4) is an earlier aminoglycoside somewhat akin to neomycin. Its usefulness has been greatly curtailed because of the introduction of more recent aminoglycosides.

Gentamicin is a mixture of aminoglycoside molecules and has a fairly broad spectrum of activity against a number of Gram-positive and Gram-nega-

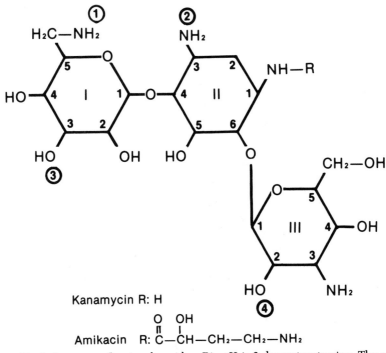

Figure 16–4. Structure of aminoglycosides. Ring II is 2-deoxystreptamine. The resemblance between kanamycin and amikacin can be seen. The circled numerals on the kanamycin molecule indicate points of attack of plasmid-mediated bacterial enzymes that can inactivate this drug: ① and ②, acetylase; ③, phosphorylase; ④, adenylylase. (Adapted from Jawetz, E: Aminoglycosides & Polymyxins. In Katzung, BG [ed]: Basic and Clinical Pharmacology, ed 3. Appleton & Lange, Norwalk, CT, 1987, p 534.)

tive bacteria including staphylococci, *E. coli, Klebsiella, Enterobacter, Pseudomonas, Proteus,* and *Serratia.* It is most useful as a bactericidal agent in severe Gram-negative infections with bacteria that are resistant to less toxic drugs. Its topical use is restricted to serious burn infections, as it is too important to use topically for anything else.

As noted in the penicillins discussion, gentamicin and other newer aminoglycosides may be synergistic with carbenicillin/ticarcillin against *Pseudomonas;* however, they should never be in the same solution, because their opposing multiple charges will render them ineffective.

Some streptococci that are resistant to gentamicin or another aminoglycoside may be killed by the synergistic effect of adding an inhibitor of cell wall synthesis such as a penicillin. This form of resistance is based on lack of aminoglycoside transport into the cell, and this transport is promoted by the action of the penicillin on the cell wall.

Gram-negative organisms resistant to gentamicin are usually cross-resistant to neomycin and kanamycin. Plasmid-transmitted inactivation of the drug by metabolism is the mechanism of this resistance.

Tobramycin is similar to gentamicin in many ways. It is believed to be less nephrotoxic than gentamicin and to have greater activity against *Pseudomonas*. It can be somewhat less active toward other bacterial species. Organisms resistant to gentamicin may still be susceptible to tobramycin, but the individual strain must be tested.

Amikacin is a semisynthetic derivative of kanamycin that became available after gentamicin and tobramycin. It is resistant to metabolic inactivation at sites two, three, and four shown in Figure 16–4. Although individual strains must be tested, amikacin may therefore still be effective against organisms that are resistant to either or both gentamicin and tobramycin. In fact, much of the development of aminoglycosides is based on attempting to produce molecules that can overcome resistance developed to previous drugs. To minimize the hazards of resistance in both the individual and the population, good judgment precludes using the most recently developed drug if an earlier drug will suffice. The newer drug is then still available if necessary.

Netilmicin is the most recent addition to this group. Like amikacin, it is protected from metabolism at a number of sites. It is also alleged to be somewhat less ototoxic and less nephrotoxic than other aminoglycosides.

Inhibitors of Cell Membrane Function

The *polymyxins* are the historical progenitors of aminoglycosides in terms of their systemic use in Gram-negative bacteremias. Their marked potential for nephrotoxicity and neurotoxicity when used parenterally has led to the use of aminoglycosides for this purpose.

The polymyxins are basic polypeptides of approximately 1400 daltons that alter the permeability of the cell membranes in susceptible bacteria and are bactericidal in such organisms. Polymyxin B (Aerosporin) and polymyxin E (also called colistin; Coly-Mycin) are the only two commercially available. They are effective against a number of Gram-negative bacteria, and there is essentially complete cross-resistance between the two.

The most popular current use for polymyxins is topically for Gram-negative infections. Because topical infections are usually mixed infections, either polymyxin is often used in conjunction with bacitracin or neomycin, or both.

Competitive Antagonists

The Sulfonamides

The **sulfonamides** resulted from the chemical intermediates used for various dyes that bound to proteins in wool. Their demonstrated use in mice and later in patients by Gerhard Domagk in the early 1930s initiated modern-day chemotherapy for systemic infections.

Modern medical use of sulfonamides is mostly limited to the treatment of urinary tract infections and other special uses. Because they are relatively inexpensive, more prominent use occurs in some areas of the world.

Most sulfonamide derivatives in use are based on the sulfanilamido or sulfanilyl radicals (Fig. 16–5), and they must have a free para-amino group to be active *in vivo*. Differing substituents on the molecule will give compounds of diverse features. This has made available drugs that (1) are more slowly absorbed from the gastrointestinal tract and therefore serve as intestinal antiseptics, (2) are more soluble at the pH of urine and therefore minimize drug crystallization in the urinary tubule, and (3) have longer persistence in the body.

The sulfonamides are bacteriostatic against many Gram-positive cocci and also some Gram-negative organisms. They compete with para-amino benzoic acid in the synthesis of folic acid. As mammals require preformed folic acid, this has no direct consequence on the patient.

Metabolism. Absorbed sulfonamides are well distributed throughout body tissues and usually have free access across the blood-brain barrier. Serum protein binding varies from 20 to 90 percent, and the recommended dosages take this protein-binding figure into account for the specific drug. The para-amino group may be acetylated and the metabolite may be more or less soluble than the parent drug (in addition to losing bacteriostatic activity).

Systemically used sulfonamides are highly concentrated in urine (20 to 25 times the blood level). This is beneficial in the treatment of urinary tract infections but potentially harmful in that the sulfonamide may crystallize out in the renal tubule, causing physical damage.

Because sulfonamides act as weak acids owing to the dissociation of the sulfamyl ($-SO_2NH-$) or comparable group, compounds with substituents on the sulfamyl nitrogen have been produced, to make the compound more acidic. This results in more drug being excreted as the more soluble salt. To further

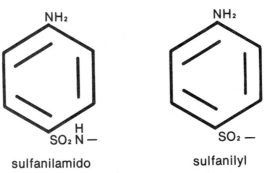

sulfanilamido   sulfanilyl

Figure 16–5. Structural basis of sulfonamides.

minimize crystalluria, one should promote fluid intake and also prevent the urine from becoming too acidic. Lower doses of several sulfonamides in combination can be used to produce an additive bacteriostatic effect while minimizing the solubility problem. The bacteriostatic effect is additive, but the solubility product of each compound does not change, which is the basis for so-called "triple sulfa" therapy.

Adverse Effects. The adverse reactions to sulfonamides may involve nearly every organ system and have an overall incidence of about 5 percent. Cross-sensitivity is common between sulfonamides, and a number of drug interactions may occur (e.g., sulfonamides can cause an increase in the hypoglycemic effect of antidiabetic sulfonylureas such as tolbutamide).

It is not always possible to discriminate between an allergic basis or a dose-related toxic basis for the adverse effects of sulfonamides. Other than the urinary tract difficulties, the most common adverse effects are skin rashes, fever, photosensitivity, and gastrointestinal symptoms such as vomiting and diarrhea. Hemolytic anemias, agranulocytosis, aplastic anemia, hepatitis, allergic toxic nephrosis, and various central nervous system symptoms are much less common.

Proteinuria and hematuria are toxic effects attributable to the crystalluria discussed earlier. Methemoglobinemia can occur with older sulfonamides, and acute hemolytic anemia may occur in patients with erythrocyte deficiency of glucose-6-phosphate dehydrogenase (discussed with the antimalarial agent primaquine). Sulfonamides should not be used to treat the pregnant woman at term or the newborn infant, because of the possibility of producing kernicterus in the newborn.

The contention that long-acting sulfonamides cause the Stevens-Johnson syndrome (erythema multiforme exudativum) was a factor in the withdrawal of those drugs from the market. The syndrome has allegedly been associated with a number of other drugs, including other antimicrobial drugs.

Choice of Sulfonamides. The "classic" sulfonamides listed in Table 16–5 are sulfadiazine and the combination of **sulfadiazine, sulfamerazine,** and **sulfamethazine.** They are still in use in economically underdeveloped countries. Trisulfapyridines or triple sulfas is a combination of equal parts of the three aforementioned sulfonamides. The combination has been used to minimize crystalluria.

Sulfisoxazole is a prominent sulfonamide with a $t_{1/2}$ of 5 to 7 hours used to treat urinary tract infections. **Sulfacytine** and **sulfamethizole** are likewise used in this fashion. *E. coli* is often the causative organism.

Special use sulfonamides have been devised for particular purposes. Some of these are noted in the table. The efficacy of **sulfasalazine** (Azulfidine) appears to be related to the release of the anti-inflammatory agent 5-aminosalicylate. Recently, 5-aminosalicylate as mesalamine (Rowasa) has become available for enema therapy of ulcerative colitis.

Cotrimoxazole is a combination consisting of **trimethoprim** and **sulfamethoxazole** in fixed-dose combination.

Table 16–5. SULFONAMIDES

Generic Name	Trade Name(s)	Comments
Clinically useful spectrum includes uncomplicated urinary tract infections with *E. coli, Enterobacter, Proteus, Klebsiella,* and G+ cocci. Also *Nocardia, Toxoplasma gondii,* and alternative in trachoma and lymphogranuloma venereum.		
sulfadiazine		Good penetration into CSF; acetyl derivative more soluble
trisulfapyridines (triple sulfas)		Equal parts of sulfadiazine, sulfamerazine, and sulfamethazine
sulfisoxazole	Gantrisin	Quite soluble at neutral and acidic pH; acetyl derivative tasteless and used orally for children. Sulfisoxazole + phenazopyridine HCl (Azo Gantrisin) also urinary antiseptic
sulfamethoxazole	Gantanol	
sulfacytine	Renoquid	
sulfamethizole	Thiosulfil	
Special Use		
mafenide	Sulfamylon Acetate Cream	Topical use in burns; painful
silver sulfadiazine	Silvadene Cream	Topical use in burns, less painful
sulfisoxazole diolamine	Gantrisin diolamine	Topical eye use
sodium sulfacetamide	Sodium Sulamyd	Topical eye use
sulfasalazine	Azulfidine	Used in ulcerative colitis; releases sulfapyridine and 5-aminosalicylate in gut
Combination Therapy		
co-trimoxazole (= trimethoprim + sulfamethoxazole)	Bactrim Septra	See text
Sulfones		
Clinically useful in leprosy (*Mycobacterium leprae*).		
dapsone or DDS	Avlosulfon	
acedapsone		Repository form of dapsone

G+ = Gram-positive.

Trimethoprim

Trimethoprim is a methotrexate analog, which in turn is a pyrimidine analog. Trimethoprim has been found to be antibacterial for a number of Gram-positive and Gram-negative bacteria and is not antagonized by para-amino

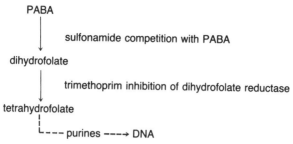

Figure 16–6. Sequential inhibition by sulfonamide and trimethoprim.

benzoic acid. It is well absorbed from the gastrointestinal tract and has prominent distribution to tissues and urine, with the urinary concentration reaching 100 times that in the blood. It reversibly inhibits dihydrofolate reductase and is 10,000 to 50,000 times more effective against the bacterial enzyme than the mammalian enzyme. The side effects of trimethoprim include skin rashes and a potential antifolate action on the hematopoietic system.

Although trimethoprim alone can be effective in urinary tract infections, it has a synergistic action when used with sulfonamides (Fig. 16–6), which is the basis of its combination with sulfamethoxazole sold as co-trimoxazole. The fixed-dose combination achieves a 20:1 ratio of sulfamethoxazole to trimethoprim in blood and tissue for maximal antimicrobial effect. It is believed that resistance is less likely to occur with the combination. It has been used in urinary tract infections, typhoid, and other conditions. It should be remembered that the potential adverse effects of both drugs can occur when the combination is used. To the sulfonamide-induced rashes, nausea, vomiting, and so forth, can be added trimethoprim's antifolate effects such as megaloblastic anemia, granulocytopenia, and leukopenia. Skin eruptions with the co-trimoxazole combination are unusually common in patients with HIV infection.

The Sulfones

The sulfones are chemically related to the sulfonamides, and their use is limited to the therapy of leprosy and some uncommon dermatological conditions. They have adverse effects comparable to those of the sulfonamides. Nonsulfone drugs also useful in leprosy include rifampin, clofazimine, and thiacetazone (amithiozone).

Nonsulfonamide Urinary Antiseptics

Nitrofurantoin and nalidixic acid (Fig. 16–7) are among the more prominent nonsulfonamide urinary tract antiseptics. **Nitrofurantoin** has relatively broad-spectrum antimicrobial activity in urinary tract infections, but *Pseudo-*

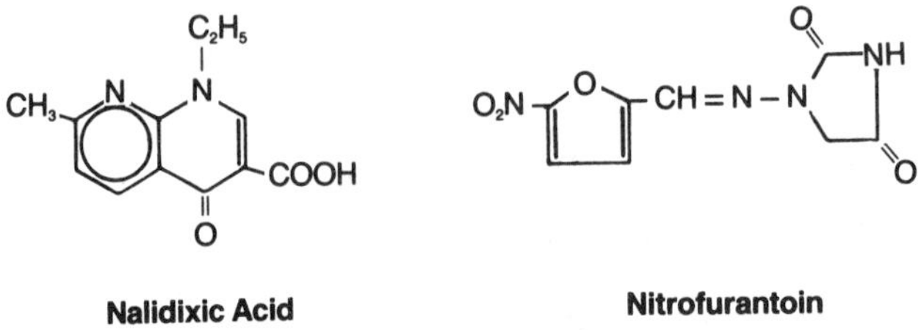

Nalidixic Acid **Nitrofurantoin**

Figure 16–7. Structure of nalidixic acid and nitrofurantoin.

monas is resistant. There is usually no cross-resistance with other antibiotics for susceptible organisms. Nitrofurantoin is well absorbed from the gut and rapidly excreted by the kidney. Gastric upset with nausea and vomiting can be minimized by taking the oral preparation with food or milk or by using the macrocrystal capsules. Skin rashes, peripheral neuropathies, hepatic necrosis, and hemolytic anemia in glucose-6-phosphate dehydrogenase–deficient individuals can occur. A variety of pulmonary signs and symptoms attributable to pulmonary hypersensitivity reactions are also known to occur. Owing to its various side effects, nitrofurantoin is contraindicated in patients with severe renal insufficiency: toxic drug levels are more likely to occur in such patients.

The structurally related nitrofurazone is a synthetic antimicrobial used as an impregnated gauze dressing on severe burns.

Nalidixic acid (Neg Gram) is another synthetic agent used for Gram-negative urinary tract infections. It is known to inhibit DNA gyrase (topoisomerase II), thereby inhibiting DNA synthesis in *E. coli*, but it is not known if this is the sole *in vivo* mechanism of action. Like nitrofurantoin, there is no cross-resistance with other antimicrobials. Skin rashes, gastrointestinal upset, drowsiness, and eosinophilia can occur.

More recently, **norfloxacin** (Noroxin) and ciprofloxacin (Cipro), fluoroquinolone compounds structurally related to nalidixic acid and cinoxacin (Cinobac), have become available. Like the latter two drugs, they too inhibit bacterial DNA gyrase and are bactericidal. Because almost all of the usual urinary tract pathogens are susceptible and bacterial resistance development is not frequent, norfloxacin or ciprofloxacin may be particularly useful in complicated urinary tract infections with organisms resistant to older, cheaper, and more proven drugs. A variety of central nervous system, gastrointestinal, skin, renal, musculoskeletal, and hematological side effects are under evaluation.

Methenamine mandelate and **methenamine hippurate** are nonspecific inhibitors of bacteria used as urinary antiseptics. Methenamine acts *via* the release of formaldehyde in urine below pH 5.5. The mandelic acid and hippuric acid moieties act by acidifying the urine. Sulfonamides and methanamine are incompatible, as the sulfonamides can form insoluble compounds with the released formaldehyde.

Antitubercular Drugs

Two important features in the treatment of tuberculosis are (a) the poor blood supply to the organism in the tubercule and (b) the rather frequent and relatively rapid development of drug resistance by the organisms. The poor blood supply necessitates long-term therapy to prevent recurrence, but the chronic drug therapy requires relatively nontoxic drugs. The potential resistance problem necessitates giving two or three drugs simultaneously to prevent the development of resistance.

Isoniazid, rifampin, and ethambutol are the three most prominent antitubercular drugs currently in use. Streptomycin is of lesser value, and a variety of secondary drugs are of occasional use. The secondary drugs can be more toxic or less effective and will not be discussed herein.

Isoniazid (abbreviated INH, for isonicotinic acid hydrazide) has an ill-defined mechanism of action against *Mycobacterium tuberculosis* related to inhibiting synthesis of mycolic acids used in cell walls of the bacilli. It is bactericidal against growing mycobacteria but less active against resting mycobacteria. It is a structural analog of pyridoxine (vitamin B_6), and pyridoxine can antagonize the neurotoxic effects of INH in the patient, but the vitamin will not antagonize the antitubercular effect of INH on the mycobacterium. As well as being used therapeutically, INH is the usual drug for prophylaxis against tuberculosis.

INH is readily absorbed from the gut, well distributed to all tissues and fluids, and excreted unchanged by the kidney. The acetylation of INH is a classic example of pharmacogenetics. People are either fast or slow acetylators of the drug, with many native Americans, Eskimos, and Orientals being rapid acetylators. This knowledge may influence dosage regimens for certain populations.

The adverse effects of INH usually appear to be of a toxic nature. Neurotoxicity is less than 5 percent and can be anything from headaches to convulsions. As noted earlier, pyridoxine antagonizes this neurotoxicity. Occasional bone marrow or liver effects are seen. Biochemical evidence of mild hepatic dysfunction is common; some progress to hepatitis, and occasional severe and even fatal hepatic necrosis may occur. The potential for liver damage seems to increase with age and it is not clear whether this represents a direct toxicity or a hypersensitivity phenomenon.

Rifampin acts by inhibiting nucleic acid synthesis in susceptible organisms *via* the inhibition of RNA polymerase. It is active against a number of Gram-positive and Gram-negative bacteria, in addition to being used in tuberculosis therapy. Because of its effective bactericidal activity against tuberculosis, it should not be used in common infections when other drugs would suffice. It should not be used alone in the treatment of tuberculosis because of rapid development of resistance by the organism.

Adverse effects include infrequent gastrointestinal symptoms, rashes, reversible leukopenia, and rare—but potentially lethal—liver dysfunction.

Headache, drowsiness, dizziness, and other central nervous system signs and symptoms may also occur. Intermittent high-dose therapy may cause a flu-like syndrome.

Ethambutol has an unknown bacteriostatic mechanism of action in tuberculosis. It should be given with one or more other drugs simultaneously because of the potential for resistance development by the organism. It is readily absorbed by the gut and rapidly excreted in the urine. Adverse effects include the rare development of either anaphylaxis or peripheral neuritis. A potential major toxic effect is a retrobulbar neuritis, which is dose related, usually reversible, and causes decreased visual acuity and decreased ability to see the color green.

Streptomycin, formerly the most important drug in the treatment of tuberculosis, is still useful in this condition and also in other circumstances, as it is an aminoglycoside. It can be useful in special situations such as plague and tularemia. Streptomycin causes a misreading of mRNA in susceptible bacteria, in turn causing the formation of nonfunctional proteins. It is used by injection, has a good distribution in extracellular fluids, and is readily excreted in the urine. Because resistance to streptomycin can occur rapidly, it is used in short-term special situations or in long-term therapy of tuberculosis with a combination of drugs.

The most prominent toxic effect of streptomycin is eighth nerve toxicity, causing both vestibular and auditory damage. The loss of hearing, balance, or both may or may not return in weeks, months, or years. Consequently, a hearing test should be administered prior to the initiation of any long-term streptomycin therapy. This toxicity is positively correlated with (1) age, (2) blood level, and (3) duration of therapy. Streptomycin is less likely to reach high concentrations in the renal cortex and therefore is less nephrotoxic than other aminoglycosides.

Various hypersensitivity reactions such as rashes can be fairly frequent (especially in people who handle streptomycin) but are usually not particularly serious.

The treatment of atypical mycobacterial infection (i.e., not *M. tuberculosis* or *M. leprae*) is a specialized area and careful attention must be paid to susceptibility testing for individual cases. The organisms may be susceptible to antituberculosis drugs but may also be resistant. Other antibiotics may be useful in individual cases.

Therapy for *M. leprae* includes dapsone and other sulfones, rifampin, and **clofazimine**. Recent research has raised hopes for the development of a vaccine for leprosy.

ANTIFUNGAL DRUGS

The antifungal drugs have no effect on bacteria. Generally speaking, these agents also should not be used systemically to treat topical fungal infections; these should be treated topically when possible.

The **polyenes** (e.g., **nystatin, amphotericin B,** and **candicidin**) act directly on fungal cell membranes to cause pore formation, with consequent alteration of permeability.

The **imidazoles** (e.g., **ketoconazole, miconazole,** and **clotrimazole**) act on fungal cell membrane synthesis by inhibiting the synthesis of fungal lipids, especially ergosterol.

Orally used antifungal agents include nystatin (Mycostatin), griseofulvin (Fulvicin, Grifulvin, Grisactin), and ketoconazole (Nizoral). Nystatin is given orally for nonsystemic use (i.e., to treat *Candida albicans* infections in the mouth or gastrointestinal tract) and is not meant to be absorbed. Griseofulvin is given orally, but is used in this fashion to treat dermatophyte infections in the hair and nails. Ketoconazole was the first antifungal agent given orally for the treatment of systemic fungal infections.

Parenterally used antifungal agents include amphotericin B (Fungizone), flucytosine (Ancobon), and miconazole (Monistat), which are all given intravenously for systemic fungal infections.

Nystatin is an important drug for the treatment of nonsystemic *C. albicans* (i.e., monilial) infections. It is poorly absorbed from the skin and mucous membranes. Therefore, it is useful for topical infections of *Candida* in the mouth (thrush), the gastrointestinal tract, and the perineum including the vagina. Besides being rather nontoxic, nonirritating, and eliciting very few local allergic reactions, acquired resistance by *Candida* to nystatin is not particularly a problem.

Griseofulvin is of no value in *Candida* infections but is quite useful in dermatophyte infections with *Trichophyton* and *Microsporum* (e.g., ringworm). Therapy for skin takes weeks; therapy for hair and nails takes months—and it is very expensive. As previously noted, griseofulvin is not effective topically and is used orally. It is well absorbed and has a propensity for concentrating in newly formed keratin. The new keratin is disease-free and explains the protracted therapy period. The drug acts by inhibiting fungal mitosis. Side effects include headaches in 15 percent (which tend to dissipate with time) and the potentiation of the effects of ethanol. Griseofulvin decreases the activity of warfarin-type anticoagulants, and phenobarbital is known to stimulate the metabolism of griseofulvin.

Amphotericin B is a relatively toxic drug used to treat seriously ill patients with systemic fungal infections by intravenous drip in the hospital. Toxic effects include anorexia, chills, fever, electrolyte disturbances, local thrombophlebitis, and potentially anaphylaxis. Greater than 80 percent of those treated will show signs of renal dysfunction. The toxic effects are seen during the course of therapy and are usually reversible. The drug is heat-labile and light-sensitive.

Amphotericin B is particularly useful in systemic therapy of *Aspergillus* species, *Blastomyces dermatitidis, Coccidioides immitis, Histoplasma capsulatum, Mucor* species, *Paracoccidioides brasiliensis,* and (with or without flucytosine) both various *Candida* species and *Cryptococcus neoformans.*

Because these and other systemic fungal infections can be complex and life threatening, they should be treated by those with expertise in both the disease and drug information that goes well beyond the usual pharmacological treatise.

Flucytosine, which is related to the cancer chemotherapy agent 5-fluorouracil, is used to treat systemic fungal infections. The flucytosine is converted to 5-fluorouracil by fungal cells, but not to a significant degree by the host mammalian cells. The 5-fluorouracil inhibits thymidylate synthetase and DNA synthesis. The development of resistant mutant fungal cells can be a problem. Uracil can impede the hematopoietic toxicity of flucytosine, while not interfering with the antifungal activity. In addition to its use with amphotericin B noted earlier, flucytosine is considered by some to be a primary drug choice in chromomycosis.

Among the imidazoles, **clotrimazole** is considered too toxic for systemic use but is useful in various topical preparations for superficial *C. albicans* infections. **Miconazole** is used topically in nystatin-resistant situations and to some degree for intravenous use. Potential adverse effects with intravenous use of miconazole include nausea, vomiting, CNS toxicity, anemia, thrombocytosis, hyponatremia, and anaphylactoid reactions; additional effects may occur from the vehicle used.

Ketoconazole is usually well tolerated orally and has a broad spectrum for a variety of fungi, including systemic mycoses. It is much less toxic than amphotericin B. Daily oral doses over several weeks can control *Candida* in the mouth, vagina, and skin. Gastrointestinal side effects and gynecomastia have been noted, as has the occurrence of liver dysfunction with high doses.

For systemic infections, ketoconazole competes with amphotericin B as a first choice for *Blastomyces dermatitidis* and *Paracoccidioides brasiliensis*. It is a primary choice for *Pseudallescheria boydii* and an alternative for *Candida* species, *Coccidioides immitis*, *Cryptococcus neoformans*, *Histoplasma capsulatum*, and *Sporothrix schenckii*.

Topical preparations for *Candida* include miconazole, clotrimazole, **butoconazole, terconazole,** nystatin, amphotericin B, candicidin, and others. Topical therapy for *Tinea* includes miconazole, clotrimazole, tolnaftate, **naftifine,** undecylenic acid, among others; some *Tinea* preparations are available without prescription.

ANTIVIRAL DRUGS

Effective drug intervention in viral infections (Table 16–6) is extremely difficult, as the viruses are intracellular parasites and their replication requires active participation of the host cell metabolic processes. The therapeutic objective is to have maximal effect on the virus-infected cells with minimal toxic effects on other host cells.

Table 16–6. ANTIVIRAL DRUGS

Generic Name	Trade Name	Primary Uses	Comments
Inhibitor of adsorption/penetration. Headache, dizziness, insomnia, and other CNS side effects commonly seen with oral dosage.			
amantadine	Symmetrel	Influenza A prophylaxis	
Inhibitors of intracellular synthesis. Toxicity varies with drug and route of administration. Ophthalmic and topical irritation and burning sensation may be associated with vehicles used. As expected, these purine and pyrimidine analogs may be toxic to rapidly proliferating tissue (e.g., bone marrow, GI tract, gonads) when used systemically.			
idoxuridine (IDU)	Herplex	Herpes simplex keratitis	Alternate to trifluridine
trifluridine	Viroptic	Herpes simplex keratitis	
vidarabine	Vira-A	Herpes simplex keratitis; Herpes simplex encephalitis, neonatal, adult disseminated	Alternate to trifluridine; alternate to acyclovir
zidovudine (azidothymidine, AZT)	Retrovir	Autoimmune deficiency syndrome	
acyclovir	Zovirax	Herpes simplex genital, encephalitis, neonatal, adult disseminated; varicella-zoster	Hydration and careful infusion can avoid drug precipitation in renal tubules
ribavirin	Virazole	Severe respiratory syncytial virus in infants and young children	
Inhibitor of late protein synthesis. Human pharmacology/toxicology of methisazone largely unknown since smallpox eliminated according to WHO.			
methisazone	Marboran	Smallpox prophylaxis	

Amantadine (Symmetrel) is used prophylactically for Asian A2 influenza, as it can prevent the penetration of cells by this virus. It is administered orally and can be beneficial in institutional environments and high-risk groups. Adverse effects include a variety of central nervous signs and symptoms including nervousness, dizziness, convulsions, and neuropsychiatric disorders.

A positive aspect of amantadine's CNS effects is its occasional use for short-term therapy of parkinsonism, presumably *via* influencing dopaminergic systems.

Both **idoxuridine** (5-iodo-2′-deoxyuridine, IDU) and **trifluridine** (trifluorothymidine, Viroptic) are used topically to treat *Herpes simplex* keratitis. The topical application to the avascular cornea keeps the drug present at a relatively high concentration to effectively inhibit DNA synthesis and viral replication. Although local toxicity and allergic contact dermatitis can occur, nontreatment can result in possible blindness.

Vidarabine (adenine arabinoside, Vira-A) is the least toxic of the purine/pyrimidine analogs and is therefore used parenterally for the treatment of systemic herpes virus infections, including encephalitis. It is phosphorylated within the cell and the triphosphate derivative is more potent in its effect on the viral DNA polymerase than on mammalian DNA polymerase.

Acyclovir (acycloguanosine, Zovirax) is available for therapy of genital herpes (type II). It is an acyclic nucleoside related to guanine that is metabolized to its triphosphate by virus-coded thymidine kinase. The triphosphate in turn inhibits viral DNA synthesis. The acyclovir is much more readily phosphorylated in viral-infected cells and the phosphorylated product is much more effective as an inhibitor of viral DNA polymerase than of host DNA polymerase. In the presence of acyclovir, the virus therefore promotes its own destruction. The drug has been considered relatively nontoxic and is useful for limited (i.e., not life-threatening) cutaneous herpes in the immunocompromised and also for first-time genital herpes. More recent uses include keratitis and *Herpes simplex* encephalitis

Zidovudine (azidothymidine, AZT, Retrovir) is available for autoimmune deficiency syndrome (AIDS) and causes headaches, particularly initially, and significant hematopoietic toxicity, which may require transfusions.

Although not an antiviral drug *per se*, pentamidine has been used as an aerosol and intravenously (Pentam 300) to prevent or treat *Pneumocystis carinii* pneumonia in AIDS patients. Trimethoprim-sulfamethoxazole (co-trimoxazole), pyrimethamine-sulfadoxine, or dapsone have also been used.

Interferons are species-specific glycoproteins produced by cells infected with viruses (type I; more recently termed IFN-α from leukocytes and IFN-β from fibroblasts) and from lymphocytes during the immune response (type II or IFN-γ). Cell-released or administered interferons induce a broad-spectrum resistance to viral infection in other cells and also affect other cellular functions. The antiviral effect, which is associated with the synthesis of new cellular mRNA and protein, appears to interfere with viral RNA and protein production rather than cell penetration.

The production of endogenous IFN-α and IFN-β can be induced by microorganisms (and components thereof) and various synthetic compounds; endogenous IFN-γ by sensitized lymphocytes on exposure to specific antigens and by mitogen-exposed lymphocytes. Exogenous human interferons have been produced by human cells in culture and more recently by bacterial recombinant DNA preparations.

The pyrogenic, hematological, CNS, gastrointestinal, and cardiovascular toxic manifestations of synthetic interferon inducers tested to date make them unlikely candidates for systemic antiviral therapy. Until the advent of recombinant DNA technology, the cost of exogenous human interferon from pooled leukocytes or cultures made this approach also unlikely. Studies with the pooled lymphocyte or culture preparations indicate potential usefulness in both topical and systemic viral infections of a chronic or recurrent nature. Interferon's usefulness in acute viral infections may be limited to prophylaxis.

Once perceived as a potential panacea, careful evaluation will determine interferon's eventual role in antiviral therapy as well as other possible medical uses.

ANTIMALARIAL DRUGS

The therapeutic use of antimalarial drugs is dependent on the type of malaria, the potential drug resistance of the organism, and whether the objective is suppression of symptoms or cure of the disease. *Plasmodium falciparum* does not have an exoerythrocytic cycle, whereas *P. vivax*, *P. ovale*, and (possibly) *P. malariae* do have such a tissue cycle.

Quinine is readily absorbed and excreted, has analgesic and antipyretic effects, is only suppressive, and can elicit various CNS manifestations including cinchonism (ringing in the ears, headache, nausea, visual disturbances) and even convulsions in high doses. Although it binds to DNA, interacts with membranes, and inhibits numerous enzymes, the specific mechanism of action of quinine in malaria is still a subject of debate.

Chloroquine, the prototypical 4-aminoquinoline, is markedly more concentrated in erythrocytes containing the malarial parasites. Like quinine and primaquine, it too intercalates between the malarial DNA strands, but other mechanisms are also proposed to explain the inhibition of nucleic acid synthesis and killing of the parasite. Chloroquine-resistant *P. falciparum* appears to be related to a decrease in the transport of drug into the resistant parasite and has been an ever-increasing problem since the mid-1960s. Numerous gastrointestinal, CNS, skin, and hematological signs and symptoms may occur with higher doses in malaria or with its use in certain connective tissue diseases. Suppressive malarial doses are usually not a problem.

Primaquine, as well as aspirin, phenacetin (acetophenetidin), nitrofurantoin, and various other agents, can have adverse effects in individuals with deficient erythrocyte glucose-6-phosphate dehydrogenase (G-6-PD). The enzyme deficiency is a sex-linked dominant disease prevalent in dark-skinned people and those of Mediterranean descent. The enzyme may be unable to regenerate enough NADPH to maintain the reduced glutathione level in erythrocytes when such drugs or metabolites are present. The consequence may be hemolytic anemia, methemoglobinemia, or both.

Although primaquine (and other 8-aminoquinolines) can intercalate between malarial DNA strands, it does not inhibit parasite nucleic acid synthesis as the 4-aminoquinolines do. The fact that primaquine metabolites are involved in its G-6-PD action raises questions on *in vitro* antimalarial mechanism studies where metabolites are not present. The true antimalarial mechanism is therefore still not clear.

More recent therapies for **chloroquine**-resistant *P. falciparum* are the combination of **sulfadoxine plus pyrimethamine** sold as Fansidar and the drug **mefloquine**. The combination of sulfadoxine plus pyrimethamine is reminiscent of that in co-trimoxazole. Cases of the Stevens-Johnson syndrome have been reported in patients using Fansidar.

AMEBICIDAL DRUGS

The major infective agent for amebiasis is *Entamoeba histolytica*. It infects as the nonmotile cyst, whereas the motile trophozoite form causes the tissue damage. The trophozoite form is the form on which the amebicide drugs act.

Amebicidal drugs can affect ameba in the gut (intraintestinal or luminal), ameba that have penetrated into body tissues (extraintestinal or systemic), or both (mixed). The nature of the disease dictates that when an extraintestinal agent is necessary, an intraintestinal agent should be administered concurrently.

Except for emetine, all of the amebicides are given orally. All may have significant toxicity associated with them.

Intraintestinal amebicides include the iodoquinolines **iodoquinol** (diiodohydroxyquin) and **clioquinol** (iodochlorhydroxyquin). These should not be used if the patient is sensitive to iodine; they are also known to alter thyroid function tests. **Diloxanide furoate** (Furamide), which is not an iodoquinoline, is used to treat asymptomatic patients who pass cysts.

Extraintestinal amebicides include emetine and chloroquine. **Emetine** is a potent emetic alkaloid which is toxic to heart tissue and whose use is generally confined to the hospital environment. **Chloroquine** is an antimalarial that is also occasionally useful in certain dermatological conditions.

Metronidazole (Flagyl) has both extraintestinal and intraintestinal effectiveness. This drug was originally (and is currently) used to treat *Trichomonas vaginalis*. It has now also been found useful in the therapy of *Giardia lamblia* and also certain anaerobic bacterial infections. Because of a high failure rate when used alone in amebiasis, metronidazole is usually used in conjunction with an intraintestinal agent. A variety of reversible toxic effects including nausea and vomiting, neurotoxicity, and leukopenia may occur. Alcohol is contraindicated when taking metronidazole, as a disulfiram-like reaction may occur. Because laboratory data indicate that metronidazole is a potential teratogen/mutagen, the drug should be avoided in pregnant or nursing women unless absolutely necessary.

ANTHELMINTIC DRUGS

As many anthelmintic drugs have significant toxicity, definitive diagnosis should be established before any are used. Many are contraindicated in patients with obstruction or ulcers and in pregnant patients.

The information needs of the individual practitioner are dependent on the nature of the practice and its geographical locale. The following constitutes only a brief comment on some of the more prominent anthelmintic drugs. A number of them interfere with the worm's energy metabolism or neuromuscular junction.

Pyrantel pamoate (Antiminth) is effective therapy for *Ascaris* (roundworm) and pinworm infestations. It causes neuromuscular paralysis in the worm, with the worm then being expelled from the intestine. A variety of infrequent and reversible gastrointestinal and CNS symptoms may occur.

Mebendazole (Vermox), which inhibits glucose uptake in worms, has a rather wide spectrum of effectiveness against pinworm, roundworm, hookworm, and *Trichuris* (whipworm). It is relatively nontoxic but is teratogenic in rats.

Thiabendazole (Mintezol), which inhibits fumarate reductase and impairs energy production in *Strongyloides,* is useful in this and some other infestations. Other than its use in treating *Strongyloides* and cutaneous larva migrans infestations, its variegated toxic manifestations make it a secondary drug choice.

Niclosamide (Niclocide) is effective in a variety of tapeworm infestations. Gastrointestinal, central nervous system, and allergic phenomena may be associated with its use.

Metrifonate (Bilarcil) is effective in *Schistosoma haematobium;* **oxamniquine** (Vansil) in *S. mansoni;* and **praziquantel** (Biltricide) is effective in all three forms of schistosomiasis, including *S. japonicum.* The adverse effects, contraindications, and cautions for these and other anthelmintics should be reviewed prior to use.

The reader is referred to standard works in pharmacology and infectious disease, as well as the annual summaries of infectious disease therapy in the *Medical Letter,*[31, 32] for current therapy of such conditions as trypanosomiasis, kala azar, and so forth.

USE AND MISUSE OF ANTIMICROBIAL DRUGS

Although the remainder of this chapter relates to antibiotics, the general principles may often be applicable to the therapy of other infectious diseases.

Combinations

When antibiotics are combined, one of three outcomes may ensue: (1) indifference, (2) synergism, or (3) antagonism. Indifference, or addition, occurs when each drug acts on the bacterial population with no interactive effect between drugs. Synergism implies an effect greater than addition, but is often difficult to prove. Some experts believe that what is termed synergism may often be due to the prevention of resistance development.[33] Antagonism is unfortunately not always thought of and can have a catastrophic outcome for the patient.

The sequential inhibition of the folic acid pathway by sulfamethoxazole and trimethoprim is an often-quoted example of synergism. An even more convincing example of synergism is the simultaneous use of a penicillin and an aminoglycoside; in which the penicillin can inhibit cell wall synthesis in certain streptococci, thereby allowing cellular penetration of the aminoglycoside, with an effective outcome that would not occur if either drug were used alone.

A classic example of antagonism was the tragic use of chlortetracycline and penicillin in treatment of patients with newborn pneumococcal meningitis. Because penicillins are most effective against multiplying bacteria, the inhibition of protein synthesis by the tetracycline impaired the effectiveness of the penicillin.

It is usually impossible to know whether a pair of antibiotics acting in combination will be either antagonistic or synergistic without reference to testing the particular strain of bacteria in the specific case. Likewise, the presence of *in vitro* synergism or antagonism does not necessarily mean that *in vivo* synergism or antagonism will be that prominent. Unpredictability of outcome and additional drug hazard to the patient has led to the withdrawal from the market of many fixed-dose antibiotic combinations in the past. The practitioner can still prescribe combinations but must do it actively and therefore with more responsibility and awareness of the combination.

Simultaneous administration of more than one antimicrobial agent has been suggested in some situations: (1) in treatment of certain mixed infections, (2) for reduction of the incidence of toxic drug reactions (by giving smaller doses of two compounds), (3) in treatment of superficially located bacteria (invariably mixed infections), (4) to delay the rate of emergence of bacterial resistance (e.g., combination therapy in tuberculosis), (5) to enhance the therapeutic activity of the particular drugs against a given organism, and (6) occasionally in treatment of severe, life-threatening infections when the etiology has not been adequately established.

Prophylaxis

When antimicrobial prophylaxis is used for the prevention of infection by a specific organism, it is usually effective.[34, 35] When prophylaxis is used for the generalized prevention of all infections, it is almost always a failure.[34, 35] In spite of this knowledge, it has been estimated that 30 to 50 percent of antibiotics prescribed in the United States are used for prevention.[35]

In surgical procedures, it is reasonable to use prophylaxis in (1) dirty or contaminated cases (less than 10 percent of all operations) or (2) prosthetic implantations. The justification of the latter is that the sequelae could be devastating if an infection occurred.

Surgical wound infections occur if there is a critical number of bacteria in the wound at the time of closure. Antimicrobial activity must therefore be present at the time of incision, during the procedure, and at closure. Antimicrobial therapy anticipated to be effective against the most expected contaminants should therefore be administered in amounts adequate to provide an effective blood level at the time of surgery and should not be continued after the first day or so. Unless one is treating an established infection, continuing therapy is only promoting the possibility of resistance development. This knowledge does not justify the 7-day median noted in one study.[36]

Misuse

Antibiotics have been called "drugs of fear"[37] because they are often misused in well-intentioned reaction to a patient's deteriorating condition from unknown causes.

Antibiotics should not be used to treat viral infections such as measles, chickenpox, mumps, and 90 percent of upper respiratory infections. They should likewise not be used to treat fever of unknown origin, which can arise from hepatitis, cancer, and so on.

Excess dosage should be avoided, but enough antibiotic should be used for a long enough period of time to avoid recurrent infection or resistance development. This requires patient cooperation and compliance.

When applicable, surgical drainage to remove pus, necrotic tissue, foreign bodies, stones, and so on, is necessary to get effective antibiotic therapy.

In addition to general guidelines such as Table 16–7, effective use of the bacteriology laboratory is imperative for proper drug selection. Except in extremely serious or life-threatening infections when empiric therapy must be initiated immediately, one should know the organism and its drug sensitivity. In spite of this, one source estimates that half of the antibiotics used in United States hospitalized patients are given without any data from the bacteriology laboratory.[38]

The bacteriology laboratory will report antibiotics to which the pathogen is sensitive and sensitivity to a given antibiotic in terms of its minimum inhibitory concentration (MIC), which is the minimum drug concentration necessary to inhibit growth of the specific organism under the given laboratory conditions. This information, combined with distribution and pharmacokinetic data, can be useful in planning dosage amount and dosage interval for the spe-

Table 16–7. USEFUL ANTIMICROBIAL SPECTRA
(SIMPLIFIED)

Gram-Positive Cocci
  penicillins
  cephalosporin (second choice)
  erythromycin
  vancomycin
  bacitracin (topical)
Gram-Negative Cocci
  penicillins
  ceftriaxone (β-lactamase resistant gonococcus)
Gram-Negative Bacilli
  aminoglycosides (coliforms; + antipseudomonal penicillin for *Pseudomonas*)
  penicillins (coliforms and ampicillin for *Haemophilus*)
  co-trimoxazole (*Shigella* + uncomplicated urinary tract)
  third-generation cephalosporin
  chloramphenicol (*Salmonella* and *Haemophilus*)
  erythromycin (*Legionella*)
  tetracyclines (*Brucella, Vibrio sp.*, and so forth)
  polymyxins (topical)
Anaerobes
  penicillin (*Bacteroides fragilis* often resistant)
  clindamycin (non-CNS *Bacteroides*)
  chloramphenicol (CNS)
  (also consider cefoxitin or metronidazole)
Spirochetes
  penicillin
Mycoplasma, Chlamydia, Rickettsia
  tetracycline
Tuberculosis
  isoniazid
  rifampin
  ethambutol
  streptomycin
Fungi
  amphotericin B
  ketoconazole
  flucytosine
  griseofulvin
  nystatin (topical)

cific anatomical site(s) of infection. For some infections, a sustained plasma level versus intermittent bolus peaks and troughs is still subject to debate as to the best therapeutic approach.

It was noted earlier that the most narrow-spectrum antibiotic that is effective for the individual case should be used. This maximizes therapeutic effectiveness while minimizing potential adverse effects on the patient and resistance development. The history of antimicrobial therapy is rampant with examples of drugs losing their usefulness due to overuse and the consequent development of resistance by organisms.

In this regard, it should be remembered that antibiotic therapy is different from the use of other pharmacological agents in that the use of an antibiotic influences resistance development and therefore affects not only the treatment of that patient but also the future treatment of all people living in the world and all of their progeny ever to come into being in the future. Additionally, patients do not make the decisions on antibiotic usage, practitioners do—and the first rule of health professionals is "Primum non nocere (First do no harm)."

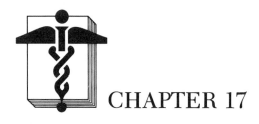

CHAPTER 17

Antitumor and Immunomodulatory Agents

THOMAS K. SHIRES, Ph.D.

ANTITUMOR AGENTS

The chemotherapeutic approach to neoplastic disease employs the strategy of **selective toxicity**. Successful drugs destroy target tissue, sparing the non-neoplastic tissue. Four useful principles illustrate the task of the anticancer drug. First, patient survival is inversely correlated with the size of the tumor burden, expressed as the total number of neoplastic cells in the host. Second, at a given dose, the killing of tumor cells by cancer chemotherapeutic drugs is fractional (the **"log kill" hypothesis**). The most effective agents in a single dose can kill in the vicinity of 99.99 percent of the body burden of tumor cells. A neoplastic mass weighing 1 kg and containing 10^{12} cells, thus, could be chemotherapeutically reduced to 10 mg containing 10^8 tumor cells, a "log kill" of 4. Third, tumor cell populations are heterogeneous. Some subpopulations of tumor cells will be more sensitive to a particular agent than others. Fourth, small numbers of tumor cells survive even the most effective available therapy. These cells are capable of clonal multiplication and may regenerate the neoplastic tissue mass. Thus, unlike antibacterial chemotherapy where restraint of a target organism's growth may be sufficient for a clinical cure, cancer chemotherapy ideally must aim at complete eradication of all the cells in its target tissue.

Also, unlike antibacterial drugs, anticancer agents must distinguish among target cell populations that are biologically part of the host, rather than foreign organisms. Selective **toxicity** must be based on some difference between neoplastic and non-neoplastic cells. In the absence of any single invariant feature distinguishing the cancer cell, relative differences have been exploited. From the perspective of chemotherapy, the most significant of these has been the greater **proliferative activity** of tumor cells compared with non-neoplastic cells in same tissue.

Cell proliferation results in the doubling of the amount of DNA in the cell ("S-phase") and the division of that DNA into daughter cells by mitosis ("M-phase"). In a proliferative cell population, the doubling and redoubling of cells results in a logarithmic increase in population. Three general kinetic parameters influence the net rate of proliferation: (1) the duration of the cell cycle, (2) the proportion of cells actually engaged in a proliferative cycle in a given tissue (the so-called growth fraction), and (3) the rate of cell death. **Proliferative cycles** may last from less than 24 hours to days or even weeks. Most of the variation occurs in the length of the phase dividing "M" from "S," the G-l phase. In non-neoplastic tissues, cells seem to require signals from external growth factors such as the leukotrienes and lymphokines of lymphocyte populations, epidermal growth factor, and nerve growth factors. Even highly proliferative populations such as those in the bone marrow, the basal cell layer of stratified squamous epithelium, and the neck cell population of intestinal glands appear subject to external regulation. Tumor cells are relatively less dependent on **proliferation controls**. Studies with tumor cell populations show that (1) cells in neoplastic tissue are highly desynchronized with respect to their position in the cell cycle, (2) population expansion is exponential, but with a growth constant that is simultaneously exponentially slowing (so-called Gompertzian growth), and (3) population expansion is generally associated with a decline in the growth fraction of that population, perhaps partially explaining the Gompertzian phenomenon. Virtually all clinically useful antitumor drugs are preferentially cytolytic for cells in the growth cycle ("**cycle dependent**"), and some act only on cells going through a specific phase of the growth cycle ("**phase specific**"). In general, rapidly growing tumors tend to be sensitive to chemotherapy; slowly growing tumors less so.

Several practical considerations influence the clinical use of chemotherapeutic agents. First, individual agents are active against specific types of tumors but not neoplastic tissue in general. The distribution of administered drug or the particular metabolic features of specific tumors may partly explain this, but overall it is not always clear why some drugs act against certain tumors in a clinically significant way and not against others. Second, undesirable **side effects** of chemotherapeutic agents (**toxicity**) occur with all agents given at useful dosages. Particular side effects tend to be dose-dependent and place a cap on the highest dose that may be administered. A frequent dose-limiting **toxicity** with many drugs is inhibition of the cytopoietic functions of the bone marrow that may result in leukopenia, thrombocytopenia, or anemia. Third, the development of tumor resistance to particular chemotherapeutic agents is a common limitation of the effectiveness of agents. The failure of particular drugs to maintain remissions can arise not only from drug-insensitive subpopulations of tumor cells but also from adaptive responses to multiple drug doses by formerly sensitive cells. These responses include decreased drug uptake by tumor cells, increased levels of enzymes that catabolyze the drug, and increased levels of drug target molecules. There is evidence that resistance is a *de novo* response that sometimes involves nonmutational changes in the tumor cell genome. One such documented change is an increase in resistant cells in the number of gene copies (gene amplification) for drug target molecules.

In the chemotherapy of cancer, tumor type (and its stage and grade) and the patient's condition (status of bone marrow or the immune system, the excretory capacities of the liver and kidney, and so forth) determine (1) whether or not to employ drug therapy, (2) the choice of drugs, if indicated, and (3) the therapeutic regimen. Certain agents achieve far better results than do other agents with a particular tumor type. This benefit can be enhanced by linkage of chemotherapy with other treatment modalities (surgery and/or radiation), with concurrent use of other antitumor drugs, and with dosage protocols that optimize drug effect (while minimizing unwanted side effects). Oncology has developed a great variety of therapeutic approaches for treatment of different types of tumors. For any one kind of neoplasia, evaluations of likely outcome for a given therapeutic approach allow ranking of different approaches to particular clinical settings. For a given situation, the best available therapy may be categorizable as able to produce (1) a cure (the achievement of a neoplasia-free state), (2) the prolongation of a cancer patient's life (by temporary induction of remission and its maintenance), or (3) palliation of the symptoms of terminal disease. The best treatment for some tumors may involve surgery and/or radiation and not drugs. In some situations, drug therapy may be a useful adjuvant following surgery and/or radiation. Tumors that are dispersed such as leukemias, lymphomas, and metastatic stages of solid tumors are treated principally with drugs or drug combinations. Solid tumors, such as carcinomas or sarcomas, are more likely to be reduced in bulk first by surgery or radiation, followed by chemotherapy to control remnants of neoplastic tissue. This chapter will not deal with specific treatments of particular tumor types. Table 17–1 lists the role different agents play in current antineoplastic chemotherapy.

Alkylating Agents

Nitrogen Mustard Derivatives

Clinically useful antitumor agents whose mechanism involves intracellular **alkylation** (Fig. 17–1) include the **nitrogen mustards,** the methane sulfonate derivative **busulfan,** the **nitrosoureas,** and a heterogeneous group of **cisplatin, dacarbazine,** and **procarbazine** (Fig. 17–2). The **mustards** are all derivatives of bis(chloroethyl)-amine. In water, the chloroethyl arms of each undergo spontaneous internal nucleophilic displacement (see Fig. 17–2). Displacements result in the loss of a chlorine, cyclization of the alkyl group whose α-carbon becomes an electrophilic reactor, and conversion of the tertiary amine into a quaternary amine. Both chloroethyl groups come to contain electrophilic centers, making each molecule a bifunctional alkylating agent with two electrophilic sites capable of cross-linking nucleophilic centers on macromolecules. Intracellular **nucleophiles** with which these activated drug electrophiles react are abundant in the cell. A particularly important nucleophile is the N^7 position of guanine in DNA or RNA. The methane sulfonate ester, **busulfan,** also undergoes spontaneous nucleophilic displacement and acts as

Table 17-1. ANTINEOPLASTIC AGENTS

	Administration Route	Major Route of Excretion/ Elimination	CNS Penetration	Cycle Specificity*	Toxicity†	Clinical Uses
I. Alkylating Agents						
A. Nitrogen Mustards						
1. Mechlorethamine (Nitrogen mustard, Mustargen)	iv	None (little leaves body)	Poor	NS	N, v, leukopenia, thrombocytopenia, vesicant, amyloidosis	Palliative in treatment of Hodgkin's (stages III, IV), lymphosarcoma, chronic myelocytic leukemia, chronic lymphocytic leukemia
2. Chlorambucil (Leukeran)	po	Renal	Poor	NS	N, v, leukopenia, thrombocytopenia, anemia	Palliative in treatment of chronic lymphocytic leukemia, malignant lymphomas, including Hodgkin's disease, lymphosarcoma
3. Melphalan (Alkeran, L-PAM, L-phenylalanine mustard, L-sarcolysine)	po	Renal	Poor	NS	N, v, leukopenia, thrombocytopenia, anemia	Palliative for multiple myeloma and nonresectable adenoma of ovary
4. Cyclophosphamide (Cytoxan, Endoxan)	iv/po	Renal	Poor	NS	N, v, stomatitis, leukopenia, thrombocytopenia, anemia, alopecia, hyperpigmentation, cystitis	Chronic myelogenous leukemias (nonblastic phases)
B. Busulfan (Myleran)	po	Renal	Poor	NS	Leukopenia (delayed 2 weeks), thrombocytopenia, anemia, alveolitis, gynecomastia, amenorrhea, Addison's disease-like syndrome	Alone or in combination with other agents for malignant lymphomas; multiple myeloma; neuroblastoma; adenoma of ovary; retinoblastoma; breast adenocarci-

412

						noma; leukemias: chronic lymphocytic and granulocytic leukemia; acute myelogenous, monocytic, and lymphoblastic
C. Nitrosoureas						
1. Carmustine (BCNU, BiCNU)	iv	Renal	Good	NS	N, v, hepatotoxicity, leukopenia (delayed 6 weeks)	In combination with other agents for glioblastoma, medulloblastoma, astrocytoma, ependymoma, brainstem glioma, multiple myeloma, Hodgkin's and non-Hodgkin's lymphomas; palliative by itself for all of these
2. Lomustine (CCNU, CeeNU)	po	Renal	Good	NS	N, v, leukopenia (delayed 6 weeks), anemia, thrombocytopenia, alopecia	In established combination therapy for brain tumors (same as carmustine), Hodgkin's lymphomas
3. Semustine (methyl CCNU)	po	Renal	Good	NS	N, v, leukopenia (delayed 6 weeks), anemia, thrombocytopenia, alopecia	Same as carmustine, but palliative only
4. Streptozotocin (Zanosar)	iv	Renal	Poor	NS	N, v, hepatotoxicity, leukopenia, anemia, nephrotoxicity (tubular necrosis, azotemia) hypoglycemia	Islet cell carcinoma
D. Cisplatin (Platinol, Platinum, CDDP [cis-diammine dichloroplatinum II])	iv	Renal	Poor	NS	N, v, leukopenia, thrombocytopenia, anemia, nephrotoxicity (acute tubular necrosis), ototoxicity	Palliative in established combinations for metastatic testicular tumors, metastatic ovarian tumors, transitional cell carcinoma
E. Dacarbazine (Imidazole, Carboximide, DTIC, DIC)	iv/po	Renal	Poor	NS	N, v, hepatotoxicity, leukopenia, anemia, thrombocytopenia, alopecia, flulike syndrome	Indicated for metastatic malignant melanoma, and in combination with other agents as second-line ther-

Table 17–1. (*Continued*)

	Administration Route	Major Route of Excretion/ Elimination	CNS Penetration	Cycle Specificity*	Toxicity†	Clinical Uses
F. Procarbazine (Matulane)	iv/po	Renal	NS		N, v. stomatitis, leukopenia, anemia, thrombocyto-penia, monoamine oxidase inhibitor, disulfiram-like effect, convulsions, peripheral neuropathy	apy for Hodgkin's disease Palliative management of generalized Hodgkin's disease
II. Antimetabolites						
A. Pyrimidine Antimetabolites						
1. 5-Fluorouracil (5-FU, Adrucil, Efudex, Fluoroplex)	iv	Lungs/renal	Poor	S	N, v, stomatitis, diarrhea, leukopenia (delayed 2 weeks), anemia, thrombocytopenia, alopecia, hyperpigmentation, cerebellar, ataxia	Palliative only, for advanced carcinomas of colon, rectum, breast, pancreas, considered incurable by surgery/other means
2. Cytosine arabinoside (ara-c, cytarabin, Cytosar)	iv/sc	Renal	Fair	S	N, v, stomatitis, leukopenia, anemia, thrombocytopenia, hepatotoxicity	Established in combination therapy for acute myelocytic and lymphocytic leukemia, non-Hodgkin's lymphoma in children
3. 5-Azacytidine	iv	None	Poor	G₁-S	N, v, leukopenia, anemia, thrombocytopenia fever (4 hours after admin), hypotension	Acute granulocytic leukemia

	Route	Excretion			Toxicity	Indications
B. Purine Antimetabolites						
1. 6-Mercaptopurine (6-MP, Purinethol)	po	Renal	Poor	S	N, v, stomatitis, leukopenia, anemia, thrombocytopenia, cholestatic jaundice	Acute lymphocytic, lymphoblastic and myelogenous leukemias, chronic myelogenous leukemia—remission induction and maintenance
2. Thioguanine (6-TG)	po	Renal	Poor	S	N, v, leukopenia, thrombocytopenia, anemia	Acute nonlymphocytic leukemia, in young patients—remission induction and maintenance
C. Folate Antagonist						
1. Methotrexate (MTX)	iv/po/it	Renal	Fair	S	Stomatitis, diarrhea, leukopenia, anemia, thrombocytopenia, renal necrosis, alopecia, hepatotoxicity	Indicated for choriocarcinoma, chorioadenoma destruens, and hydatidiform mole; used in combination for epidermoid cancers of head and neck, squamous and small cell lung cancer, breast cancer, stages III and IV lymphosarcomas; palliative for acute lymphocytic and lymphoblastic leukemias
III. Antineoplastic Alkaloids						
A. Vinca Alkaloids						
1. Vincristine (Oncovin)	iv	Bile	Poor	M	N, v, stomatitis, diarrhea, alopecia, neuropathy (paresthesias)	Acute leukemias, Hodgkin's disease, lymphosarcoma, reticulum cell sarcoma, rhabdo-

415

Table 17–1. (Continued)

	Administration Route	Major Route of Excretion/ Elimination	CNS Penetration	Cycle Specificity*	Toxicity†	Clinical Uses
						myosarcoma, neuroblastoma, Wilms' tumor (in combination with other agents)
2. Vinblastine (Velban)	iv	Bile	Poor	M	Leukopenia (unusual), alopecia, neuropathy (paresthesias)	Palliative for generalized Hodgkin's disease (stages III and IV), lymphocytic and histiocytic lymphomas, cancer of testis, mycosis fungoides (advanced)
B. Podophyllotoxins						
1. Etoposide (VePesid, VM-16)	iv/po	Renal	Poor	S/G_2	N, v, leukopenia, thrombocytopenia, anemia, alopecia, bronchospasm, flushing hypersensitivity	Testicular tumors refractory to prior chemotherapy, surgery, or radiation; in combination with other drugs
2. Teniposide (VM-26)	iv/ia	Renal	Fair	S/G_2	N, v, leukopenia, bronchospasm, flushing hypersensitivity	Primary CNS tumors and metastases, small cell tumors or lung
IV. *Antineoplastic Antibiotics*						
A. Intercalating Agents						
1. Dactinomycin (Actinomycin D, Cosmegen)	iv	Renal	Poor	NS	N, v, diarrhea, stomatitis, leukopenia, hyperpigmentation, alopecia, erythematous rashes	In combination with other agents for Wilms' tumor, rhabdomyosarcoma, and cancer of testis and uterus

416

2. Doxorubicin (Adriamycin)	iv	Bile	Poor	NS	N, v, diarrhea, stomatitis, leukopenia, anemia, thrombocytopenia, congestive heart failure, alopecia	Acute lymphoblastic and myeloblastic leukemias; Wilms' tumor; neuroblastoma; soft tissue and bone sarcomas; cancer of breast, bladder, ovary, and thyroid; lymphomas; bronchogenic adenoma of lung
3. Daunorubicin (Daunomycin Cerubidine)	iv	Bile	Poor	NS	N, v, stomatitis, leukopenia, anemia, thrombocytopenia, congestive heart failure, alopecia	Alone or more usually in combination for acute myelogenous and monocytic leukemias
B. DNA Scission and Intercalating Agent						
1. Bleomycin (Blenoxane)	iv/im	Renal	Poor	S, G_2	N, v, stomatitis, diarrhea, alopecia, hypotension, hyperpyrexia, pulmonary fibrosis, hyperpigmentation	Palliative for squamous cell cancer of head and neck; testicular carcinomas; lymphomas: Hodgkin's, reticulum cell, and lymphosarcoma
C. Nonintercalating Agents						
1. Mitomycin (Mutamycin, Mitomycin C, Mutamycin)	iv	Renal	Poor	NS	N, v, diarrhea, stomatitis, leukopenia, anemia, thrombocytopenia, alopecia	In combination with other agents for adenocarcinomas of stomach and pancreas
2. Mithramycin (Mithracin, Plicamycin)	iv	Renal	Fair	NS	N, v, hepatotoxicity, leukopenia, anemia, thrombocytopenia, nephrotoxicity, epistaxis, and spontaneous bleeding	Adjuvant to surgery/radiation for testicular tumors

Table 17–1. (Continued)

	Administration Route	Major Route of Excretion/ Elimination	CNS Penetration	Cycle Specificy*	Toxicity†	Clinical Uses
V. Antitumor Enzymes						
A. L-asparaginase (Elspar)	iv	None	Poor	NS	Pancreatitis, hypofibrinogenemia, hepatotoxicity, allergic reactions	In combination with other agents for acute lymphocytic leukemia
VI. Antitumor Hormonal Agents						
A. Androgens						
1. Methyldihydrotestosterone (Dromostanolone, Drolban)	im	Renal	None	NS	Hypercalcemia, edema in extremities, virilization, acne	Avanced and disseminated breast cancer in postmenopausal women or premenopausal women in whom ovarian function has been terminated—palliative only
2. Nandrolone phenpropionate (Durabolin)	im	Renal	None	NS	Hypercalcemia, edema, virilization, acne	Postmenopausal breast cancer; palliative only
3. Testolactone (Teslac)	po	Renal	None	NS	Hypercalcemia, edema, increased blood pressure, glossitis, maculopapular erythema, acne	Postmenopausal mammary carcinoma; palliative only
4. Testosterone cypionate (Depo-Testosterone)	im	Renal	None	NS	Hypercalcemia, virilization, edema, with/ without congestive heart failure, acne	Advanced postmenopausal mammary carcinoma; palliative only
B. Estrogens						
1. Diethylstilbestrol (Stilphostrol, DES)	po/iv	Bile/renal	Fair	NS	*In women:* hypercalcemia, hypertension, gallbladder disease, uterine bleeding, edema,	Advanced prostatic carcinoma, advanced inoperable breast cancer in postmenopausal

Agent	Route	Excretion			Toxicity	Uses
					thromboembolic disease. *In men:* gynecomastia, thrombo-embolic disease, edema	women; palliative only
2. 17-Ethinylestradiol (Norinyl, Demulen, Norlestrin, Modicon, Brevicon, Ortho-Novum)	po/iv	Bile/renal	Fair	NS	Thromboembolic disorders, hypercalcemia, hypertension, bleeding irregularities	Palliative for breast cancer
3. Mestranol (Enovid, Ovulen)	po/iv	Bile/renal	Fair	NS		Palliative for breast cancer
C. Estrogen Antagonists						
1. Tamoxifen (Nolvadex)	po	Bile/feces	NA	NS	N, v, hypercalcemia, transient thrombocytopenia, hot flashes	Palliative for advanced breast adenocarcinoma in postmenopausal women
D. Progestins						
1. Medroxyprogesterone (Depo-Provera, Provera)	po/im	Renal	Fair	NS	Hypertension	Adjunctive or palliative for renal carcinoma and metastatic endometrial carcinoma
2. Megestrol Acetate (Megace)	po	Renal	Fair	NS	Hypertension	Adjunctive or palliative for renal carcinoma and metastatic endometrial carcinoma
3. Hydroxyprogesterone Caproate (Delalutin)	im	Renal	Fair	NS	Hypertension	Adjunctive or palliative for renal carcinoma and metastatic endometrial carcinoma
E. Glucocorticoids						
1. Prednisone	po		Fair	NS	Fluid retention, hypertension	In combination with other agents for treatment
F. GnRH Agonists						
1. Leuprolide	sq	None	?	NS	Hot flashes	Prostatic cancer

*NS = Not cycle specific. †n = Nausea; v = vomiting.

419

Mustard Derivative

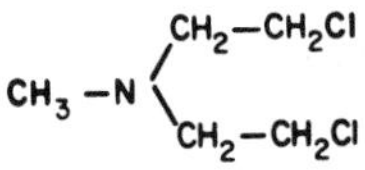

Mechlorethamine
(Nitrogen Mustard)

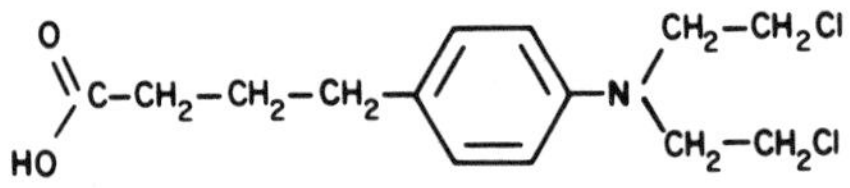

Chlorambucil Leukeran

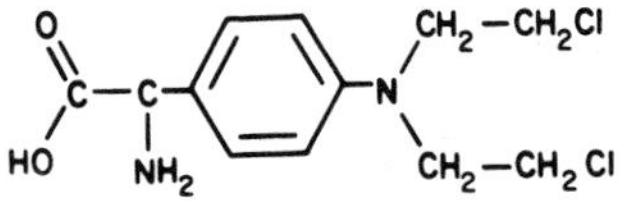

Melphalen
(phenylalanine mustard)

Methane Sulfonate

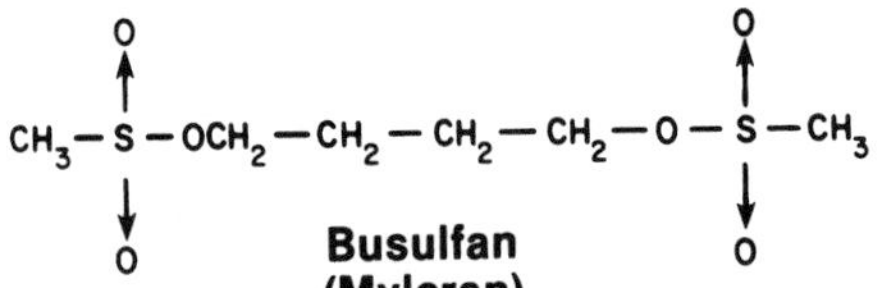

Busulfan
(Myleran)

Nitrosoureas

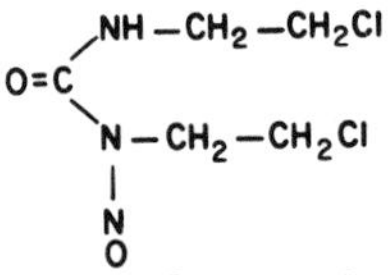

Carmustine
(BCNU, bischlorethyl-nitrosourea)

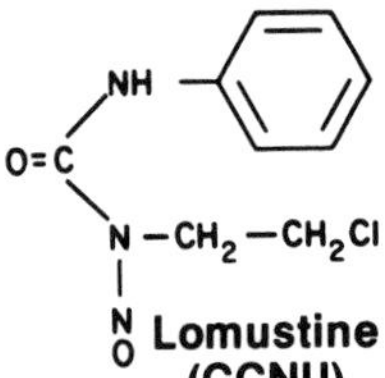

Lomustine
(CCNU)

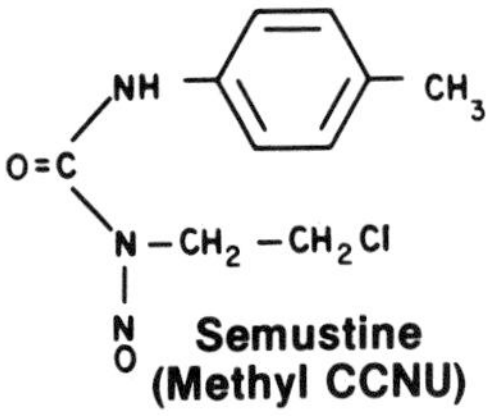

Semustine
(Methyl CCNU)

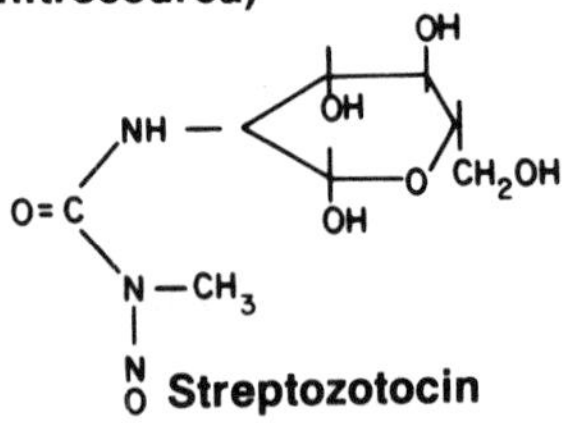

Streptozotocin

Figure 17–1. Alkylating agents.

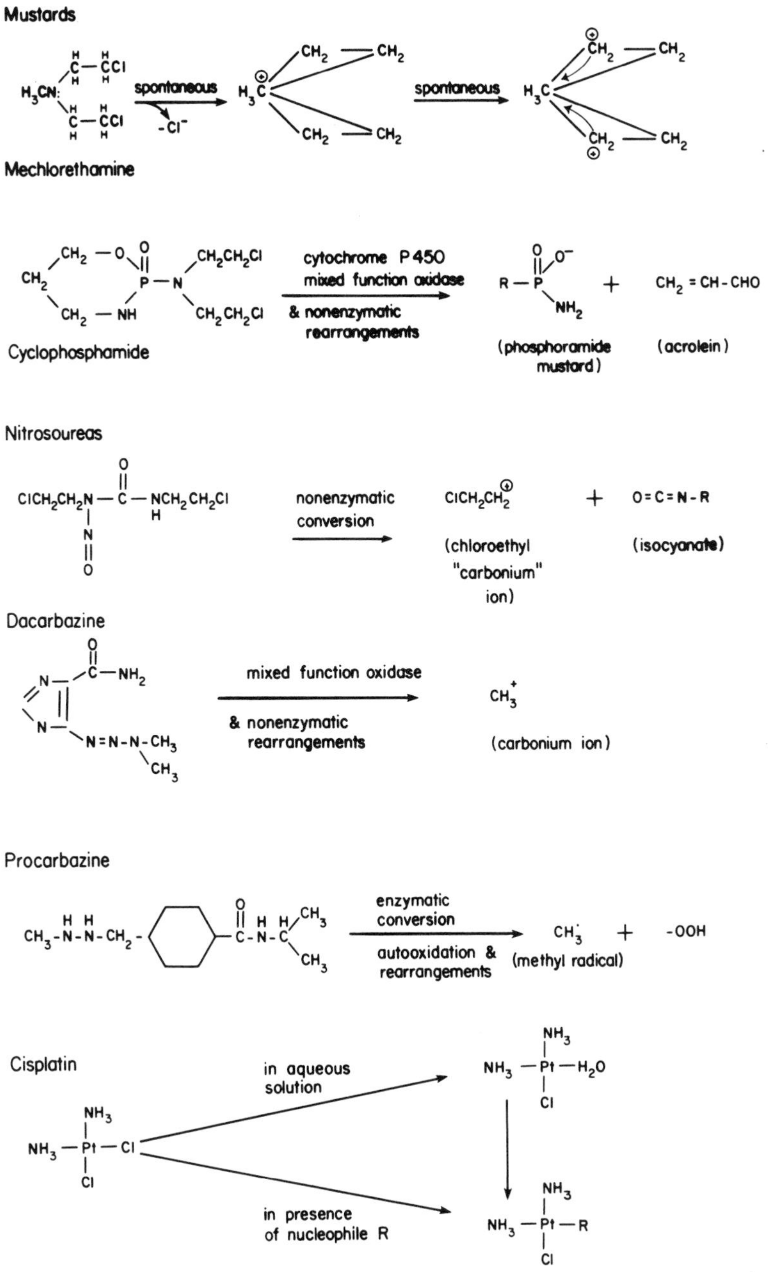

Figure 17–2. Formation of reactive forms of alkylating agents.

a bifunctional alkylator. **Cyclophosphamide** differs from other **mustards** in its requirement for enzymatic activation (see Fig. 17–2). **Cyclophosphamide** seems to increase its own rate of metabolism as evidenced by the decline in the plasma $t_{1/2}$ after third and fourth doses compared with that with the first.

Alkylation of nucleic acids by **cross-linking agents** causes loss of their template function. DNA and RNA polymerase activities on the damaged templates are inhibited. The addition of alkylators at N^7 or O^6 positions of guanine bases causes their abnormal base-pairing. DNA repair systems are stimulated in surviving cells and will replace the alkylated bases but with a risk (albeit a low one) of inappropriate base replacement and possible resultant mutation. **Alkylation of nucleophiles on proteins** probably also occurs. When the protein is an enzyme, loss of enzymatic activity may result.

The speed of spontaneous activation of **mechlorethamine** is so rapid the drug must be administered intravenously. Little parenterally administered mechlorethamine is excreted unchanged. Drug adducts (complexes of drug and various nucleophile-bearing chemical structures) are excreted, sometimes long after drug administration. Mustards like **melphalan** and **chlorambucil** activate at a much slower rate than **mechlorethamine** and, therefore, may be successfully administered orally. They have longer serum half-lives, and small portions of administered drug may be recovered unbound and unchanged in urine. **Cyclophosphamide,** because of its complex and tissue-dependent activation, has the most prolonged residence in serum of all the mustard group. As a group, the **alkylating mustards** fail to cross into the cerebrospinal fluid. Intrathecal **cyclophosphamide** has little antitumor activity because of the need for its access to the liver.

Unwanted side effects of **mustard therapy** usually include depression of bone marrow functions. Granulocytopenia is the dose-limiting toxicity for most of these compounds. Anemia and thrombocytopenia may also be seen. Nausea, vomiting, anorexia, and diarrhea, though unpleasant, are self-limiting. **Cyclophosphamide** toxicity is peculiar in a number of respects. Alopecia occurs regularly with the use of cyclophosphamide but not usually with the other mustards. Thrombocytopenia is observed only with very high doses of cyclophosphamide and is frequently absent even in the presence of profound drug-induced leukopenia. Sterile hemorrhagic cystitis occurs in 10 to 20 percent of patients receiving cyclophosphamide, but good patient hydration tends to reduce its severity and incidence. **Immunosuppression** occurs with all the alkylating agents but is reversible. **Carcinogenicity** of the compounds is a long-term outcome of mustard use. Cyclophosphamide is one of only a handful of proven human chemical carcinogens.

Clinically, cyclophosphamide is the most frequently employed alkylating agent. In addition to a variety of solid tumors (e.g., neuroblastoma; adenocarcinomas of ovary, breast, and lung; rhabdomyosarcoma; and Ewing's sarcoma), it is important in treatment of lymphomas (Hodgkin's and non-Hodgkin's types), acute and chronic lymphocytic leukemias, and multiple myeloma.

Mechlorethamine's use against Hodgkin's lymphoma is usually in combination with **vincristine** (Oncovin), **procarbazine,** and **prednisone** (the so-called **MOPP** regimen). Some clinical effect is obtained with carcinomas of the breast, ovary, and lung. **Chlorambucil** is the drug of choice for Waldenström's macroglobulinemia and can be useful in chronic lymphocytic leukemia. **Melphalan** is principally employed for multiple myeloma. Chronic granulocytic leukemia is the main use for **busulfan** (see Table 17–1).

Nitrosoureas

These antitumor **alkylating agents** are analogs of **mechlorethamine.** Nitrosourea replaces ethylamine and, except for **streptozotocin,** one of the two substituents on the nitrosourea is a 2-chloroethyl group (see Fig. 17–1). **Streptozotocin** differs in having methyl and glucose substituents on the **nitrosourea** configuration. In aqueous solution, the nitrosoureas spontaneously undergo nucleophilic rearrangement that splits the molecule into 2-chloroethyldiazine and isocyanate (or carbamoyl) derivatives (see Fig. 17–2). The latter interacts with ϵ-amino groups on lysine. The chloroethyldiazine derivative undergoes further spontaneous rearrangements that result in the formation of an alkylating chloroethyl carbonium ion. This group appears to be responsible for the antitumor cytotoxicity of the nitrosoureas.

All nitrosoureas disappear rapidly from serum after administration. In the case of **BCNU** and **streptozotocin,** this forces the use of an intravenous route of administration. **CCNU** and **methyl-CCNU** are therapeutically effective *per os.* Because they are lipid soluble, BCNU, CCNU, and methyl-CCNU achieve clinically useful concentrations in cerebrospinal fluid and find specific utility in the treatment of primary brain tumors. As with the mustards, the antitumor activity of the nitrosoureas is cycle-dependent but not cycle-specific. The most significant clinical toxicity of the antineoplastic **nitrosoureas** is their depression of marrow cytopoiesis. This depression is delayed in onset by about 1½ weeks and reaches its nadir 4 to 6 weeks after administration. Severe nausea and emesis are also usual. Pulmonary fibrosis is an occasional consequence of treatment with the nitrosoureas, as it is with busulfan and cyclophosphamide.

The use of streptozotocin is virtually restricted to treatment of β-cell tumors in the pancreatic islets of Langerhans. The other nitrosoureas have a broad spectrum of clinically useful activity. In addition to primary tumors of the central nervous system (CNS), they are employed against melanomas, Hodgkin's and non-Hodgkin's lymphomas, and against colorectal adenocarcinomas.

Procarbazine

Procarbazine is a drug clinically effective against Hodgkin's and non-Hodgkin's lymphomas and some primary brain neoplasms (see Table 17–1). A chemical derivative of methylhydrazine (see Fig. 17–2), procarbazine is enzymatically demethylated to azoprocarbazine in liver and erythrocytes. Azoprocarbazine undergoes spontaneous auto-oxidation in the presence of oxygen, producing hydrogen peroxide. The peroxide formation may have some significance in the drug's antitumor activity. Azoprocarbazine is further metabolized to a methyl radical (probably the utlimate cytolytic derivative of the drug) and to N-isopropylterephthalanic acid, which is excreted by the kidneys.

Procarbazine is rapidly absorbed from the gastrointestinal (GI) tract and disappears rapidly from the serum. It crosses the blood-brain barrier easily. The drug is cycle dependent but does not act by inhibiting any particular phase of the cycle.

Procarbazine was originally developed as a monoamine oxidase inhibitor, and hypertension is a risk with this drug in patients who have eaten tyramine-rich foods (bananas, cheeses). A variety of neurotoxicities occur with the use of procarbazine: depression or agitation, sedation, ataxia, hypotension, and peripheral neuropathy. The drug has a disulfiram-like effect, and it potentiates the depressive effects of phenothiazines, barbiturates, and narcotics. Altogether, neurotoxic side effects occur in about 5 to 10 percent of patients. The principal clinical toxicity (50 to 75 percent of all patients) is a dose-limiting marrow depression. Leukopenia and thrombocytopenia are most frequent results of this inhibition of the marrow cytopoiesis.

Cisplatin

Cisplatin is a coordination complex of platinum with two ammonium and two chloride groups (see Fig. 17–2). Activity requires that these groups be *cis* to each other, the *trans* configuration being inactive. The compound is water soluble and is stable as a dry powder for long periods of time. In aqueous solution, water adds to the complex and in the presence of nucleophiles the chloride-leaving group is displaced. Because there are two chloride-leaving groups per *cis*platin molecule, the agent is bifunctional and capable of **cross-linking** DNA.

*Cis*platin is given intravenously and is rapidly distributed to tissues, with less than 10 percent of the drug remaining in the serum after 1 hour. What remains in the serum is virtually all bound to protein and inactive. Most of the platinum is eventually secreted by the kidney as a variety of low molecular weight complexes. About 50 percent of the administered platinum is recoverable in urine 24 to 48 hours after administration.

A notable side effect of *cis*platin treatment is severe vomiting, usually within 1 hour of the drug's administration (see Table 17–1). Emesis is not dose dependent and is not suppressed by antiemetic drugs. Irreversible tubular necrosis in the kidney is not uncommon in patients with poor urine output. Renal **toxicity,** which like emesis is not dose dependent, may be avoided by good patient hydration prior to drug administration and perhaps the use of diuretic agents. **Myelosuppression** by *cis*platin tends to be delayed, the leukopenic nadir taking place 2 to 4 weeks after drug administration. Marrow depression and two other occasional side effects—tinnitus and high-frequency hearing loss—are reversible and dose dependent.

*Cis*platin administered with **vinblastine** and **bleomycin** against disseminated testicular tumors produces about a 75 percent complete remission rate. The drug is very active against bladder cancer and epidermoid carcinomas of the head and neck. The drug also is valuable in treating cancers that have failed to respond to other agents or have relapsed after treatment, as in the case of ovarian adenocarcinoma.

Dacarbazine

Dacarbazine is a structural analog of 5-aminoimidazole-4-carboxamide (AIC), a natural intermediate in **purine biosynthesis** (see Fig. 17–2). Antitumor effects of dacarbazine do not seem to arise from its interference with **purine metabolism** but from an **alkylating action**. The drug is oxidatively demethylated by the P-450-dependent mixed function oxidase system primarily in the liver. The *N*-demethylated product nonenzymatically decomposes into AIC and diazomethane. The latter is further transformed to the monofunctional free carbonium ion.

Dacarbazine is administered as a saline infusion, and all unaltered drug is gone from the serum in about 6 hours. The AIC metabolite is secreted by the kidneys. Dacarbazine is cell cycle dependent but not phase specific. Myelosuppression is relatively mild with dacarbazine. A flulike syndrome with myalgia and malaise may occur 7 to 10 days after the drug's administration. Its greatest value has been in its combined use with BCNU and vincristin against malignant melanoma, with doxorubicin against various sarcomas, and with cyclophosphamide against neuroblastoma (see Table 17–1).

Antimetabolites

Antimetabolites are chemical analogs of naturally occurring intermediates in cellular metabolism. Enzymatic recognition of these false substrates results in inhibition of the enzymes. Current, therapeutically useful, antitumor antimetabolites are directed against synthetic pathways of **purine** and **pyrimidine precursors** of RNA and DNA.

Purine Antimetabolites

6-Mercaptopurine and **6-thioguanine** are analogs of inosine and guanine, respectively (Fig. 17–3). Both are converted to their monophosphates by hypoxanthine-guanine phosphoribosyl transferase (6-thioguanidylic acid and 6-

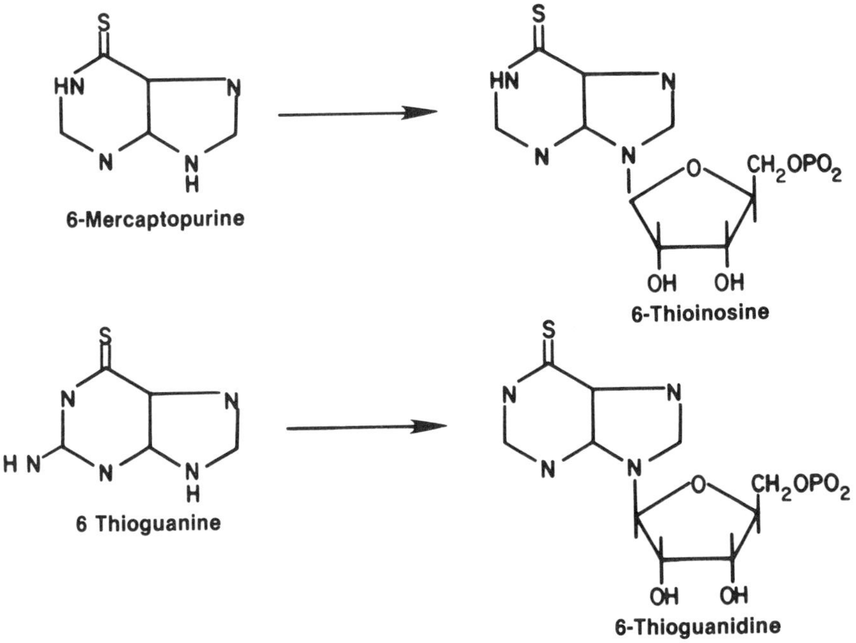

Figure 17–3. The purine antimetabolites.

thioinosinic acid, respectively), and these metabolites competitively inhibit the first enzymatic step in **purine synthesis** (ribosylamine 5-phosphate:pyrophosphate phosphoribosyl transferase) as well as two key enzymes in the synthetic pathways for AMP (IMP-aspartate ligase) and GMP (inosinic acid–NADP-oxidoreductase). Both drugs depress **RNA** and **DNA synthesis** and block the S phase of the cell cycle. 6-Thioinosinate is catabolized to 6-thiouric acid *via* a pathway that includes xanthine oxidase. Xanthine oxidase is not involved in the catabolism of 6-thioguanylate. Allopurinol concurrently administered with 6-mercaptopurine reduces the risk of toxicity.

Although both drugs are administered *per os* (see Table 17–1), absorption by the GI tract of 6-thioguanine is erratic compared with that of 6-mercaptopurine. About 50 percent of an oral dose of mercaptopurine passes from the GI tract into the circulation. **Thioguanine** lasts somewhat longer in serum than mercaptopurine. Gastrointestinal toxicity associated with both drugs is relatively mild, and the **suppression of marrow cytopoiesis** is only moderate.

The **purine antimetabolites** were among the earliest cancer chemotherapeutic agents employed clinically. They found special success in primary remission of acute lymphocytic leukemia in children and also had some efficacy against both acute and chronic forms of myelogenous leukemia.

Pyrimidine Antimetabolites

5-Fluorouracil ("Fluorouracil," FU) is readily metabolized to diphosphate and triphosphate derivatives and to deoxy monophosphates and diphosphates by most cells in the body (Fig. 17–4). The ultimate **antitumor metabolite** is FdUMP (fluorodeoxyuridylic acid). FdUMP binds tightly to the active site of thymidylate synthetase, a rate-limiting enzyme in thymidine synthesis, which converts dUMP (dexyuridylic acid) to dTMP (thymidylic acid). Because thymidylic acid is one of the four major bases composing DNA, inhibition of dTMP synthesis inhibits the formation of new DNA. 5-FU, thus, blocks the S phase of the cell cycle. Death in 5-FU–treated cells results from a thymine-depleted state whose mechanism for lethality is currently not well understood.

Fluorouracil was one of the first chemotherapeutic agents to show useful activity against solid tumors, particularly adenocarcinomas of the breast and colon. The drug is administered intravenously. GI side effects predominate with continuous intravenous infusion; with bolus intravenous administration, depression of bone marrow function is most pronounced. The bone marrow effects develop 9 to 25 days after administration of the drug. Other toxic reactions such as alopecia and neurotoxicity are less common than the GI and marrow problems (see Table 17–1).

Substitution of arabinose for ribose in cytosine gives a drug that has become important for induction of remission in acute myelogenous leukemia. **Cytosine arabinoside (araC)** is converted in cells first to its monophosphate and then to its triphosphate derivative (Fig. 17–5). **araC triphosphate** is a potent competitive inhibitor of DNA polymerase, competing with dCTP; there-

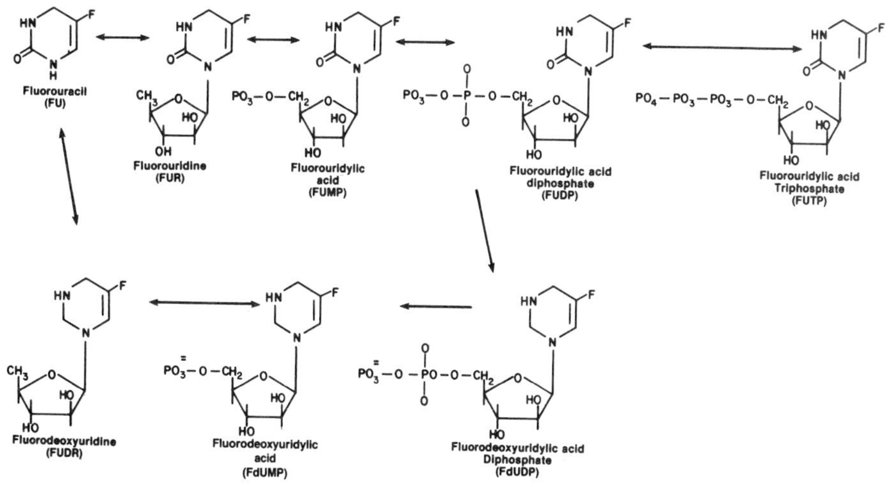

Figure 17–4. Metabolism of 5-fluorouracil (5-FU).

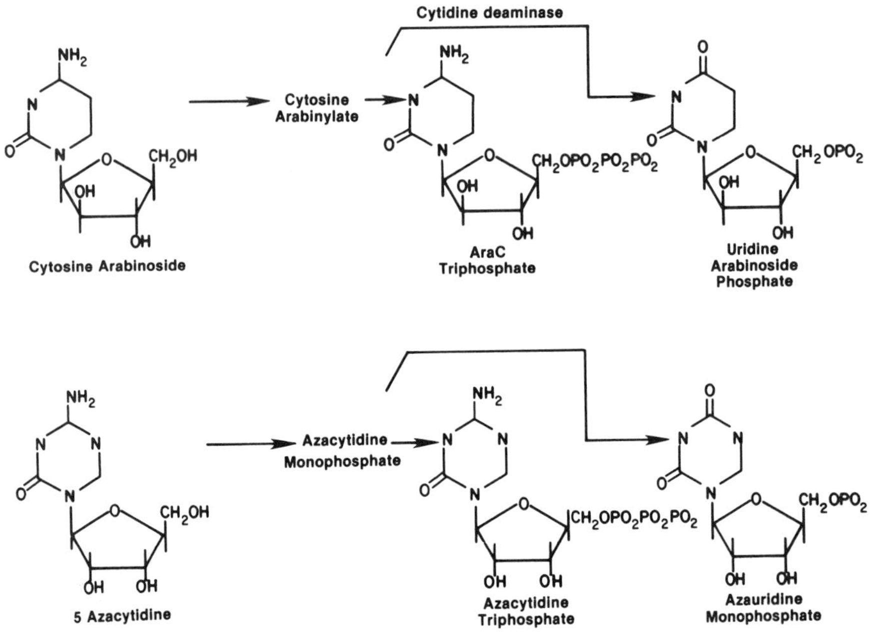

Figure 17–5. Metabolism of cytosine arabinoside (araC) and 5-azacytidine (AZA).

fore, it specifically inhibits the S phase of the cell cycle. Inactivation of araC is rapid. A widely distributed enzyme, cytidine deaminase, converts araC monophosphate to uridine arabinoside monophosphate, which is secreted in the urine. The abundance of this enzyme in the GI epithelium precludes oral administration of araC. The drug crosses the blood-brain barrier. Cerebrospinal fluid (CSF) levels peak at about 50 percent of those in serum. Better levels in the CSF are achieved by intrathecal administration. Toxic side effects of this drug are all relatively mild.

5-Azacytidine (AZA) is a cytidine derivative in which the C-5 carbon has been replaced with a nitrogen (see Fig. 17–5). This drug has proven to be particularly useful against acute myelogenous leukemia. Like araC, AZA must be activated to its triphosphate, but unlike **araC** the mechanism of its action is unclear. As AZA triphosphate, the drug is incorporated into RNA as a fraudulent base. Total cellular RNA synthesis and DNA synthesis are inhibited, as is the post-transcriptional processing of ribosomal RNA. The rate-limiting enzyme in pyrimidine synthesis, orotidylate decarboxylase, is also inhibited. AZA is S-phase specific. Like araC, AZA is metabolized by cytidine deaminase. The product of this conversion, azauridine monophosphate, has no antitumor activity.

Azacytidine is administered by intravenous infusion. Thirty minutes after intravenous bolus administration, 2 percent of the drug remains in the serum unaltered. Inhibition of bone marrow function is the usual problem with aza-cytidine. Hypotension is an occasional side effect whose likelihood is diminished by administering the drug by intravenous infusion instead of intravenous bolus injection.

Methotrexate (MTX)

Methotrexate (MTX), an N^{10}-methyl derivative of folic acid (Fig. 17–6), is considered an antimetabolite because of its action as a fraudulent substrate for the enzyme dihydrofolate reductase. This enzyme catalyzes the second of two reducing steps that convert folic acid to tetrahydrofolic acid (FH_4) (see Fig. 17–6). FH_4 is, in turn, converted to a variety of cofactors, such as N^5,N^{10}-methylene-FH_4 (required for thymidylate synthetase) and N^5,N^{10}-methenyl-FH_4 and N^{10}-formyl-FH_4 (required by enzymes in the purine synthetic pathway).

MTX is taken up into cells by an energy-dependent transport system that appears to be identical with that transporting folate. Inside cells, MTX binds irreversibly to the dihydrofolate reductase molecule protein and remains with the protein until it is degraded. However, MTX may be antagonized by repletion of intracellular pools of FH_4 derivatives with **citrovorum factor**. This factor, also called **folinic acid,** has the structure of N^5-formyl-FH_4 (see Fig. 17–6). Administration of citrovorum factor after MTX can replenish intracellular FH_4 pools to levels sufficient to allow survival of cells until resynthesis of new dihydrofolate reductase can replace MTX-inactivated enzyme. Because of

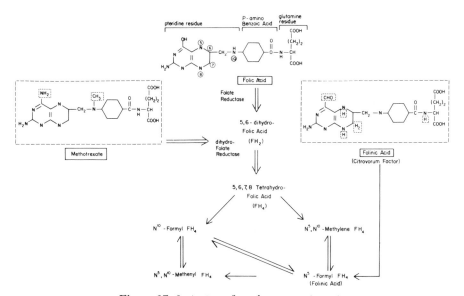

Figure 17–6. Action of methotrexate (MTX).

the importance of folate derivatives to nucleic acid synthesis, MTX tends specifically to block the S phase of the cell cycle.

MTX may be administered either intravenously or by mouth (see Table 17–1); higher serum levels are achievable by the former route. Saturation of the MTX transport system in the gut limits absorption. CSF levels of parenterally administered MTX are only 0.1 percent of serum levels, and better CSF levels are obtained by intrathecal injection. Toxicity of MTX involves tissues with high growth fractions—GI tract, bone marrow, and skin. High doses of the drug can precipitate renal tubular necrosis or, after intrathecal administration, neurotoxicity. Repeated low doses may provoke hepatotoxicity, including cirrhosis.

Cure of choriocarcinoma is achievable with MTX. The drug also is used for a variety of adenocarcinomas in a number of combinations with other chemotherapeutic agents. It is used in maintenance regimens for acute lymphocytic leukemia and for prophylaxis and control of meningitic phases of that disease. Responses of various lung tumors, epidermoid carcinoma, and osteogenic sarcoma are reported for MTX. MTX has an **immunosuppressive effect,** and a number of diseases of immunological origin have been treated with the drug, including chronic rheumatoid arthritis, systemic lupus erythematosus, and Wegener's granulomatosis.

Antineoplastic Alkaloids

Clinically useful antineoplastic plant derivatives generally act by inhibiting mitosis and sometimes have been called "spindle poisons" because of the deterioration of the mitotic spindle and metaphase arrest caused by most of them. The **vinca alkaloids vincristine** and **vinblastine** are imidazole derivatives extracted from periwinkle plants *(Vinca)* (Fig. 17–7). Structurally, vincristine differs from vinblastine by a single carboxyl substituted for a methyl group. They avidly bind to specific receptors on the 6S dimer of α- and β-1 tubulin, preventing the dimer from assembling into a microtubular structure. Microtubular arrays such as the mitotic spindle are in a state of continuous assembly and disassembly. In the presence of vinca alkaloids, disassembly goes on unabated while assembly is prevented. Microtubular structures not only underlie the karyokinesis and cytokinesis of mitosis but also support general cell functions like secretion, axonal flow, and a variety of plasma membrane activities. The **podophyllin** or May apple alkaloids represented by the well-studied laboratory chemical podophyllotoxin (see Fig. 17–7) act in a manner similar to that of the vinca alkaloids. Podophyllotoxin has not proven to be a useful chemotherapeutic agent. Two of its semisynthetic analogs, **etoposide** and **teniposide** (see Fig. 17–7), have clinical efficacy but do not cause metaphase arrest. They act in late S phase or early G2 and prevent entry into **M phase;** their mechanism is currently not understood.

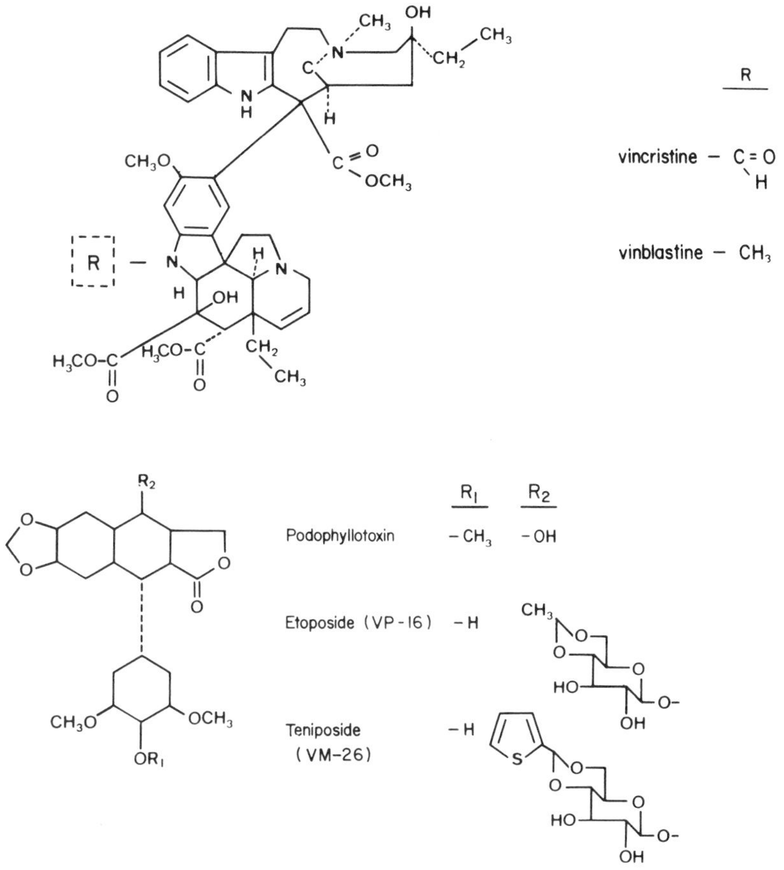

Figure 17–7. Antineoplastic alkaloids.

Vincristine and vinblastine are erratically absorbed from the GI tract and consequently are administered intravenously (see Table 17–1). Both are metabolized to desacetyl forms, which are as active as the parent compound. Slightly more than half of the excretion of both drugs takes place through the biliary tract, the rest by the kidney. About three quarters of a dose of either drug becomes protein bound in the plasma. Vincristine disappears from the serum more rapidly than vinblastine. Vincristine has a notable synergism with methotrexate that apparently arises from the alkaloid's enhancement of the cellular uptake of MTX.

The vinca alkaloids are remarkably different in their human toxicity, given their seemingly minor molecular differences. About 30 percent of the patients receiving vincristine develop neurotoxicity, compared with 5 to 10 percent for vinblastine. A greater than 30 percent incidence of leukopenia follows vinblastine administration, while white cell counts remain within normal limits after vincristine. Anorexia and nausea are practically absent after vincristine but occur in better than 30 percent of patients receiving vinblastine. The neurotoxicity associated with vincristine may be manifested in a spectrum of not always reversible symptoms including paresthesias, loss of deep tendon reflexes, foot drop, and ataxia. Decreased nerve conduction, axonal degeneration, and demyelination may be observed along with these effects. Because both vincristine and vinblastine cross the blood-brain barrier poorly, it is hard to ascribe neurotoxicity simply to tissue distribution.

Advantage has been taken of the nonmyelosuppressive characteristics of vincristine in the multiple drug regimens for Hodgkin's disease (MOPP, previously mentioned), for acute lymphocytic leukemia (with prednisone), and for pediatric tumors like Wilms' tumor, Ewing's sarcoma, and neuroblastoma (with cyclophosphamide or dactinomycin). Vinblastine is commonly employed in combinations for some leukemias (with doxorubicin [Adriamycin], bleomycin, and dacarbazine—the ABVD combination) or testicular tumors (with bleomycin and *cis*platin).

Etoposide is valuable for its induction of remission of small-cell lung carcinomas and, to a lesser extent, of various nonlymphocytic leukemias. **Teniposide** is effective as a single agent against reticulum sarcomas and, to a lesser extent, Hodgkin's disease and lymphosarcoma. These drugs are excreted in the urine and have a longer duration of residence in serum than either of the two vinca alkaloids. The dose-limiting side effects of these podophyllin derivatives involve the bone marrow and result in leukopenia and thrombocytopenia.

Antineoplastic Antibiotics

Intercalating Agents

The successful members of this class of antineoplastic drugs are obtained from microbial sources. The mechanisms of all entail interaction with DNA, yet none have cell cycle **phase-specific cytotoxicity**. Three have planar regions in their molecular structures and **intercalate** between stacked base-pairs of the DNA double helix. Dactinomycin (Actinomycin D) (Fig. 17–8) preferentially inserts between guanosines of guanosine-cytosine pairs. The phenoxazone chromophore of dactinomycin slips between the deoxyguanosines, and its two peptide-containing tails run in opposite directions up and down the minor groove of the helix. Doxorubicin and daunorubicin (see Fig. 17–8) intercalate without base preference. None of these three intercalators interact with single-stranded DNA or RNA. Intercalation causes local structural distortion of the DNA that inhibits both DNA and RNA polymerases. Transcriptional inhibition is not uniform. With low doses of dactinomycin, transcription of

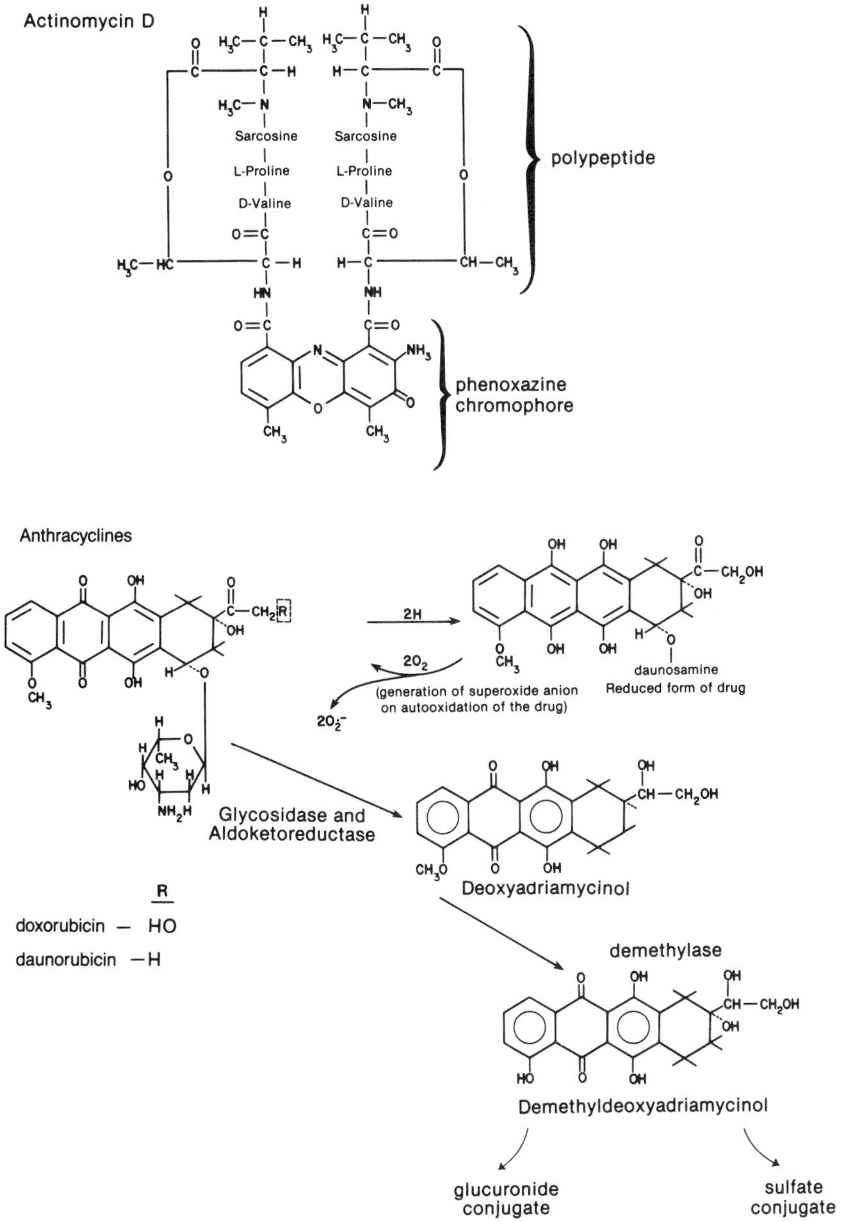

Figure 17–8. Antineoplastic antibiotics: intercalating agents.

rRNA is selectively inhibited. General depression of transcription requires high doses of the intercalators.

Dactinomycin is administered intravenously and is taken up by the cells by passive diffusion. Because of the drug's tight binding inside the cell, tissues retain the drug for long periods. Nine days after administration only about 30 percent of the drug has been excreted *via* renal or biliary routes. Metabolism is limited to addition of lactone to a small percent of the administered dose. Dactinomycin enhances the results of x-ray treatment of tumors by inhibiting the repair of radiation-damaged DNA. It is included in several different combined-drug modalities effective against Wilms' tumors and Ewing's sarcomas. Used by itself, the drug causes regression of rhabdomyosarcoma, metastatic testicular tumors, Kaposi's sarcoma, and choriocarcinoma. Myelosuppression is the toxicity that restricts the size of dactinomycin doses. Dactinomycin is also immunosuppressive.

Doxorubicin and **daunorubicin** are anthracycline antibiotics that differ significantly in antineoplastic spectra but only slightly in molecular structure. Both consist of an anthracycline nucleus and a glycosidically linked amino sugar, daunosamine (see Fig. 17–8). Doxorubicin is active against a larger number of tumor types (both hematogenous and solid) than daunorubicin. Daunorubicin's usefulness is largely limited to acute myelogenous and lymphocytic leukemias. Aside from these differences, the two drugs seem very much alike. Both have about the same affinity for DNA and share similar metabolic fates. For doxorubicin, successive action of glycosidase and an aldo-ketoreductase converts the parent compound into the still active adriamycinol. Adriamycinol is then O-demethylated, conjugated with either sulfate or glucuronide, and excreted in the bile. Daunorubicin is a somewhat better substrate for aldo-ketoreductase than doxorubicin, but overall the plasma half-lives and metabolic conversion rates of both compounds are relatively rapid. Both compounds are concentrated in spleen and kidney but neither cross into the CNS well. The toxicities of both are similar (see Table 17–1). Myelosuppression results in a neutropenic nadir about 2 weeks after administration. Anemia and thrombocytopenia are much less severe. The marrow effects are dose-related and dose-limiting. Nausea, vomiting, stomatitis, and, in virtually all patients, alopecia also occur. Cardiotoxicity occurs after total cumulative doses of 550 mg per m^2. Electrocardiographical changes occur shortly after administration followed by the development of cardiomyopathy. At its worst, an irreversible congestive heart failure can occur that is refractory to digitalis and diuretics. The ejection fraction of patients undergoing doxorubicin treatment should be measured prior to and at regular intervals during therapy (e.g., MUGA scan). Restriction of total drug during the course of therapy to less than 550 mg per m^2 reduces the incidence of cardiac problems. It has been suggested that cardiac tissue damage caused by doxorubicin involves redox cycling of the drug back and forth between its quinone and dihydroquinone forms. Auto-oxidation of the reduced form in the presence of oxygen generates two molecules of superoxide anion that, in turn, may give rise to more reactive oxygen radicals that abstract hydrogen from unsaturated fatty acid double bonds. Fatty acid lipoperoxidation is deleterious to the function of membranes and appears to be cytolytic when it reaches sufficient magnitude.

Nonintercalating Antibiotics

Mitomycin (mitomycin C) reacts as an alkylating agent and displays bifunctional activity in cross-linking DNA (Fig. 17–9). Unlike other antineoplastic alkylators, it favors the O^6 position of guanine over the N^7 position. In the cell, mitomycin is metabolized from its parent quinone to dihydroquinone by an NADPH-dependent quinone reductase. The tertiary methoxy of the dihydroquinone becomes a spontaneous leaving group, after which the aziridine ring spontaneously opens, generating one electrophilic center (A, Fig. 17–9). A second center arises in the carbamate region of the molecule (B, Fig. 17–9). As with other alkylators, mitomycin causes chromosome breakage and acts as a mutagen and a carcinogen.

Although mitomycin has activity against a broad spectrum of tumors, significant myelosuppression by the drug clinically limits its usefulness (see Table 17–1). The frequent leukopenias and thrombocytopenias associated with the drug reach their height of severity 5 to 6 weeks after a single dose. Marrow depression is cumulatively worsened by increased dose size and frequency of administration. Mitomycin is also responsible for an unpredictable and unexplained pulmonary fibrosis, fortunately of infrequent occurrence. The drug can be used by itself effectively against superficial bladder carcinomas by intravesical administration. Little drug escapes from the lumen of the bladder. Combination therapy of mitomycin with bleomycin is employed against disseminated uterine cervical carcinoma and with doxorubicin (and sometimes 5-FU) against gastric, lung, and pancreatic adenocarcinomas. Mitomycin is so erratically absorbed from the GI tract that it is usually administered intravenously despite the risk of cellulitis at the injection site. A relatively rapid disappearance from serum is not explained by poor recoveries of the drug from urine, suggesting an as yet unknown metabolism of the compound or a slow release of drug adducts from tissues.

Mithramycin is a member of the chromomycin group of **streptomyces** antibiotics that reversibly bind to DNA in the presence of Mg^{2+} (see Fig. 17–9). RNA synthesis is depressed to a greater extent than DNA synthesis. Although mithramycin can displace already bound dactinomycin from DNA, it is not an intercalator. On the other hand, like dactinomycin, mithramycin seems to have a preference for regions of DNA rich in deoxyguanosine. The chemical nature of the antibiotic's reaction with DNA is not clear. Use of mithramycin in clinical oncology is largely limited to treatment of metastatic testicular tumors and of hypercalcemia of neoplastic origin. The drug appears to have no effect on either parathormone secretion or renal excretion of CA^{2+}, but in-

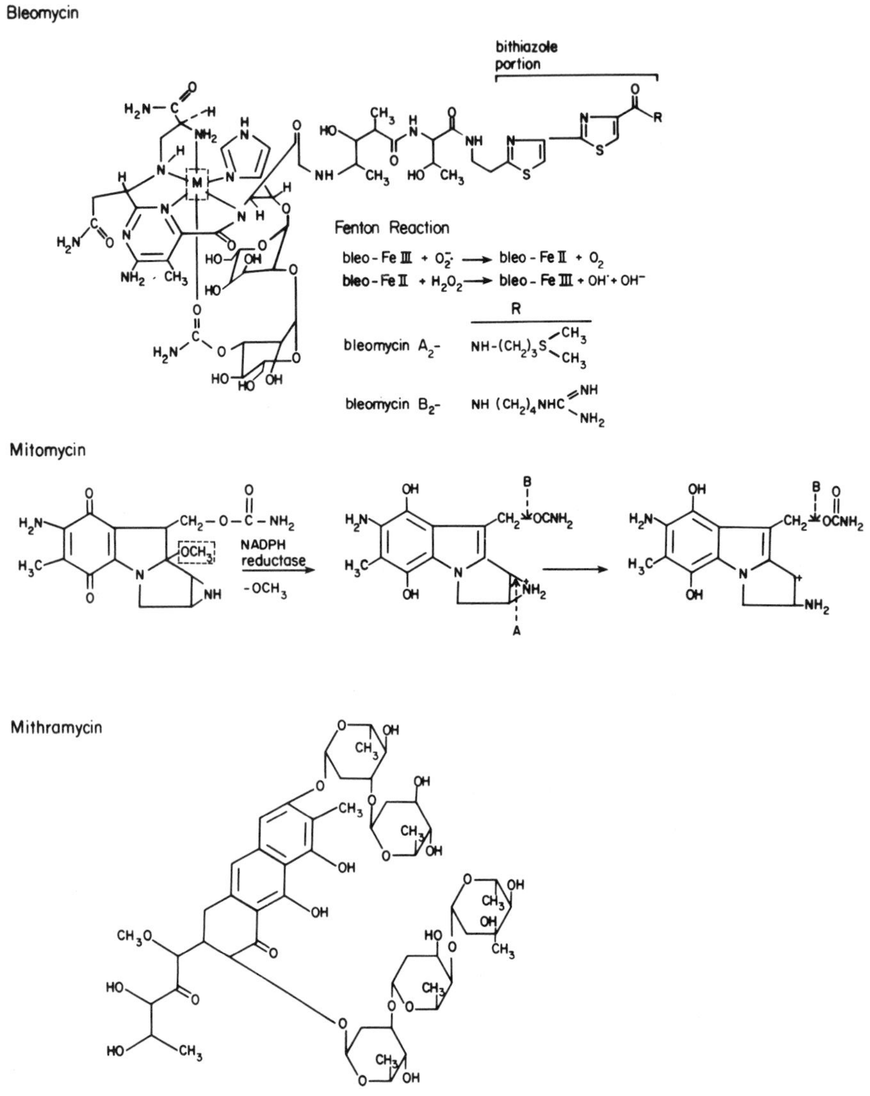

Bleomycin

Mitomycin

Mithramycin

Figure 17–9. Antineoplastic antibiotics: nonintercalating agents.

stead inhibits bone resorption due to osteoclasia. The basis for this effect is not understood.

Limited data from humans suggest that mithramycin is cleared almost completely from the blood in 2 hours after intravenous administration. About half the drug is recovered in urine 4 hours after administration. The drug concentrates in liver and kidney and a small amount enters the cerebrospinal fluid. Toxicity includes thrombocytopenia, hepatotoxicity, nephrotoxicity, and spontaneous bleeding.

Bleomycin

Bleomycin is unusual in that its attack on DNA combines intercalation and catalysis of oxygen-dependent reactive intermediates. The bleomycin molecule (see Fig. 17–9) is a water-soluble basic glycopeptide with a pyridine-containing core that chelates a metal ligand (usually copper or iron), amino acid and sugar side chains, and a planar bithiazole group responsible for DNA intercalation. Bleomycin causes both DNA single- and double-strand scissions by a mechanism in which the drug-metal complex may activate the ground-state oxygen molecule by a series of one-electron reductions producing super-oxide anion, hydrogen peroxide, and hydroxyl radical (the iron-catalyzed Fenton reaction, see Fig. 17–9).

Parenterally administered drug reaches its highest concentrations in skin and lungs and is virtually absent in CSF. Both renal excretion and metabolism contribute to the relatively quick clearance of the drug from serum. Bleomycin hydrolase inactivates the drug. Tissues that have low levels of this enzyme (such as lung and skin) show high accumulations of the drug, and *vice versa*. In some studies, tumors with low levels of the enzyme are more responsive to the drug than those with higher levels.

The GI tract, liver, kidneys, immune system, and CNS generally escape unwanted side effects of bleomycin therapy. More importantly, the drug has virtually no myelosuppressive action. Oral mucositis, alopecia, and hyperpigmentation occur. A diffuse interstitial fibrosis of the lungs is dose-limiting for bleomycin and is irreversible. The development of toxicity in lungs and skin correlates with high accumulations of drug in these tissues. The lungs are also associated with high tissue concentrations of the major component required for bleomycin action, oxygen.

Current antitumor therapy with bleomycin principally entails its use in drug-combination regimens: against histiocytic lymphoma (BACOP—bleomycin, doxorubicin, cyclophosphamide, vincristine, and prednisone), Hodgkin's lymphoma (ABVD—doxorubicin, bleomycin, vinblastine, and dacarbazine), and various testicular tumors (bleomycin, vinblastine, and *cis*-platin). The drug also is used to treat squamous cell carcinomas of the genitalia, face, and neck.

Antitumor Hormonal Agents

Hormonal therapy of neoplastic disease is predicated on the dependence of some tumors on particular hormones for growth. Roughly 80 percent of adenocarcinomas of the prostate contain cells sensitive to **androgens**. Prostatic cancer that has spread through the capsule of the prostate and therefore not certain to be completely removed by surgery may be treated by androgen depletion. This is effectively achieved by administration of androgen counterhormones like **diethylstilbestrol (DES)** often combined with orchiectomy (see Table 17–1). Large doses of DES (5 mg per day) plus gonadectomy produce overall remission rates of 70 to 88 percent for 2 to 3 years. Long-term survival is limited by the development of insensitive cell populations in the tumor and by the side effects of the high-dose regimens of the **estrogens**—pulmonary emboli and other thrombotic complications. Small doses of DES (1 to 2 mg per day) plus orchiectomy will not suppress extratesticular sources of androgens such as the adrenal gland. Surgical ablation of the adrenal gland and/or the hypophysis coupled with low-dose DES and orchiectomy has had disappointing results, but suppression of the adrenal gland with high doses of **dexamethasone** or **aminoglutethimide** has been more promising.

Prostatic cancer also responds well to treatment with agonist analogs of **gonadotropin-releasing hormone** (GnRH agonists). At least six of these modifications of the GnRH peptide are commercially synthesized (leuprolide, buserelin, lutrelin, nafurelin, decapaptyl, and Zoladex) for subcutaneous depot injection or nasal insufflation. GnRH analogs cause atrophic changes in the prostate secondary to suppression of testicular function and reduction in circulating levels of testosterone. Adrenal production of androgens is not influenced by decline in LH and FSH. Therefore, GnRH analog therapy is best accompanied by a blocker of androgen synthesis such as **flutamide**. The course of antineoplastic therapy with GnRH agonists lasts several years. Major side effects are decline of libido and vasomotor hot flashes. The hormonal approach to advanced forms of prostatic carcinomas can forestall use of the less desirable cytotoxic chemotherapeutic agents.

Determining candidacy of prostatic cancer patients for androgen-deprivation therapy by the measurement of **androgen receptor** levels in tumor tissue is often ignored in light of the relatively high incidence of responsiveness for the tumor in general. For another type of tumor, breast adenocarcinoma, determination of sensitivity is more important. It is estimated that only between one quarter and one third of breast tumors have some degree of dependency on estrogen. Ovarian ablation has long been known to reduce the size of tumor masses, especially in premenopausal patients. Adrenalectomy or hypophysectomy or both are more effective with postmenopausal patients. These procedures are more advisable for patients whose biopsy specimens show the presence of specific **estrogen receptors** by radioimmunoassay.

Beside the irreversible surgical methods of achieving estrogen depletion in breast cancer patients, there are four alternative approaches. The first employs counterestrogenic androgens (see Table 17–1). Virilizing androgens like **methyldihydrotestosterone** (dromostanolone) or **7-β, 17-α, dimethyltestosterone** (calusterone) produce remission rates about equal to those of testosterone or **fluoxymestrone** (judged by studies in which 20 to 25 percent of patients were unscreened for estrogen sensitivity). In the second approach, massive doses of estrogens (50 to 100 times those used in maintenance regimens) gave overall remission rates of about 38 percent. High levels of estrogen probably act by inhibiting secretion of prolactin. Diethylstilbestrol, mestranol, and 17 β-ethinylestradiol are commonly used estrogens. High-dose estrogen therapy is thought to be less effective in premenopausal patients than androgens. It carries the considerable risk of thromboembolic disease, fluid retention, and uterine bleeding. The third approach employs estrogen antagonists like **tamoxifen** or **nafoxidine**. Remissions are most frequent in cases of advanced, estrogen-sensitive breast cancer in postmenopausal women. Estrogen antagonists compete for estrogen receptors with natural ligands, and the drug-receptor complex can be demonstrated to block repletion of receptor protein. Both tamoxifen and nafoxidine cause hypercalcemia, nausea, and hot flashes. Nafoxidine is also associated with dermatological problems such as photosensitivity and ichthyosis. All four of these approaches to breast cancer are reserved for advanced forms of the disease, often adjuvant to prior surgical excision of the main tumor masses.

Progesterone, a hormone that stimulates the differentiation of mammary epithelium, can produce regression of breast adenocarcinomas. In postmenopausal women with advanced tumors, a 30 percent response rate is achieved with daily doses of 1 g of medroprogesterone (MPA). At this dosage, MPA acts directly on progesterone receptors in the neoplastic tissue. MPA also causes decreased adrenal production of hydrocortisone and androgen and a decline in the levels of circulating ACTH. A serious drawback to MPA is the need to replace hydrocortisone during therapy. A particularly successful use of MPA is with endometrial carcinoma. In this tumor, progesterone (and estrogen) receptors occur with fairly high frequency, and MPA achieves response rates approaching 50 percent. The combination of tamoxifen with MPA in treatment of endometrial carcinoma heightens effectiveness. It is reported that tamoxifen stimulates the frequency of progesterone receptors.

Glucocorticoids are known to cause involution of the thymus and other lymphoid tissues. Prednisone has an established use in controlling chronic lymphocytic leukemia. Circulating tumor cell counts are reduced by the drug, and erythropoiesis and thrombocytopoiesis are stimulated. This later effect is especially desirable when myelophthistic anemia and thrombocytopenia occur. Prednisone inhibits patients' immune responses, and its use must take into account the risk of intercurrent infection. Prednisone is also used against Hodgkin's disease and non-Hodgkin's lymphomas as part of combination chemotherapeutic regimens. The basis for its contribution in treatment of these lymphomas is uncertain. No clear relationship between therapeutic antitumor effect and the levels of corticosteroid receptors in tumor cells has been consistently demonstrated.

Antitumor Enzymes

Asparaginase

Asparaginase is the only enzyme with a currently established use in cancer chemotherapy (see Table 17–1). A number of tumor types possess demonstrably low levels of the enzyme asparagine synthetase. Low levels of this enzyme reduce tumor cell capacity to transaminate aspartic acid and thus synthesize the amino acid asparagine, forcing them to rely on nutritional sources of asparagine. Deprivation of asparagine blocks protein synthesis and causes tumor cell lysis. In cancer patients, deprivation can be achieved by injection of the catabolic enzyme asparaginase which hydrolyzes asparagine to aspartate and ammonium ion. Although asparaginase occurs widely in nature, only those forms of the enzyme having a K_m value low enough to hydrolyze asparagine rapidly at the usually low concentrations at which it is found in the serum are useful. Asparaginase for therapeutic use is commercially prepared from either *E. coli* or *Erwinia carotova*.

Intravenous injection of the enzyme lowers both serum asparagine and serum glutamine levels. Virtually none of the enzyme escapes from the vascular compartment. None is found in the CSF. The plasma half-life of the injected enzyme is 6 to 30 hours. The serum proteases apparently responsible for turnover of the enzyme are not well understood. Asparaginase is a rare example of a chemotherapeutic agent whose action is independent of the cell cycle.

The use of asparaginase is centered on acute lymphoblastic leukemia, frequently in combination with vincristine and prednisone. Remission rates of greater than 90 percent are achieved with this combination. The most common side effect of asparaginase is hypersensitivity. About one fourth of patients receiving the enzyme develop urticarial reactions and, much less frequently, anaphylactoid responses. Next in frequency is neurotoxicity: patients show confusion, somnolence, and even coma. The EEG changes that accompany these symptoms are reversible on withdrawal of the drug. Acute hemorrhagic pancreatitis is an occasional grave side effect, as is liver toxicity. The mechanisms underlying brain, pancreatic, and hepatic toxicities associated with administration of antitumor preparations of this enzyme are not understood. L-asparaginase causes only minimal myelosuppression.

IMMUNOMODULATORY AGENTS

Immunomodulatory agents are used therapeutically to influence the course of disease processes involving immune reaction. They are classifiable either as enhancing agents (those heightening immune response) or as suppressors (those depressing immune response). Each class may be subdivided into specific and nonspecific agents. Specific immunomodulatory agents are those that act to alter the immune response to particular antigens; nonspecific agents influence immune responses to a broad spectrum of antigens. Within the full range of current therapeutically useful immunomodulatory agents, there occur examples of all categories of agents with the exception of specific immunoenhancers.

Nonspecific Immunosuppressive Agents

Antilymphocyte Serum (ALS)

Equine ALS developed against peripheral human lymphocytes was, for many years, a principal means of curtailing transplant rejection. Depending on the particular immunizing antigens involved in the development of ALS antibodies, administration of ALS could sharply reduce host-versus-graft cells and allow homologous foreign tissue to be sustained by the host. Successful induction of tolerance requires cross-matching of a patient's cell type with particular ALS preparations. ALS also strongly depresses the primary, humoral immune response. The ability of ALS to maintain graft tolerance is limited by its side effects of serum sickness and idiosyncratic patient intolerance of the heterologous serum. The use of ALS currently has been largely replaced by newer agents although it remains an option.

Glucocorticoids (Prednisone-Deltasone, Meticorten; Prednisolone-Deltacortef)

The lymphocyte targets of glucocorticoids are T cells. In animals, prednisone causes thymic involution, but in humans no such widespread lymphocytolysis seems to occur. A small subset of theta-positive, **phytohemagglutinin-responsive cells,** sometimes termed unsensitized T cells, may be vulnerable to glucocorticoids; however, the main immunodepressive effect of steroids stems from depression of effector systems. The cytotoxicity of T-killer cells is markedly reduced by **prednisone,** and the induction of tolerance by systems involving the action of T-suppressor cells is blocked. Prolongation of graft survival is enhanced by prednisone, but part of this effect may be due to the anti-inflammatory action of the steroid. The primary humoral immune response, the anamnestic response, and the established immunity will all be reduced by prednisone.

Prednisone is used for autoimmune diseases (e.g., lupus erythematosus, idiopathic thrombocytopenia), for various forms of arthritis, and for the prevention of allograft rejection. Dosage and regimens are variable. Initial daily dosages commonly are 2 to 10 mg/kg with later reduction to 1 mg/kg/day, but up to 1×10^3 mg/kg/day may be employed in certain situations such as graft rejection crises. It should be noted that prednisone doses of the caliber used for immunosuppression initially cause marked decreases in circulating white cell counts. Glucocorticoids stimulate emigration of leukocytes from vascular compartments and sequestration of circulating lymphocytes at sites such as the bone marrow. No cytolysis seems to be involved, and circulating counts return to normal in about 24 hours if steroid is discontinued.

Alkylating Agents

The immunosuppressive side effect of some antitumor drugs has been exploited in therapeutic situations in which restraint of the immune system is desired. **Cyclophosphamide (Cytoxan)** or, rarely, busulfan (Myleran) is occasionally used for treatment of chronic arthritis. Primary humoral immune responses are chiefly affected, with lesser influences on the anamnestic reaction, established immunity, or graft rejection. Cyclophosphamide must be administered before or during exposure to antigen. The value of this drug must be weighed against its side effects of marrow depression, carcinogenicity, and teratogenicity.

Antimetabolites

Methotrexate has been occasionally used as an immunosuppressive agent, but the most widely employed antimetabolite is **azathioprine**. Azathioprine is a form of 6-mercaptopurine in which the sulfhydryl group of the mercaptopurine is blocked with a nitroimidazole derivative. The first step in its metabolism is the removal of the nitroimidazole group leaving 6-mercaptopurine. Azathioprine has considerably less antitumor activity than does 6-mercaptopurine but much greater immunosuppressive activity. Primary and secondary humoral immune responses are strongly suppressed, as is host-versus-graft reaction. The compound may be administered up to several hours after exposure to antigens and still be effective. As with other antimetabolites, toxicity is a severe problem and includes sterility, intercurrent infections, neoplasia, and teratogenesis. Its primary use has been to prevent organ transplant rejection, usually in concert with other immunomodulatory agents. For instance, in kidney transplantation graft recipients will receive ALS several days prior to transplantation. Shortly before the actual surgery azathioprine treatment will be started and will be continued on a daily dosage regimen for up to 200 days. The regular administration of ALS will typically last 100 days after transplantation. Last, prednisone administration will begin approximately 30 to 40 days after transplantation and be continued as long as azathioprine is given.

Cyclosporine

Cyclosporine (Cyclosporin A) is an antibacterial product of the fungus *Trichoderma polysporum.* Like the polysporin group of antibiotics, it is a circular polypeptide, composed of 11 amino acids including two rarely described in nature, *N*-methyl leucine and methyl valine. The action of this highly lipid soluble compound is discrete and nonlympholytic. Cyclosporine acts against cytotoxic and T-helper cells as they are being sensitized by antigen. The drug appears to suppress the synthesis and secretion of interleukin II (IL-2) by T-helper cells, and it inhibits the formation of IL-2 receptors on maturing cytotoxic T cells. The effect of this two-pronged attack is to prevent the proliferation of T cells sensitized by the particular antigen. Coincidence of cyclosporine administration with antigen presentation and lymphocyte sensitization is crucial. There is also evidence that T-suppressor cell maturation may be suppressed by this drug.

Cyclosporine is administered orally in olive oil or IV in polyoxyethylated castor oil. It is distributed to most parts of the body and its plasma $t_{1/2}$ equals 17 to 40 hours. It is inactivated by metabolism primarily in the liver by hydroxylation and methylation. Metabolites are excreted *via* the bile and feces, and only 0.1 percent of the excreted drug is unchanged. Dose-limiting toxicity of cyclosporine is renal failure. The drug is also associated with an increased incidence in B-cell lymphomas, and it has been speculated that the drug may activate oncogenic viruses such as the Epstein-Barr virus. Cyclosporine is widely used to suppress the rejection of bone marrow, kidney, liver, and heart transplants. The risk associated with the use of the drug is considerably less than that associated with the use of drugs such as azathioprine, and cyclosporine has become the drug of choice for preventing homologous graft rejection.

Specific Immunosuppressive Agents

Erythroblastosis fetalis is a perinatal immunohemolytic anemia. The disease develops during a pregnancy in which an Rh-negative mother bearing an Rh-positive fetus becomes immunized with fetal red cells. Such immunization may occur as a result of amniocentesis, cesarean surgery, or hemorrhage during parturition. Maternal anti-Rh IgGs can cross the placenta, enter the fetal circulation, interact with red cell antigen, and thus activate complement with consequent red cell lysis. Full-blown erythroblastosis fetalis usually occurs in the Rh-positive offspring of Rh-negative mothers who have previously delivered several Rh-positive infants and who have presumably been immunized during each of the pregnancies and deliveries.

Erythroblastosis fetalis can be prevented by administration of Rh immune globulin (RhoGAM, or HypRho-D). This is a human IgG preparation against Rh antigens taken from $Rh_o(D)$-negative and D_u-negative human donors who have been immunized with $Rh_o(D)$ and D_u-positive blood. An immunoglobulin fraction is prepared by ethanol precipitation to a specified high final titer of anti-Rh antibodies. Rh immune globulin suppresses the formation of maternal anti-Rh antibody. The preparation is administered intramuscularly at the time of delivery of each Rh-positive offspring or after any event in which sensitization might occur (e.g., amniocentesis). The suppression of autogenous immune response to a particular antigen by concomitant passively acquired antibodies to the same antigen is a well-known but not well-understood phenomenon. Widespread use of Rh immune globulin has markedly reduced the incidence of erythroblastosis fetalis. The incidence of reported side effects of this preparation is very low. The most common complaints are discomfort at site of injection and slight fever; less commonly, various types of allergic reactions may occur, especially in patients who received multiple injections.

Nonspecific Immunoenhancing Agents

Naturally Occurring Factors Having Immunoenhancing Effects

Interleukin II. The lymphocyte growth factor and lymphokine, interleukin II, is a polypeptide available commercially and produced by recombinant DNA technology. Interleukin II stimulates (1) T-cell growth and differentiation, (2) anti-tumor activity of cytotoxic T-cells, (3) antitumor activity of NK cells (neutral killer cells), and (4) the secretion of interferon. It is usually administered by intravenous infusion and disappears from the serum in a biphasic fashion with a $t_{1/2}$ of 6.9 minutes and 30 to 60 minutes. Intravenous infusion causes an initial decline in the number of circulating lymphoid cells followed by an expansion of 2 to 12 times the number of circulating cells over pretreatment levels. IL-2 causes regression in human T-cell leukemia (hairy cell leukemia) and in preliminary trials appears to be effective against several different metastatic tumors.

Interferons (IFN). Interferons are a family of polypeptides secreted by a variety of cell types: α-IFNs from leukocytes, β-IFNs from fibroblast and epithelial cells, and γ-IFNs from T-lymphocytes. Interferons strongly depress viral replication but, in addition, have a number of other functions directed against cells of the immune system:

1. B-cell differentiation and production of antibodies are stimulated by all interferons.
2. The activity of cytotoxic T-cells is enhanced.
3. The cytotoxicity of the NK cells (neutral killer cells) is enhanced.
4. A number of macrophage activities are stimulated, including phagocytosis, the presentation of antigen, tumor-killing capacity, prostaglandin synthesis, oxidative metabolism, and the intracellular killing of parasites.
5. Differentiation of bone marrow stem cells is stimulated.
6. IgE-mediated histamine release by basophils is stimulated.

Production of interferon is subject to a large number of stimuli in addition to viral infection, as outlined in Table 17–2. Interferon-producing cells stimulated by any of these agents respond by increasing the rate of synthesis and secretion of interferon. The secreted interferon then attaches to surface receptors that may be on the secreting cell itself or on others nearby. The receptor-bound interferon is then internalized and stimulates at least three separate systems in target cells. First of these is a system that degrades messenger RNA and involves ribonuclease L (RNAase L). Central to this system is a poly-adenosine intermediate 5'-0-triphosophoryladenyl [2'-5' adenyl] 2'-5'-adenosine (2'-5' A). This intermediate at extremely low levels (10^{-9} M) causes a 50 percent inhibition of translation of messenger RNA and protein synthesis. It is of interest that some patients with autoimmune disease such as lupus erythematosus have detectable levels of 2'-5' A in serum, and administration of interferon to these patients carries a heightened risk of toxic side effects. Interferon stimulates the RNAase L system by inducing the enzyme 2'-5' A synthetase. This enzyme appears to occur in most cells of the body.

A second intracellular system stimulated by interferon is the interferon-induced, double-stranded RNA-activated protein kinase system. In addition to 2'-5' A synthetase, interferon also activates a protein kinase, which requires activation by double-stranded RNA (dsRNA), the protein kinase P_1. P_1 phosphorylates two proteins, protein P_1 (which has no known function) and the

Table 17–2. INTERFERON-INDUCING AGENTS

Class I Inducers (of α and β INFs only)

Microorganisms:
    Viruses, mycoplasma, rickettsiae, protozoa chlamydiae, some bacteria (e.g., *Brucella*)
Microbial components:
    dsRNA (from viruses or virally infected cells) endotoxins and bacterial lipopolysaccharides (LPSs) antibiotics:
    Glutarimides (e.g., cycloheximide), kanamycin
    Surface glycoproteins (e.g., envelopes from viruses, hemagglutinins)
Polyanions (mostly synthetic):
    Polyvinylsulfate, dextran, polynucleotides polyI:polyC
Synthetic low MW compounds:
    Tilorone (fluorene and fluorenone derivatives)

Class II Inducers (of γ INFs only)

    Antigens (Ag)
    Interleukin 2 (IL-2)
    Antibody-Ag complexes
    Mitogens (concanavalin A, phytohemagglutinin, pokeweed antigen)
    Antilymphocyte antiserum (ALS)

translation initiation factor eIF-2 (which when phosphorylated becomes inactive). Thus, the effect of interferon stimulation of kinase P_1 is to inhibit protein synthesis, thereby also reinforcing the effect of the RNAase L system.

A third effect of interferon is to enhance the presentation of class 2 histocompatibility antigens. Class 2 antigens (e.g., HLA-DR and Ia) are expressed on B-cells, activated T-cells, and macrophages and assist cells in processing antigen. Increased levels of these surface glycoproteins would appear to stimulate immune response and to underly some of the major immunoenhancing effects of interferons.

All three classes of interferons (α, β, and γ), are now produced in commercial quantities using recombinant DNA technology. Interferon is approved for use against advanced forms of **Kaposi's sarcoma,** when the patient suffers immune deficiency. Antitumor activity by interferon has been reported for a large number of different types of neoplasms. The most frequent side effect of interferon in clinical use has been a flulike syndrome characterized by fever, rigors, fatigue, malaise, anorexia, and myalgia. Less frequently mental confusion, nausea, and liver function abnormalities may occur. Antibodies to interferons have been found in some patients.

Drugs Having Immunoenhancing Activity

A number of drugs have been reported to have **immunoenhancing activity** as a side effect of their action, including levamisole and inosiplex (Isoprinosine). Characteristics of these effects and the conditions under which they occur are obscure. **Levamisole** is an established antihelmintic that is known to delay the progress of systemic lupus erythematosus, rheumatoid arthritis, and aphthous stomatitis and to be of benefit in chronic influenza, acute hepatitis, and herpetic infections. Levamisole stimulates precursor T-cells to differentiate by modulating cyclic AMP levels. It also stimulates activity of macrophages engaged in immune responses. Levamisole appears not to have distinct anti-inflammatory action nor does it stimulate B-cell proliferation or antibody production. Its value seems to be limited to immunodeficiency situations, and its action in enhancing immune responses is merely to increase their activity to a near-normal level. A severe drawback in the use of any immunoenhancing agent for diseases involving immunodeficiency is the general lack of understanding of the cause of immunodeficiency in any condition.

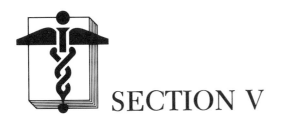

SECTION V

Toxicology

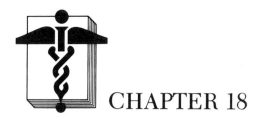

CHAPTER 18
Toxicology

THOMAS R. TEPHLY, M.D., Ph.D.

Toxicology is the study of adverse effects of chemical substances on biological systems. Toxicology embraces the understanding of the toxicity of drugs and drug combinations, abuse agents, studies on food additives, pesticides, industrial chemicals, accidental poisonings, and applications in forensic medicine. Beyond the consideration of a given substance in a specific individual and an understanding of the principles of action of a given agent in a given

449

biological system, toxicology invokes a broader definition when the system includes the community or an ecosystem.

All chemical substances can exert harmful effects at some dose. Therefore, dose-response or dose-toxicity relationships are a key to understanding
the relative safety or hazards of chemical agents. At some point risks are acceptable even when toxicity is evident, as, for example, in the treatment of
cancer when the use of potent drugs is required. The function of normal as
well as invading cells may be altered by these potent agents, but selective
toxicity toward cancer cells is expected to be greater and forms a rational approach to therapy. Although all drugs may be considered as poisons, not all
poisons are drugs. There are many chemicals that have no therapeutic benefit
(e.g., lead, methanol, mercury, dioxin, carbon tetrachloride). Substances that
are not beneficial or therapeutic are often imposed on an environment in the
home, in the community, or in a given individual. In such cases regulations
must be imposed and risk assessments are made in order to derive concentrations that may be acceptable for economic use and that pose only a low and
acceptable degree of hazard in a given environmental situation.

PRINCIPLES OF TOXIC ACTIONS

The term **xenobiotic** is used extensively to define substances that are foreign to the animal organism. This term ignores therapeutic usefulness or economic benefit and includes all exogenous substances, irrespective of their
effects in a biological system. Certain principles governing the effects of xenobiotics in biological systems have been useful in describing the interaction of
chemical substances on living systems.

During an **exposure phase,** a xenobiotic gains access to the organism and
usually (except when dermatotoxicity occurs) must be absorbed into the organism to produce a response. The routes of absorption include the oral, inhalational, or dermal route. Direct injection may also be considered as a possible
but uncommon means of entry of the chemical agent into the body. It is important to note that most substances do not transfer directly to the site of toxicity once they are absorbed into the body. Instead, they enter into one or
more compartments where they may be stored or transported to sites distant
from their site of attack in the **toxicodynamic phase.**

There are a number of processes by which the organism can deal with a
xenobiotic (**dispositional phase**). This phase includes metabolism (biotransformation), excretion, and storage. Most xenobiotics are weak electrolytes and
are lipid soluble at physiological pH. Because **excretion** (the final phase of disposition) from the body is slow for most lipid-soluble substances, they must
be metabolized to more water-soluble metabolites before they can be eliminated by the kidney. Metabolic reactions include oxidation, reduction, conjugation, and hydrolysis and are located primarily but not exclusively in the

liver. Conversion of a xenobiotic to a metabolite does not always lead to detox-ification; in fact, many agents are converted to more toxic substances. Carbon tetrachloride conversion to the trichloromethyl radical, methanol conversion to formaldehyde and formate, acetaminophen conversion to a reactive metabo-lite, and benzo(a)pyrene conversion to a diol epoxide represent only a small number of such examples. Activation of chemical substances by the metabolic systems in the animal usually leads to the production of an agent with greater water solubility and, therefore, one more readily excretable. On the other hand, some metabolites may be more active and may bind covalently (irre-versibly) to a critical cell constituents important for cell viability. An **active metabolite** of a xenobiotic is a product of metabolism that exerts a positive or negative effect on a biological system. A **reactive metabolite** formed from metabolic reactions is a substance that can react with cell constituents and can exert an irreversible and possibly lethal effect.

Transport of xenobiotics and metabolites within the organism occurs through the blood and lymphatic systems. Within the blood most substances have the capability of binding to blood proteins—primarily albumin—and, as such, may remain in storage where a potentially releasable pool may be avail-able for an extended period of time. Other sites of storage within the organism are also important. Lipid-soluble substances are distributed to tissues that have high concentrations of lipid, and some metals have specific sites of stor-age (e.g., lead in cancellous bone). Silent stores can serve as detoxifying sites in certain cases (such as with DDT) where lipid deposition in mammals gov-erns its very long half-life. Excretion may be through renal, biliary, or salivary routes or even through the sweat glands; however, the rate of excretion is usu-ally determined by biotransformation processes.

The toxic response (**toxicodynamic phase**) of a given xenobiotic can be specific or general. Substances that interfere with cellular energy production of the cell can be expected to exert toxicity in a generalized fashion through-out the animal. Such examples include cyanide, arsenic, and hydrogen sulfide. Agents with specific organ toxicities include carbon tetrachloride (liver), para-quat (lung), and cadmium (kidney).

Quantification of a toxic effect is determined by measuring the intensity of the effect versus the dose of a specific substance (the **graded dose-effect relationship**). Also, specific effects (such as death) within a given population can be recorded and related to the dose producing that effect (**quantal dose-effect relationship**). The LD_{50} is defined as the dose producing death in 50 percent of the population. This dose is often used to assess the toxicity and is determined in experimental animals. It provides a rough estimate of toxicity taken into consideration as part of the total and overall risk assessment of a substance. One of the most troublesome problems in risk assessment is relat-ing the toxicity of substances in experimental animals to humans.

Other considerations in determining the toxicity of a given substance in-clude the animal's age, sex, nutritional status, and species. Ionizing radiation is a much more serious consideration in the very young animal; perturbation of the pituitary-steroidogenic end-organ tissue relationship by steroid therapy is important in determining the the type of alteration of secondary sex characteristics brought on by therapy. Nutritional deficiency can enhance the effects of agents acting on biochemical pathways utilizing certain vitamin-dependent reactions.

HOUSEHOLD POISONS

Drugs and chemicals found in the home often serve as a source of poisoning for young children. Aspirin was once the most common intoxication seen in young children until the advent of special packaging for this type of medication. This is no longer a serious problem in childhood poisoning. However, many other medications that do not have child-proof containers may still be available. In addition, many household products contained in boxes or bottles often serve as a source of potential hazard. Cosmetics are usually readily available to a young child but do not serve as a serious problem, and only a small percentage of children who ingest cosmetics are hospitalized. Pesticides in or around the home are much more serious. Chlorinated pesticides are not usually a serious problem, but organophosphate pesticides can produce toxicity which is difficult to treat. The basis of organophosphate poisoning resulting in the inhibition of cholinesterases is described in Chapter 3. Carbamate insecticides act in a fashion similar to organophosphates.

Poisoning by petroleum products such as gasoline, kerosene, and furniture polish are some of the most difficult intoxications to treat. The viscosity of the petroleum product determines the type and seriousness of toxicity; there is an inverse relationship between viscosity of petroleum products and the degree of toxicity that they produce. These substances produce (1) mucous membrane irritation, (2) central nervous system (CNS) depression, and (3) severe pulmonary toxicity (chemical pneumonitis and pulmonary edema). When ingested, light petroleum products are often aspirated and pneumonias are seen as a serious complication with these substances. The treatment of such an intoxication should be handled with care, and it is recommended that no lavage procedures be employed. It is doubtful that emesis would be useful in such a situation, although it should be seriously considered with large overdoses or when other toxic agents may be present in the product.

Corrosive agents are commonly found in or around the home. Alkaline substances such as those used in dishwasher detergent and products designed to free drainage systems (Liquid-plumr, Drano, potassium hydroxide, sodium hydroxide, sodium hypochloride, and so on) produce severe damage to mucous membranes. These situations should be considered emergencies and should not be treated by lavage or emesis. Acidic substances such as those present in storage batteries, toilet bowl cleaners, and swimming pool cleaners are somewhat less dangerous and damaging than alkaline substances. These injuries should not be treated with emesis or lavage and often are managed with large volumes of water or milk in order to reduce the local and gastrointestinal corrosive attack. Every attempt should be made to prevent aspiration.

ENVIRONMENTAL TOXICOLOGY

Many thousands of chemicals are synthesized in large quantities in order to produce the many products that we have easy access to and that have made our lives comfortable. In addition, many products have been synthesized for selective toxic effects on animals and plants. A by-product of the chemical revolution promoting economical agricultural development is the increased burden of chemicals on the environment (ecosystem). A number of pesticides have proven to be less selective in their action than was hoped for. Thus, DDT was a very useful pesticide and an important preventative in diseases produced by insects. Substances such as DDT have a high level of persistence in the environment and have generally proven to be harmful to some segment of the ecosystem. **Biological magnification** occurs with DDT and other substances that are highly lipid soluble and highly resistant to biological decay. DDT has been demonstrated to accumulate in the food chain in a pyramidal fashion from plankton, to small bait fish, to ducks, and to the peregrine falcon with successive increases in concentration. This magnification of concentration has led to disturbances in the reproduction of the peregrine falcon (the peak of the pyramid), and it has undergone a radical diminution in numbers owing to the accumulation of DDT. DDT has been banned from usage in this country because of its harmful effects on these species and others. Polyhalogenated biphenyls also represent a class of chemicals that are highly lipid soluble, persist in the environment, and tend to accumulate in the food chain.

Biological toxification can also occur in the environment. Mercuric ion (Hg^{2+}) has been demonstrated to be converted to methyl mercury in rivers, lakes, and larger bodies of water. The methylation of mercury changes the substance to a highly lipid-soluble chemical that may undergo biological magnification in a fashion similar to that described for DDT.

Air Pollutants

Carbon Monoxide

Carbon moxoxide (CO) is a product of the incomplete combustion of carbon matter and constitutes the most prevalent contaminant in the environment—probably over 50 percent. Most of it is generated from automobile exhausts, with about 10 percent contributed from industrial waste. Carbon monoxide is also produced endogenously as a result of the catabolism of heme and may contribute as much as 1 percent of the carboxyhemoglobin normally present in human blood. Cigarette smoke is also another source of carbon monoxide, and heavy smokers may have as much as 5 percent of their hemoglobin as carboxyhemoglobin.

In addition to general contamination in the environment, carbon monoxide is a common and serious suicidal agent, its emission from automobile exhausts causing as much as 50 percent of all fatal poisonings. Carbon monoxide is an odorless gas that is extremely stable in the atmosphere and that can quickly serve as an intoxicant in situations when its concentration may increase rapidly. In addition to automotive exhausts, well-insulated homes that use fossil fuels or wood as a major source of heating can achieve high concentrations of carbon monoxide.

The mechanism of toxicity of carbon monoxide depends on its interaction with reduced hemoglobin (ferrous form). Carbon monoxide competes with oxygen for reduced hemoglobin and has an affinity approximately 240 times that of oxygen. Thus, 0.1 percent carbon monoxide in the atmosphere is equivalent to 21 percent oxygen and, at equilibrium, 50 percent of the hemoglobin in the blood can be saturated with carbon monoxide at 0.1 percent concentration in the air. Because of its interaction with hemoglobin, there is a reduced oxygen-carrying capacity of the blood. In addition, carbon monoxide produces a reduction of dissociation of oxygen from oxyhemoglobin and perturbs the oxyhemoglobin dissociation curve. An individual who ordinarily would survive with 50 percent hemoglobin saturated with oxygen in the absence of carbon monoxide would not survive for long in a case of carbon monoxide poisoning, in which 50 percent of hemoglobin is present as carboxyhemoglobin. Therefore, the decrease in releasability of oxygen from hemoglobin in carbon monoxide intoxication leads to a further and often lethal complication.

The major organ systems affected by carbon monoxide are the central nervous and cardiovascular systems. These vital systems possess a high rate of oxygen utilization and would be expected to be most sensitive to lack of oxygen. Therefore, common symptoms of carbon monoxide poisoning are most easily referable to the central nervous and cardiovascular systems. CNS effects range from confusion, headaches, and dizziness at 10 to 20 percent blood saturation to nausea, decreased vision, and coma with 30 to 50 percent blood saturation. Cardiovascular effects are associated with symptoms of disturbed cardiac rhythm, tachycardia, syncope, weak pulse, and cardiac depression. In addition, respiratory failure is seen at very high and prolonged exposure.

The first consideration in the treatment of carbon monoxide poisoning is removal of the individual from the environment, after which the administration of oxygen is mandatory. It has been demonstrated that the half-life of carboxyhemoglobin is about 250 minutes without treatment but decreases to about 40 minutes after the administration of 100 percent oxygen.

Cyanide

Carbon monoxide toxicity has been classified as an **anoxic anoxia** because of the decrease in the oxygen-carrying capacity of the blood produced by this substance. Several other agents such as **cyanide** (CN⁻) and **hydrogen sulfide** also perturb oxygen metabolism, but in another fashion. These substances interact with oxygen utilization through the inhibition of cytochrome oxidase activity. In contrast to carbon monoxide, which binds primarily to ferrous heme proteins, cyanide combines with ferric heme proteins. In its interaction with cytochrome oxidase, there is an inhibition of oxygen utilization and the development of a cellular anoxia (**histotoxic anoxia**). In this state the blood's oxygen-carrying capacity may be normal, and increased oxygen levels in the blood may even be observed. As with carbon monoxide intoxication, the cardiovascular and central nervous systems are most sensitive to the effects of cyanide.

The treatment of cyanide poisoning depends on (1) treatment with sodium thiosulfate and (2) conversion of hemoglobin to methemoglobin (ferric hemoglobin) with agents such as sodium nitrite. The administration of sodium thiosulfate takes advantage of the high level of the enzyme rhodanese in the liver, which is capable of detoxifying cyanide in a reaction yielding sodium thiocyanate, a substance that is much less toxic than cyanide and readily excretable by the kidney. The use of sodium nitrite to produce methemoglobin takes advantage of the conversion of hemoglobin to its ferric form. In this state cyanide can combine with a reservoir of ferric hemoglobin and thereby can allow for removal of a large quantity of cyanide that would otherwise gain tissue accessibility and produce toxicity in its combination with mitochondrial cytochromes.

Sulfur Oxides

Sulfur oxides (such as sulfur dioxide) are often termed "reducing gases" because in their interaction with aqueous systems they are converted to sulfuric or sulfurous acid. They produce serious irritation on contact with mucous membranes of the eyes and nasal mucosa. The primary source of gaseous sulfur oxides is usually the combustion of fossil fuels and emission from industrial sources that employ such fuels. Thus, coal, which contains a modest amount of sulfur, petroleum products, wood, or tobacco smoke may allow for the emission of sulfur gases. These gases have produced serious and extensive air pollution in the past when coal burning with high sulfur-containing coal was relatively common. Emissions from industrial settings today may play an important role in the generation of sulfur-containing gases, which may be deposited many hundreds or thousands of miles away through precipitation as "acid rain."

With respect to human intoxication, sulfur gases are quite water soluble, and more than 90 percent is absorbed at or above the larynx. While irritating, the sulfur gases or acids are relatively nontoxic compared with the nitrogen gases. Upon chronic exposure they lead to an alteration of the upper respiratory bronchi and bronchioles, increasing bronchial and bronchiolar constriction and the resistance of the pulmonary airway.

Nitrogen Oxides

The primary source of **nitrogen oxides** is automobile exhaust emissions. When gasoline or diesel fuels are burned, nitrogen gases are generated, which, if not properly controlled by automobile catalytic converters, can be emitted into the environment where they serve as a source of highly irritating oxidizing gases. The nitrogen gases exist in a number of oxidation states as a result of their interaction with atmospheric oxygen in the presence of ultraviolet light. Nitrogen dioxide (NO_2) may be converted to nitric oxide (NO), ozone (O_3), and atomic oxygen, which may then serve to participate in reactions catalyzed by ultraviolet light. This can lead to the oxidation of hydrocarbons emitted coincidentally, with the ultimate generation of active aldehydes (peroxyaldehydes) and ozone.

These oxidizing substances and gases can produce marked irritation and mucous membrane toxicity. The nitrogen gases are not readily soluble in water; they penetrate to alveolar sites and may produce toxicity in the lower respiratory tract. Thus, pulmonary edema is more commonly observed with the nitrogen gases than with sulfur gases. Nitrous oxides, ozone, aldehydes, and peroxyradicals make up the components of photochemical smog and may cause marked changes throughout the respiratory tract. For example, ozone is a major by-product of photochemical smog processes and is unstable, highly oxidant, and capable of producing pulmonary edema. Chronic exposure may lead to alteration of the respiratory system with the generation of alveolar membrane damage, damage to pulmonary macrophages, and chronic lung disease. A number of hydrocarbons are also usually present in photochemical smog and some of them are also highly active substances. It is possible that nitrogen-containing substances may also contribute to the "acid rain" phenomenon.

Halogenated Aromatic Compounds

A number of halogenated substances have been used in commerce or as pesticides and, because of their stability in the environment, pose a possible hazard. They have had a wide variety of uses and have been studied extensively recently. **Polychlorinated biphenyls** (PCBs) were produced from 1948 to 1973 in the United States because of their extreme stability to heat and oxidation. They were employed as insulation in electrical capacitors and for other purposes when insulation was necessary. They have an extremely long biological half-life and have accumulated in large bodies of water such as the Great Lakes and the Hudson River. Their toxicity was first discovered in Japan in 1968 when an epidemic due to the contamination of rice oil with PCBs was observed. The major symptoms noted were acne, spontaneous abortions, abnormal skin pigmentation, and a starvation-like syndrome. Since then numerous large-scale epidemics in animals have been observed. Symptoms relating to the reproductive system and the starvation syndrome have been noted. **Polybrominated biphenyls** (PBBs) were discovered to produce a marked starvation syndrome in intoxicated animals in Michigan in the early 1970s. Chickens and cattle were exposed to PBBs, and to this day a significant population of people in Michigan possess a high level of PBBs in their tissues. This substance is also highly persistent in nature and highly lipid soluble.

Dioxin (2,3,7,8-tetrachlorodibenzodioxin; TCDD) has received a great deal of attention because of its extremely toxic effects in certain animal species. This substance has been shown to be a powerful fetocide and produces a starvation syndrome in lower animals. It is present as a contaminant of many organic synthetic reactions involving chlorinated substances and may be present as a contaminant in numerous pesticides when care has not been taken to remove it. It has been claimed to be responsible for a number of the toxicities involving other chlorinated substances. Its toxicity (LD_{50}) in certain animal species is in the order of micrograms per kilogram.

Hexachlorobenzene is another chlorinated substance that has been used as a fungicide and preservative of seed grains. It has been demonstrated to produce a chemical porphyria because of its effect on the heme biosynthetic pathway. It exerts its action by decreasing uroporphyrinogen III decarboxylase activity.

Heavy Metals

Many metals are required for life but can also produce toxicity in overdoses. With metals such as iron, a fine balance exists between the amount needed for normal physiological function and that which may be toxic. On the other hand, numerous metals have no requirements for life and appear to be only adventitious. Lead and mercury are metals that have been demonstrated to represent important problems in toxicology. On the one hand, lead is commonly present in the earth's crust and its concentration in our environment has increased greatly in the last 100 years. Mercury, on the other hand, is an example of a metal that is not present at high levels in the environment but has been associated with several epidemics of enormous magnitude because of its accidental ingestion as a contaminant in food. These metals will be compared and contrasted with respect to the populations affected and their mechanisms of toxicity.

Lead

Lead is present in the environment at very high levels owing to its extensive use in industrial processing and to automotive emission. It is 16th in the order of abundance in the earth's crust and seventh in abundance in the human body. Sources of lead include storage batteries, solders, wiring, alloys, and pigments. It is found occasionally in pottery and in glazes for ceramics, and is concentrated in the soils along major roads and highways.

Lead is present in the body and in soil primarily as the inorganic salt and is not significantly alkylated in nature. Most of the lead that is absorbed into the animal organism enters *via* the gastrointestinal (GI) route. The amount of lead ingested daily is somewhere between 1 and 5 mg. Adults absorb about 10 percent of this amount and maintain a balance by excretion in the urine and feces. This daily source may come from dirt or may be leached from eating utensils or from lead-containing containers. Interestingly, children absorb about 40 percent of a given load presented to the GI tract. This may be especially important, as children are apt to ingest more dirt (pica) or paint chips derived from environments in which paint was applied prior to the regulation prohibiting lead pigments in paints. This appears to be the most common source of intoxication in children, although not all sources of lead have been identified. In adults, an often identified source of excessive lead ingestion is illicit liquor that has been processed through automobile radiators, in which a significant amount of lead is present in the solders making up the composition of the condensers. Soft water, or water containing an acid pH, is more likely to allow for lead extrusion from solders or piping that may contain lead. The water intake derived from such piping may contain considerably more lead than water that has a neutral pH or is alkaline. Except for certain industrial situations, such as in lead refining or mining, lead inhalation is usually not a significant problem. This is due to the fact that particles of lead derived from combustion procedures must be ≤0.5 microns in order to be significantly absorbed *via* the pulmonary route. Particles larger than 0.5 microns are generally carried from the respiratory tract to the larynx through ciliary action, and swallowed. Alkylated lead, which is an octane enhancer in gasoline, is rarely a source of significant intoxication.

The body burden of lead exists primarily (>90 percent) in hard bone. Considerable quantities can be absorbed and stored in bone before lead can cause damage to soft tissues. A sudden increase in concentration or release from hard bone can lead to a significant increase in concentration of lead in soft tissues such as the CNS, liver, or kidney. Teeth may also serve as a reservoir for lead, and it has been possible to use lead concentrations in deciduous teeth as a means for estimating the body burden of lead.

Lead exerts its effects on a number of organ systems, the most important one being the CNS. Young children who have a poorly developed blood-brain barrier and in whom an increase in the amount absorbed from the GI tract is observed are especially susceptible to the CNS effects of lead. Blood lead values of 30 μg per 100 ml of blood or greater represent a state of intoxication. There is a significant amount of information to suggest that this level may be too high for children and too low for adults. In a young child, headaches and vague complaints such as nausea and general lethargy are common. Toxic symptoms and signs observed with increasing concentrations of lead in the body range from ataxia to convulsions and vomiting, coma, and death. In adults, the CNS complaints are often more vague, and higher concentrations in the body are generally required before symptoms are observed.

Another system markedly affected by lead is the hematopoietic system (Fig. 18–1). Lead exerts a profound inhibition of the enzyme delta-aminolevulinic acid (ALA) dehydratase. At very low levels of lead in the blood (10 μg per dl of blood), a significant inhibition of erythrocytic ALA dehydratase has been demonstrated. This is an enzyme of the heme biosynthetic pathway, which catalyzes the conversion of ALA to porphobilinogen. Another enzyme of the heme biosynthetic pathway that appears to be affected by lead is ferrochelatase. This enzyme catalyzes the formation of heme from protoporphyrin

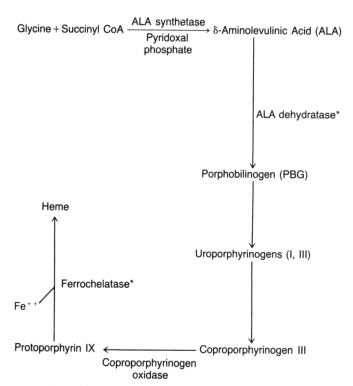

Figure 18–1. Effect of lead on heme biosynthesis (* = enzymes inhibited by lead).

IX and ferrous ion. Thus, it is possible to observe increases in ALA excretion in the urine, elevation of ALA in plasma, and increases in tissue levels of protoporphyrin IX in lead intoxication. Because protoporphyrin IX is relatively lipid soluble, it accumulates in erythrocytes and has been termed free erythrocyte porphyrin (FEP).

Heme is a critical prosthetic group for many enzymes that are necessary for life processes, and microcytic hypochromic anemias associated with lead poisoning are probably due to the inhibition of hemoglobin synthesis.

Gastrointestinal colic characterized by severe cramping abdominal pain is often reported in cases of severe lead poisoning. In addition, renal toxicity and certain endocrinopathies also have been observed in severe lead intoxication.

The treatment of lead poisoning is best accomplished by, first, removing the individual from the environmental setting. When signs and symptoms are not observed, this usually suffices to allow for the lead level in blood to decrease. When signs and symptoms are noted one should consider chelator therapy with agents such as calcium EDTA or BAL (dimercaptopropanol). Recently, it has been proposed to treat children with chelators even if overt symptoms are absent provided that blood lead values are at the intoxicating level.

Mercury

Whereas lead poisoning is commonly seen in young children and represents a relatively common intoxication, **mercury** intoxication is relatively rare except for sporadic episodes. Unfortunately, they have been major disasters. Methyl mercury poisoning in Japan and Iraq are examples of epidemics in which a large percentage of the population was affected, with disastrous results. In 1953, in Minamata Bay, mercury poisoning was discovered with a high population affected with CNS symptoms and signs. In Iraq in the early 1970s methyl mercury, which has been used as a seed grain protectant, was incorporated into flour and about 7,000 cases of poisoning occurred. This represents probably the largest toxicology epidemic in history. In Iraq, paresthesias were commonly seen and with more severe intoxication ataxia, visual changes, dysarthria, and hearing defects were observed. In this particular case, 10 percent of the affected population died and a large percentage of children born to intoxicated mothers demonstrated teratogenic effects.

Mercury has historically been an extremely valuable and useful metal. Metallic mercury (Hg°) has been used in laboratories and in industrial processes. It vaporizes at room temperature, and chronic exposure may lead to mercury poisoning. Metallic mercury absorbed across the alveolar membrane is rapidly metabolized to Hg^{2+}, and its toxicity is ascribed to the mercuric form. Mercurous mercury (Hg^+) is poorly absorbed across intact membranes and has very little effect because of its poor absorption into the animal organism. It is interesting that this form of mercury has been used for centuries in many medications for many diseases without producing any harm. Inorganic mercuric salts (Hg^{2+}) produce drastic effects on the GI tract. Once it is ingested it leads to marked GI sloughing and bloody diarrhea. That which is absorbed is transported to various tissues, especially the kidneys, where it binds and concentrates. It can produce CNS as well as renal toxicity.

Organic or alkylated mercuric salts have been a more serious source of toxicological problems. Methyl and other organic forms of mercury have been used as fungicides and employed as protectants of seed grains. When it has entered into the diets during periods of crop failures, it has produced devastating results. Occasionally, animal meat may contain methyl mercury if animals have been fed from grains treated with methyl mercury. Methyl mercury possesses properties that are quite different from the inorganic forms. It is relative lipid soluble and possesses a long biological half-life. It produces marked CNS and teratogenic effects. Thus, it may lead to paresthesias, sensory disturbances such as blindness, convulsions, and death. A large number of birth defects are seen in offspring from mothers intoxicated with methyl mercury.

Hg^{2+} exerts its toxicity as a result of its high affinity for sulfhydryl groups (-SH groups), which are necessary components of many important cell constituents, such as key enzymes of biochemical pathways. Mercury can also attack membranes where sulfhydryl groups may play important roles in cellular integrity.

There is no effective treatment of mercury intoxication. Chelating agents such as BAL have often been used without success. This may be because once mercuric ion or methyl mercuric ion has entered the system and has been distributed to the sites of toxicity and bound to important sulfhydryl groups, chelators cannot effectively remove the mercuric ion.

Asbestos

Asbestos is a tubular fibrous hydrated silicate with high levels of iron, magnesium, and zinc. Historically this substance has been considered as valuable as gold because of its unique properties of resisting fire and heat. It has been used for thousands of years as an insulator against fire and has been used extensively in concretes, paints, and pipe insulation.

Acute asbestos intoxication is characterized by a diffuse, non-nodular pulmonary fibrosis. This is relatively rare and can be prevented by appropriate masking. Chronic exposure to asbestos, however, has resulted in a number of serious problems. There is a significant association between exposure to asbestos and the occurrence of lung tumors and mesotheliomas. These neoplasms of the pleura and peritoneum occur 200 to 300 times more often in asbestos workers than in the general public. Also, there is an increase in incidence of GI tract cancers in a population of individuals who may have ingested asbestos over a long time period.

Because of the common environmental contamination of asbestos, extreme efforts are being made to remove it from general public exposure—especially in schools. Elimination of the source is the only possible management for potential toxicities resulting from exposures to asbestos.

ALIPHATIC ALCOHOLS

The low molecular weight alcohols are considered CNS depressants. The potency of CNS depression increases linearly with the length of the carbon chain so that methanol is the weakest in the series of C_1-C_4 alcohols; ethanol possesses twice the potency of methanol and n-butanol is twice as potent as ethanol. The alcohols have in common an ability to rapidly penetrate membranes and distribute to body water. Their disposition in the body through metabolism plays a major role in regulating their concentration in the animal organism as well as in governing their toxicity.

Methanol

Methanol ("wood alcohol") is widely used today. It is an important organic solvent contained in windshield cleaning fluid, duplicating machine fluids, and gasoline as an octane enhancer. As a source of energy it will probably enjoy increasing popularity. It is often added to ethanol as a denaturant.

Although methanol is the simplest of the alcohols, it is one of the most toxic because of its conversion to metabolic products that produce a characteristic poisoning syndrome in primates and in humans. Toxicity of methanol in humans is characterized by an initial mild CNS depression followed by a 12- to 24-hour latent period, during which time no signs or symptoms are noted. After this, there is marked metabolic acidosis and ocular toxicity. If untreated, marked CNS toxicity occurs with the resulting death of an individual in coma. It is not uncommon to find that it is possible to correct the metabolic acidosis and leave an individual permanently blind. This is understood by consideration of the role of metabolism in its toxicity.

Methanol poisoning is not seen in lower animals such as rats, rabbits, and guinea pigs. Studies in monkeys have demonstrated that the latent period observed following ingestion of methanol is a period of time during which compensated metabolic acidosis occurs with progressively increasing concentrations of formic acid in the blood and tissues and decreasing bicarbonate in the blood. Overt metabolic acidosis occurs with the exhaustion of blood bicarbonate and marked decreases in blood pH occur coincident with signs and symptoms of ocular toxicity. It is known that metabolic acidosis, in itself, does not produce ocular toxicity and that the blindness is due to the formic acid generated as a result of methanol metabolism. At physiological pH, formate has been demonstrated to produce ocular toxicity in primates. Lower animals such as rats and mice also metabolize methanol to formic acid but, in these species, formic acid metabolism to carbon dioxide proceeds much more rapidly than that seen in primates and humans. The accumulation of formic acid in blood and tissues in humans and primates accounts for the metabolic acidosis and blindness.

Methanol is rapidly absorbed from mucosal membranes and is uniformly distributed to body water. Its metabolism in monkeys and humans is carried out primarily in the liver through the catalysis of alcohol dehydrogenase (Fig. 18–2). Formaldehyde is formed as a result of the oxidation of methanol which, in turn, is rapidly metabolized to formate through either a specific hepatic formaldehyde dehydrogenase or aldehyde dehydrogenases present in the hepatic cell. Both formaldehyde and aldehyde dehydrogenases are NAD-dependent reactions.

The metabolism of formate to carbon dioxide is also carried out primarily in the liver. Formate is metabolized to carbon dioxide through a series of folate-dependent reactions whereby tetrahydrofolate and formate are converted to N^{10}-formyl tetrahydrofolate; this is subsequently metabolized to carbon dioxide through a formate dehydrogenase. Rates of formate metabolism to carbon dioxide are much lower in primates and in humans than in lower animals. This is due in part to a low hepatic tetrahydrofolate level and in part to decreased formyl tetrahydrofolate dehydrogenase activity. Lower animals appear to have higher hepatic tetrahydrofolate levels and a higher formate dehydrogenase activity. Studies have shown that, in monkeys, it is possible to protect or treat methanol-intoxicated animals with high doses of folate, which enhances the rate of metabolism of formate to carbon dioxide and reduces formate levels and prevents metabolic acidosis.

The treatment of human methanol poisoning depends upon reversing the metabolic acidosis and removing the methanol and formic acid from the body. Sodium bicarbonate administration restores the body bicarbonate, which has been depleted as a result of the accumulation of formic acid and reverses the metabolic acidosis. Hemodialysis is the best means available to remove methanol and formate rapidly from the body. Treatment should continue until blood levels less than 50 mg of methanol per 100 ml of blood are achieved. Because of the water solubility of methanol and formate, charcoal-filtering devices are not useful and, in fact, may hinder the hemodialysis procedure. It should be emphasized that elevated formaldehyde levels are never observed in methanol poisoning. In cases of formaldehyde poisoning it has been demonstrated that

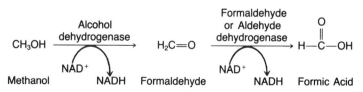

Figure 18–2. Metabolism of methanol.

there is an immediate and marked accumulation of formic acid in the blood along with an acute metabolic acidosis. Hemodialysis and bicarbonate have been useful in treating acute formaldehyde poisoning.

When hemodialysis is unavailable and when rapid therapy is required, ethanol has often been used as a treatment for methanol poisoning. Ethanol competes with methanol for hepatic alcohol dehydrogenase and, since ethanol has a much higher affinity for hepatic alcohol dehydrogenase, it inhibits the oxidation of methanol. However, ethanol is itself rapidly metabolized, and doses of ethanol should be employed to keep concentrations of ethanol at about 100 mg percent of blood until methanol blood levels are reduced to 50 mg per 100 ml of blood or below. This may take quite a long time, but it is necessary in order to prevent the oxidation of methanol. Ethanol is metabolized about 8 to 10 times faster than methanol.

The mechanism of blindness produced by formate is unknown; however, it is possible to correct the metabolic acidosis in some people and yet fail to prevent ocular toxicity. These individuals remain blind or have reduced vision for life. Correction of the metabolic acidosis does not remove formate. Every attempt to remove the formate should be made in order to preserve vision. Characteristically, in cases of methanol poisoning there is a marked optic disk edema similar to that seen in cases of acute increases in cerebrospinal fluid pressure. In methanol poisoning, however, cerebrospinal fluid pressure is not increased. Therefore, methanol poisoning is a unique chemotoxicity that is dramatically observed as a retinopathy.

Ethanol

Ethanol (ethyl alcohol, "alcohol"), though of little therapeutic value, is probably the most commonly used and abused chemical substance known. Unlike methanol and ethylene glycol, ethanol does not produce an acute toxicity, because its metabolic products, acetaldehyde and acetate, are fairly rapidly metabolized.

Ethanol is employed as an organic solvent, is added to gasoline to enhance octane, and is a significant component in wine, beer, ale, brandy, and whiskey. It can serve as a source of calories (8 calories per gram). It depresses the CNS in a concentration-dependent fashion.

Following ingestion, ethanol is rapidly and completely absorbed from the GI tract. The achievement of peak blood levels may be diminished if the stomach volume has been increased such as through the ingestion of liquids or food, but once absorbed, ethanol distributes uniformly to body water.

Metabolism

Ethanol appears to inhibit gluconeogenesis as a result of its metabolism in the liver. Inhibition of ethanol metabolism appears to decrease the accumulation of fat in the liver and prevents the inhibition of gluconeogenesis.

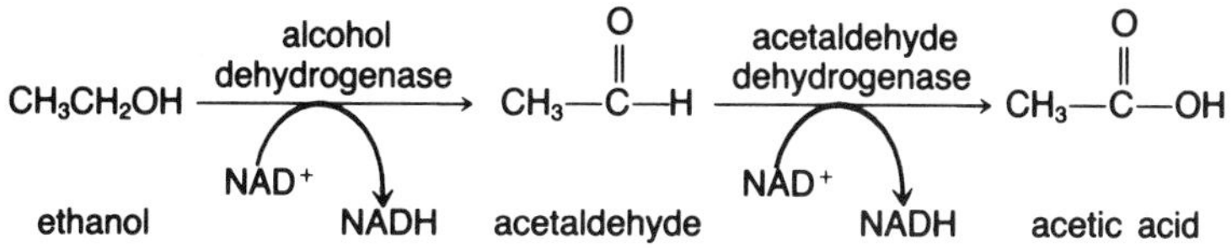

CH$_3$CH$_2$OH $\xrightarrow[\text{NAD}^+ \quad \text{NADH}]{\text{alcohol dehydrogenase}}$ CH$_3$—$\overset{\overset{\textstyle O}{\|}}{C}$—H $\xrightarrow[\text{NAD}^+ \quad \text{NADH}]{\text{acetaldehyde dehydrogenase}}$ CH$_3$—$\overset{\overset{\textstyle O}{\|}}{C}$—OH

ethanol   acetaldehyde   acetic acid

Figure 18–3. Metabolism of ethanol.

Ethanol is rapidly metabolized in the liver at rates of about 100 to 150 mg per kg per hour in humans. This is equivalent to about 7 grams of absolute alcohol or two-thirds ounce of 100-proof alcohol per hour. The rate of ethanol disappearance from the blood is approximately 15 mg per 100 ml of blood per hour. Thus, ethanol disappears by zero-order kinetics from the blood. This decrease in amount of ethanol from the blood with time is linear to approximately 10 mg per 100 ml of blood, at which time the rate of disappearance may be exponential. The rate-limiting step in ethanol metabolism in the liver is its conversion to acetaldehyde as catalyzed by alcohol dehydrogenase (Fig. 18–3). Although ethanol is rapidly metabolized to acetaldehyde, acetaldehyde is metabolized to acetate much faster than ethanol is metabolized to acetaldehyde. Acetaldehyde metabolism is carried out in the liver through acetaldehyde dehydrogenase, an NAD-dependent reaction. The acetate formed in this reaction is not metabolized primarily in the liver, and the bulk of acetate formed as a result of ethanol metabolism is converted to carbon dioxide *via* the Krebs cycle in extrahepatic organs. Thus, one would expect increases in acetate blood level following ethanol administration, and this has been demonstrated.

Acute Alcohol Intoxication

Concentrations achieved in the blood up to 50 mg percent will result in an impairment of visual activity; removal of inhibitions, usually resulting in inappropriate behavior; and production of a euphoric state. Blood concentrations higher than 50 mg percent may cause muscular incoordination characterized by impaired driving, hand unsteadiness, slurred speech, and imbalance. Generally, at levels of 100 mg percent or higher, sufficient impairment occurs that one is considered to be under the influence of alcohol if driving an automobile in most states in the United States. This concentration has been demonstrated to lead to objective deficits in function, muscular incoordination, and lengthened reaction time in greater than 99 percent of a given population. A marked increase in automobile accidents has been demonstrated in individuals at this blood level or higher. At concentrations higher than 200 mg percent an individual is usually severely affected. Anesthesia, followed by coma and death due to respiratory depression, can occur at blood concentrations of 400 to 500 mg percent. However, these blood levels are rarely reached, because an individual is usually unconscious well before achieving them. Often, an individual vomits at high blood levels; this allows for effective removal of a certain amount of ethanol from the body. The mechanism of action of ethanol on the CNS, though not well understood, may cause changes in the fluidity of neuronal lipid membranes; however, it is known that ethanol depresses also both excitatory and inhibitory synapse function and enhances presynaptic inhibition.

Tolerance

Tolerance to the central action of ethanol is well known. Naive individuals (nondrinkers) are much more sensitive to given concentrations of ethanol than are chronic alcoholics. Alcoholics probably possess some tolerance and may appear to be able to perform tasks better with the same blood level of alcohol than an individual who is naive to the substance. The mechanism of this type of tolerance is still unknown and is considered due to a "behavioral" tolerance. Although tolerance to its intoxicating effects does occur, tolerance that develops to its respiratory effects is minimal. Metabolic tolerance, although less common, may also be seen in certain individuals. In this case, the individual is able to metabolize ethanol faster.

Effects and Complications of Alcohol Abuse

The long-term heavy use of alcohol can lead to serious organ damage and central and peripheral neurological deficits, resulting in memory loss and psychotic behavior. Because the chronic ingestion of alcohol is often accompanied by poor dietary intake, severe nutritional deficiencies frequently result. Thiamin deficiency, common in chronic alcoholics, contributes to the development of Wernicke-Korsakoff syndrome. Other vitamin B deficiencies have also been described and are important in understanding the medical management of the chronic alcoholic.

Ethanol increases the production of saliva and gastric juices and may directly release gastrin as well as histamine in the stomach. Irritation of the gastric mucosa occurs, resulting in chronic gastritis. Acute ethanol ingestion produces peripheral vasodilation; chronic ingestion leads to cardiomyopathy with accompanying arrhythmias in about 10 percent of chronic alcoholics. Alcohol exerts a diuretic effect by suppressing the secretion of antidiuretic hormone from the pituitary. Recent evidence points to the production in children of alcoholic mothers of a fetal alcohol syndrome characterized by mental retardation, characteristic facial deformities, and a host of other developmental abnormalities related to disturbances of embryonic cell proliferation.

The liver is significantly affected by ethanol. At high blood alcohol levels there is an increase in fat concentration in the liver and at high doses (2 to 3 g per kg) there may be a release of catecholamines and subsequent mobilization of fatty acids from peripheral fat stores. A number of mechanisms have been offered to account for the increased fat in liver observed after chronic ingestion of ethanol. Increases in the synthesis of fat, decreased fatty acid oxidation, decreased secretion of lipids from the liver, and increased fatty acids delivered to the liver have all been demonstrated. Chronic alcoholics are subject to a hepatitis that may be due to either nutritional or genetic factors. Hepatitis is a major cause of death in chronic alcoholics, and liver cirrhosis is commonly seen in these individuals.

Inhibitors of acetaldehyde dehydrogenase such as disulfiram (Antabuse) have been used clinically in the treatment of chronic alcoholism. An individual treated with disulfiram accumulates acetaldehyde following the ingestion of ethanol, which, in turn, leads to facial flushing, headache, severe nausea, vomiting, and diarrhea. The rationale for the use of this therapy relies upon the development of an aversion to drinking alcohol because of the production of a toxic state. This treatment has been successful in a small percentage of the population of chronic alcoholics. There are other drugs commonly employed therapeutically that also are capable of inhibiting acetaldehyde metabolism and that may produce an acetaldehyde syndrome. One drug commonly associated with the production of an acetaldehyde is metronidazole. When toxicity is observed following the ingestion of ethanol, one must suspect that this agent or some similar substance inhibits acetaldehyde dehydrogenase.

Central Nervous System Alcohol Withdrawal Syndromes

Chronic ingestion of ethanol will lead to the development of physical dependence. In the physically dependent chronic alcoholic, abrupt or moderate withdrawal from alcohol leads to a series of autonomic and motor hyperactivity characterized by tremors, convulsions, and a disordered sense of perception (delirium tremens). This state of withdrawal has severe consequences if not treated. At this time, treatment with diazepam (Valium) or chlordiazepoxide (Librium) provides for adequate management and a low percentage of fatalities. Prior to the use of these agents, a 20 percent fatality rate was often observed in chronic alcoholics who experienced delirium tremens.

Ethylene Glycol

Ethylene glycol ($HOCH_2CH_2OH$) is the major component of "antifreeze" used in automobile radiators. Its toxicity is similar to methanol in that metabolic products of ethylene glycol are responsible for the toxicity seen in humans.

Characteristically, following the ingestion of ethylene glycol there is a CNS depression that may lead to marked sedation, weakness, coma, and death. After a short latent period there is a metabolic acidosis and renal toxicity that is not easily treated. Ethylene glycol is metabolized in the liver by alcohol dehydrogenase to glyoxal which, in turn, is rapidly metabolized to glycolic acid. Glycolic acid has been demonstrated to accumulate in humans owing to a low activity of glycolic acid oxidase. Thus, the metabolic acidosis observed is due to the accumulation of glycolic acid. Further metabolism of glycolic acid to oxalic acid leads to the kidney toxicity seen. Oxalic acid chelates calcium, and calcium oxalate formation in the kidney disrupts renal tubular function. It is not uncommon to observe a high concentration of precipitated calcium oxalate crystals in the kidneys of an individual intoxicated with ethylene glycol.

The treatment of ethylene glycol intoxication is difficult, but attempts are usually made to carry out hemodialysis in order to remove the ethylene glycol and glycolic acid. However, this treatment is not always successful if marked accumulation of oxalic acid has occurred and calcium oxalate crystals have already developed. Treatment with ethanol has also been employed in order to inhibit the metabolism of ethylene glycol through competition between ethanol and ethylene glycol for hepatic alcohol dehydrogenase.

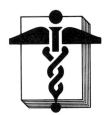

References

1. Reidenberg, MM: The discipline of clinical pharmacology. Clin Pharmacol Ther 38:2, 1985.
2. Rane, A: Basic principles of drug disposition and action in infants and children. In Yaffe, SJ (ed): Pediatric Pharmacology: Therapeutic Principles in Practice. Grune & Stratton, New York, 1981, p 70.
3. Williams, RL, and Mamelock, RD: Hepatic disease and drug pharmacokinetics. Clin Pharmacokinet 5:528, 1980.
4. Blaschke, TF: Protein binding and kinetics of drugs in liver diseases. Clin Pharmacokinet 2:32, 1977.
5. Branch, RA, Morgan, MH, James, J, and Read, AE: Intravenous administration of diazepam in patients with chronic liver disease. Gut 17:975, 1976.
6. Wilkinson, GR: Influences of liver disease on pharmacokinetics. In Evans, WE, Schentag, JJ, Jusko, WJ (eds): Applied Pharmacokinetics: Principles of Therapeutic Drug Monitoring. Applied Therapeutics, San Francisco, 1980, p 57.
7. Gibson, TP: Influence of renal disease on pharmacokinetics. In Evans, WE, Schentag, JJ, Jusko, WJ (eds): Applied Pharmacokinetics: Principles of Therapeutic Drug Monitoring. Applied Therapeutics, San Francisco, 1980, p 33.
8. Welling, GH, and Craig, WA: Pharmacokinetics in disease states modifying renal function. In Benet, LZ (ed): The Effect of Disease States on Drug Pharmacokinetics. American Pharmaceutical Association, Washington, DC, 1976, p 155.
9. Kunin, CM: A guide to use of antibiotics in patients with renal disease. Ann Intern Med 67:151, 1967.
10. Vessell, ES: Pharmacogenetics: Multiple interactions between genes and environment as determinants of drug response. Am J Med 66:183, 1979.
11. Ouslander, JG: Drug therapy in the elderly. Ann Int Med 95:711, 1981.
12. Steel, K, Gertman, PM, Crescenzi, C, and Anderson, J: Iatrogenic illness on a general medical service at a university hospital. N Engl J Med 304:638, 1981.
13. Venulet, J (ed): Assessing Causes of Adverse Drug Reactions. Academic Press, New York, 1982.
14. Spector, R (ed): The Scientific Basis of Clinical Pharmacology: Principles and Examples. Little, Brown & Co, Boston, 1986.
15. Miller, RR, and Greenblatt, DG: Drug Effects in Hospitalized Patients. John Wiley & Sons, New York, 1976.
16. Reynolds, JEF: Martindale: The Extra Pharmacopoeia, ed 28. Pharmaceutical Press, London, 1982.

17. Hutchinson, TA, et al: An algorithm for the operational assessment of adverse drug reactions. II. Demonstration of reproducibility and validity. JAMA 242:633, 1979.

18. Hutchinson, TA, et al: Reason for disagreement in the standardized assessment of suspected adverse drug reactions. Clin Pharmacol Ther 34:421, 1983.

19. Kramer, MS, Leventhal, JM, Hutchinson, TA, and Feinstein, AR: An algorithm for the operational assessment of adverse drug reactions. I. Background, description and instructions for use. JAMA 242:623, 1979.

20. Dukes, MNG: Meyler's Side Effects of Drugs, ed 10. Excerpta Medica, Amsterdam, 1984.

21. Davies, DM: Textbook of Adverse Drug Reactions, ed 2. Oxford University Press, New York, 1981.

22. Kelner, MJ, and Bailey, DN: Propylene glycol as a cause of lactic acidosis. J Anal Toxicol 9:40, 1985.

23. Griffin, JP, and Darcy, PF: A Manual of Adverse Drug Interactions, ed 2. J Wright, Guildford, England, 1979.

24. Hansten, PD: Drug Interactions: Clinical Significance of Drug-Drug Interactions and Drug Effects on Clinical Laboratory Results, ed 4. Lea & Febiger, Philadelphia, 1979.

25. Bochner, F, Hooper, WD, Tryer, JH, and Eadie, MJ: The cause of an outbreak of phenytoin intoxication. J Neurol Sci 16:481, 1972.

26. Sedman, AJ: Cimetidine-drug interactions. Am J Med 76:109, 1984.

27. Goodman, LS, and Gilman, AG (eds): Goodman and Gilman's The Pharmacological Basis of Therapeutics, ed 7. Macmillan, New York, 1985, p 392.

28. Stewart, GT: Allergy to penicillin and related antibiotics: Antigenic and immunochemical mechanism. Ann Rev Pharmacol 13:309, 1973.

29. Sullivan, TJ, et al: Skin testing to detect penicillin allergy. J Allergy Clin Immunol 68:171, 1981.

30. Spector, R: Avoidance of drug toxicity. In Spector, R, et al: The Scientific Basis of Clinical Pharmacology. Little, Brown & Co, Boston, 1986, pp 483–484.

31. The choice of antimicrobial drugs. Med Letter 30:33–40, 1988.

32. Drugs for parasitic infections. Med Letter 30:15–24, 1988.

33. Brumfitt, W: In Williams, JD (ed): Antibiotic Interactions. Academic Press, London, 1979, p 177.

34. Weinstein, L: The complications of antibiotics therapy. Bull NY Acad Med 31:500–518, 1954.

35. Sande, MA, and Mandell, GL: Antimicrobial agents: General considerations. In Goodman, AG, et al (eds): The Pharmacological Basis of Therapeutics, ed 7. Macmillan, New York, 1985, p 1089.

36. Ibid, p 1090.

37. Kunin, CM, et al: Use of antibiotics: A brief exposition of the problem and some tentative solutions. Ann Int Med 79:555–560, 1973.

38. Sande, MA, and Mandell, GL, op cit, p 1092.

39. Price, HL: A dynamic concept of the distribution of thiopental in the human body. Anesthesiology 21:40–45, 1960.

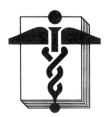

Bibliography

Abramowicz, M (ed): Medical Letter, New Rochelle, NY, 1984.

Calve, D, Chase, TN, and Barbeau, A (eds): Advances in Neurology: Dopaminergic Mechanisms. Vol 9. Raven Press, New York, 1975.

Churchill-Davidson, HC (ed): A Practice of Anesthesia, ed 5. Lloyd-Luke, London, 1984.

Crooke, ST, and Prestayko, AW: Cancer and Chemotherapy. Vol III. Academic Press, New York, 1981.

Cuddy, PG, et al: Acute drug intoxication. Emerg Dec 10:25, 1986.

D'Amoto, RJ, Lipman, ZP, and Snyder, SH: Selectivity of the parkinsonian neurotoxin MPTP. Science 231:987, 1986.

DeGroot, LJ (ed): Endocrinology, vol 2, ed 2. Saunders, Orlando, 1988.

Dripps, RD, Eckenhoff, JE, and Vandem, LD: Introduction to Anesthesia: The Principles of Safe Practice, ed 6. WB Saunders, Philadelphia, 1982.

Eger, EI: Anesthetic Uptake and Action. Williams & Wilkins, Baltimore, 1974.

Fariello, RG, et al: Neurotransmitters, Seizures, and Epilepsy II. Raven Press, New York, 1984.

Fields, HL, Dubner, R, and Cervero, F (eds): Advances in Pain Research and Therapy, Vol 9. Raven Press, New York, 1985.

Foley, KM, and Inturrisi, CE (eds): Opioid Analgesics in the Management of Clinical Pain. Raven Press, New York, 1986.

George, R, et al (eds): Annual Review of Pharmacology and Toxicology. Annual Reviews, Palo Alto (various years).

Goodhart, RS, and Shils, ME (eds): Modern Nutrition in Health and Disease. Lea & Febiger, Philadelphia, 1980.

Goodman, AG, et al (eds): The Pharmacological Basis of Therapeutics, ed 7 (and earlier editions). Macmillan, New York, 1985.

Goth, A (ed): Medical Pharmacology, ed 11 (and earlier editions). CV Mosby, St Louis, 1984.

Guzé, BH, and Baxter, LR, Jr: Neuroleptic malignant syndrome. N Engl J Med 313:163, 1985.

Hollister, LE: Drug abuse in the United States: The past decade. Drug Alcohol Depend 11:49, 1983.

Jeste, DV, and Wyatt, RJ: Dogma disputed: Is tardive dyskinesia due to postsynaptic dopamine receptor supersensitivity? J Clin Psychiatr 42:455, 1981.

Katzung, BG (ed): Basic and Clinical Pharmacology, ed 3. Appleton & Lange, Norwalk, CT, 1987 (and earlier editions, as well as antecedent Medical Pharmacology by Meyers, FH, et al).

Mathé, G, Bonadonna, G, and Salmon, S (eds): Adjuvant Therapies of Cancer. Springer-Verlag, Berlin and New York, 1982.

471

Miller, GW: Foundations of addictionology. NJ Fam Phys 3:6, Winter 1986.

Morgan, JP: Alcohol and drug abuse curriculum guide for pharmacology faculty. US Dept Health Hum Serv 5:1, 1985.

Olson, GA, et al: Endogenous opiates: 1982. Peptides 4:563, 1983.

Perry, MC, and Yarbro, JW: Toxicity of Chemotherapy. Grune & Stratton, Orlando, 1984.

Perry, PJ: Assessment of addiction liability of benzodiazepines and buspirone. Drug Intell Clin Pharm 19:657, 1985.

Picker, D, et al: Neurolept-induced decrease in plasma homovannilic acid and antipsychotic activity in schizophrenic patients. Science 225:954, 1984.

Pratt, WB: Chemotherapy of Infection. Oxford University Press, New York, 1977.

Pratt, WB, and Ruddon, RW: The Anticancer Drugs. Oxford University Press, New York and Oxford, 1979.

Pratt, WB, and Tekety, R: The Antimicrobial Drugs. Oxford University Press, New York, 1985.

Schmitt, FO, and Worden, FG (eds): The Neurosciences: Third Study Program. MIT Press, Cambridge, MA, 1974.

Siegel, RK: Treatment of cocaine abuse: Historical and contemporary perspectives. J Psychoactive Drugs 17(1):1, 1985.

Skipper, HE, Schabel, FM, and Wilcox, WS: Cancer Chemother Reps 35:1, 1964.

Skipper, HE: Cancer chemotherapy is many things: GH Clowes memorial lecture. Cancer Res 31:1173, 1971.

Sugrue, MF: Do antidepressants possess a common mechanism of action? Biochem Pharmacol 32:1811, 1983.

Sulser, F, Vetulani, J, and Mobley, PL: On the mode of action of antidepressant drugs. Biochem Pharmacol 27:257, 1978.

Wei, ET: Enkaphalin analogs and physical dependence. J Pharmacol Exp Ther 216(1):12, 1981.

Williams, JD (ed): Antibiotic Interactions. Academic Press, London, 1979.

Williams, RH: Textbook of Endocrinology, ed 6. WB Saunders, Philadelphia, 1981.

Yates, WR: The National Institute of Mental Health Epidemiology Study: Implications for family practice. J Fam Pract 22(3):251, 1986.

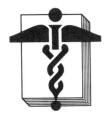

Review Questions

WILLIAM R. HUCKLE, TIMOTHY J. NESS

Answers are [A]: 1 and 3 are correct
     [B]: 2 and 4 are correct
     [C]: 1, 2, and 3 are correct
     [D]: 4 is correct
     [E]: All are correct

SECTION I
Fundamental Principles

Chapter 1

1. A competitive pharmacological antagonist acts by
   (1) activation of different receptors than does an agonist.
   (2) decreasing the affinity of the receptor for an agonist.
   (3) activation of the same receptor as does an agonist.
   (4) blockade of agonist interaction with its receptor.

2. A drug that is acid-labile or subject to extensive "first-pass" metabolism would probably not be a good candidate for
   (1) intravenous administration.
   (2) sublingual administration.
   (3) intra-arterial administration.
   (4) oral administration.

3. Renal reabsorption of a drug that is _____ will be favored by _____ the pH of the urine.
   (1) a weak base; decreasing
   (2) a weak acid; decreasing
   (3) a weak acid; increasing
   (4) a weak base; increasing

4. For a drug that shows extensive binding to plasma proteins, impaired hepatic function would most likely result in

473

(1) increased renal filtration of the drug.
(2) increased half-life of the drug in the body.
(3) increased free plasma concentration of the drug.
(4) increased active secretion of the drug.

5. Prolonged administration of phenobarbital (which induces drug-metabolizing enzymes) in combination with Drug B may result in
(1) decreased effectiveness of Drug B.
(2) increased effectiveness of Drug B.
(3) no change in the effectiveness of Drug B.
(4) altered patterns of metabolites produced from Drug B.

Chapter 2

1. Prior to FDA approval of a new drug, which of the following must be characterized and reported?
(1) clinical efficacy
(2) therapeutic and toxic dose ranges
(3) overt toxicities
(4) production and quality control procedures

2. Under current FDA drug approval procedures, which of the following characteristics is/are most difficult to identify?
(1) long-term toxic effects
(2) pharmacokinetic parameters
(3) harmful drug-drug interactions
(4) chemical composition

3. Pharmaceutical preparations that are chemically equivalent but differ in bioavailability do not exhibit
(1) chemotherapeutic equivalence.
(2) identical pharmacokinetics.
(3) bioequivalence.
(4) pharmaceutical equivalence.

4. For a drug that is largely excreted in the urine, dosage requirements may depend on
(1) prior exposure to aminoglycosides.
(2) glomerular filtration rate.
(3) pulmonary function.
(4) cardiac output.

5. Isoniazid-induced liver damage is associated primarily with
(1) hemoglobin oxidation.
(2) age-related differences.
(3) dietary deficiencies.
(4) genetic differences in rates of drug metabolism.

Chapter 3

1. Which of the following types of adverse drug reactions would be least likely to occur immediately following the **first** administration of a drug?
   (1) pharmacological (toxic)
   (2) overdose-related
   (3) genetics-related
   (4) allergic

2. After an FDA-approved drug has been in use in humans for a period of time, which of the following assessments of drug reactions becomes possible?
   (1) voluntary reporting by physicians
   (2) statistical analysis of epidemiological data
   (3) case-control studies
   (4) FDA-required drug trials

3. The standard assessment of causality (SAC) algorithm given in Table 3–7 would allow a clinician to
   (1) take into consideration a wide variety of clinical information.
   (2) predict with certainty the adverse effects of a drug prior to its administration.
   (3) integrate what is known about reactions to a given drug into a patient's unique history.
   (4) unambiguously ascribe causality for a given drug reaction.

4. Cardiac arrhythmias or heart block are frequently associated with which of the following drugs?
   (1) morphine
   (2) aspirin
   (3) gentamicin
   (4) digitalis

5. An example of an antagonistic drug-drug interaction is
   (1) alcohol + phenobarbital.
   (2) naloxone + morphine.
   (3) lithium + thiazides.
   (4) vitamin K + warfarin.

SECTION II
Pharmacology Related to the Nervous System

Chapter 4

1. Which of the following factors often frustrate attempts to modify specific peripheral nervous system functions by chemical intervention?

(1) While subclasses of receptor type have been delineated (e.g., $\alpha_{1,2}$- and $\beta_{1,2}$-adrenergic), potential drugs often show activity at more than one receptor type.

(2) A given receptor type can occur on a number of tissues; thus, a drug activating these receptors can have numerous effects.

(3) Reflex arcs exist that are capable of rapidly counteracting the effects of peripherally active drugs.

(4) All peripherally active drugs can cross the blood-brain barrier equally well, thereby causing central nervous sytem effects.

2. Which of the following agents would have the effect of activating a muscarinic cholinergic synapse?
   (1) physostigmine
   (2) atropine
   (3) carbachol
   (4) pralidoxine

3. Which of the following agents would have the effect of activating an α-adrenergic synapse?
   (1) cocaine
   (2) tyramine
   (3) phenylephrine
   (4) isoproterenol

4. Propranolol and metoprolol are thought to reduce blood pressure by
   (1) decreasing renal (DA_1) blood flow.
   (2) dilating (α_1) vessels in the skin and viscera.
   (3) activating parasympathetic (muscarinic) drive to the heart.
   (4) blocking sympathetic (β_1) drive to the heart.

5. Which of the following agents might be used to restore function at the neuromuscular junction in myasthenia gravis?
   (1) curare
   (2) chlorisondamine
   (3) succinylcholine
   (4) neostigmine

6. The parasympathetic nervous system
   (1) can be highly localized in function (e.g., act on a single organ such as the heart).
   (2) uses acetylcholine as a preganglionic neurotransmitter; hence, some (anti)cholinergic drugs affect its ganglionic transmission.
   (3) uses acetylcholine as a postganglionic neurotransmitter; hence, some (anti)cholinergic drugs affect its postganglionic transmission.
   (4) has its postganglionic cell bodies primarily in the thoracolumbar system of paraganglia.

7. The sympathetic nervous system
   (1) generally acts as an integrated system—when one part is activated, all parts may be affected.
   (2) uses noradrenaline as a preganglionic neurotransmitter; hence, adrenergic drugs will affect sympathetic ganglionic transmission.
   (3) has a great amplification (50×) of signal from the preganglionic stage to the postganglionic stage.
   (4) postdenervation does not exhibit postganglionic supersensitivity.

8. Acetylcholine acts at
   (1) A_1 and A_2 purinergic receptors.
   (2) nicotinic and muscarinic receptors.
   (3) α_1, β_2, and DA_1 receptors.
   (4) the neuromuscular junction.

9. To limit the effects of the parasympathetic nervous system on the GI tract one could administer
   (1) the acetylcholinesterase inhibitor physostigmine.
   (2) the nicotinic antagonist hexamethonium.
   (3) the muscarinic agonist pilocarpine.
   (4) the muscarinic antagonist atropine.

10. To increase heart rate, one could
   (1) administer the muscarinic antagonist atropine to remove vagal tone.
   (2) administer propranolol to activate β_2 adrenoceptors.
   (3) administer isoproterenol to activate β_1 adrenoceptors.
   (4) administer phenylephrine to activate α_1 adrenoceptors.

11. Dopamine can act
   (1) peripherally to cause vasodilation of the renal and mesenteric arteries *via* DA_1 receptors.
   (2) peripherally, to increase heart rate *via* β_1 adrenoceptors.
   (3) centrally, to modulate motor function.
   (4) centrally, to modulate affective behavior.

12. Tyramine
   (1) is an indirect-acting sympathomimetic.
   (2) is found in relatively high quantities in certain cheeses and wines.
   (3) can cause a hypertensive crisis in patients taking MAO inhibitors.
   (4) like ephedrine, may demonstrate tachyphylaxis, a quickly reduced response to repeated administration of the drug.

13. Inhibitors of acetylcholinesterase
   (1) will partially reverse the effects of competitive neuromuscular junction blockers such as curare.
   (2) can act as nerve gases or poison pills causing respiratory paralysis and consequent death.

(3) are used as insecticides; hence, anticholinergic drugs can be effective in the treatment of toxic doses of insecticides.

(4) can reverse the effects of neurotransmitter depletors such as reserpine.

Chapter 5

1. Barbiturates, but not benzodiazepines,
   (1) are general CNS depressants.
   (2) enhance membrane hyperpolarization at the GABA-associated Cl^- ionophore.
   (3) are potent inducers of hepatic drug-metabolizing enzymes.
   (4) produce tolerance and physical dependence.

2. Which of the following are correctly matched?
   (1) status epilepticus; diazepam
   (2) absence seizures; ethosuximide
   (3) grand mal seizures; primidone
   (4) reduced Na^+ and Ca^{2+} fluxes; phenytoin

3. It is thought that development of tardive dyskinesias by antipsychotic drugs reflects
   (1) blockade of dopamine receptors in the limbic system.
   (2) supersensitivity of dopamine receptors in the basal ganglia.
   (3) activation of dopamine receptors in the limbic system.
   (4) the existence of similar drug receptors in different brain regions.

4. The peripheral effects of chlorpromazine include
   (1) hypotension.
   (2) decreases in gastric motility.
   (3) blockade of multiple receptor types.
   (4) mydriasis.

5. Which of the following result from co-administration of L-dopa with the peripheral decarboxylation inhibitor carbidopa?
   (1) Peripheral metabolism of L-dopa is inhibited, such that effective CNS concentrations can be attained with a lower administered dose.
   (2) CNS side effects (abnormal movements, impaired mental status) are diminished.
   (3) Nausea and vomiting side effects are diminished.
   (4) CNS decarboxylation of L-dopa is inhibited.

6. Which of the following currently available therapies for movement disorders can be considered to stop the progression of the disease?
   (1) Parkinson's disease; L-dopa
   (2) Huntington's chorea; phenothiazines

(3) Tourette's syndrome; haloperidol

(4) Wilson's disease; penicillamine

7. Which of the following are significant effects of tricyclic antidepressants?
   (1) tardive dyskinesia
   (2) hypotension *via* peripheral α_1-adrenoceptor blockade
   (3) general CNS stimulation
   (4) increased activity at biogenic amine synapses *via* blockade of serotonin and norepinephrine reuptake

8. Which of the following are correctly matched?
   (1) phenelzine; hepatotoxicity
   (2) lithium; manic phase of bipolar affective disorders
   (3) lithium; relatively low therapeutic index
   (4) benzodiazpines; relatively low therapeutic index

9. Which of the following CNS stimulants is/are used in the treatment of narcolepsy?
   (1) methylphenidate
   (2) theophylline
   (3) pentylenetetrazole
   (4) amphetamine

10. Which of the following must be considered in the treatment of acute opioid intoxication?
    (1) Withdrawal symptoms may be precipitated by naloxone.
    (2) Naloxone is effective only for intoxication mediated by κ opioid receptors.
    (3) Naloxone has a shorter half-life than many pure opioid agonists.
    (4) Naloxone exhibits partial opioid agonist activity.

11. Benzodiazepines are used as
    (1) anxiolytics.
    (2) sedative hypnotics.
    (3) anticonvulsants.
    (4) muscle relaxants.

12. Drugs which are thought to act as CNS depressants by acting *via* GABAergic mechanisms include
    (1) bicuculline.
    (2) benzodiazepines.
    (3) picrotoxin.
    (4) barbiturates.

13. Drugs with low therapeutic indices, indicating that the toxic dose of the drug is near the effective dose, include

(1) benzodiazepines.
(2) barbiturates.
(3) furosemide.
(4) cardiac glycosides.

14. Because the drug triazolam is a rapidly metabolized benzodiazepine, the following side effects are sometimes seen:
    (1) prolonged respiratory depression
    (2) "rebound" anxiety
    (3) increased lipid solubility of the parent compound
    (4) early morning insomnia

15. Barbiturates
    (1) radically alter sleep patterns (decrease sleep latency and REM activity).
    (2) have a high therapeutic index.
    (3) cause dispositional tolerance to a variety of drugs by inducing hepatic microsomal drug-metabolizing enzymes.
    (4) are the drugs used in cases of pediatric or geriatric pain.

16. Most effective antipsychotics (e.g., chlorpromazine, haloperidol)
    (1) are "clean" drugs acting almost exclusively as dopamine antagonists.
    (2) have relatively high therapeutic indices.
    (3) can have major motor side effects but rarely affect the cardiovascular system.
    (4) often produce the side effect of tardive dyskinesia after prolonged use.

17. Tricyclic antidepressants
    (1) cause a generalized CNS stimulation.
    (2) cause increases in CNS adrenergic/serotonergic activity.
    (3) are "clean" drugs without the muscarinic cholinergic activity seen with the antipsychotics.
    (4) profoundly affect the autonomic nervous system and cardiovascular systems.

18. Postural hypotension can be a major side effect of
    (1) MAO inhibitors.
    (2) tricyclic antidepressants.
    (3) systemic vasodilators.
    (4) methyl xanthines.

19. When administering an opioid analgesic, one should be concerned with the following effects of the drug:
    (1) respiratory and gonadotrophin secretion depression
    (2) production of nausea

(3) increased tone in the gastrointestinal tract causing colic
(4) chronic pupillary dilation

20. Tolerance/dependence to the effects of narcotics
    (1) is defined by signs of withdrawal (salivation, lacrimation, perspiration, diarrhea).
    (2) leads to insufficient pain control.
    (3) develops in normal patients.
    (4) often leads to behavior interpreted as "drug craving."

21. Compared with morphine, methadone
    (1) is better for chronic pain control (e.g., with cancer) because of a higher efficacy.
    (2) acts more specifically at receptor subtypes involved in pain control and less at subtypes involved with euphoria.
    (3) is an antagonist at some opioid receptors.
    (4) is more readily absorbed from the gastrointestinal tract.

Chapter 6

1. Administration of which one(s) of the following would precipitate withdrawal symptoms in someone dependent upon heroin?
   (1) methadone
   (2) clonidine
   (3) meperidine
   (4) naloxone

2. Which one(s) of the following have actions described as sympathomimetic?
   (1) amphetamine
   (2) cocaine
   (3) isoproterenol
   (4) thiopental

3. Of the following, all but which one(s) can produce a state of euphoria?
   (1) diazepam
   (2) morphine
   (3) mescaline
   (4) fenfluramine

4. Substitute chemotherapy is appropriate for someone dependent upon which of the following drugs?
   (1) phenobarbital
   (2) diazepam
   (3) heroin
   (4) oxycodone

Chapter 7

1. Lidocaine has strong excitable membrane stabilizing effects. Because of this it is useful
   (1) in the acute treatment of arrhythmias.
   (2) in the chronic control of seizures.
   (3) as a local topical or infiltration anesthetic.
   (4) as a muscle relaxant, acting solely by directing stabilizing muscle cell membranes.

2. Use of a vasoconstrictor such as epinephrine mixed with lidocaine
   (1) results in selective cell death of excitable tissues.
   (2) can lead to tachycardia if the solution is too quickly absorbed.
   (3) is only used in emergency situations to stop arrhythmias.
   (4) allows for prolonged local action of the anesthetic by reducing absorption of the drug.

3. Lidocaine can
   (1) lead to convulsions.
   (2) lead to cardiovascular and respiratory collapse.
   (3) cause allergic reactions.
   (4) control arrhythmias.

Chapter 8

1. Inhalational anesthetics are absorbed through the respiratory system; hence, the rate at which the anesthetic builds up within the body is dependent upon
   (1) the minute volume of the ventilation.
   (2) the blood-gas coefficient of the anesthetic.
   (3) the rate of redistribution of the anesthetic from the blood to other tissues.
   (4) the concentration of the anesthetic in the respired air.

2. The minimum alveolar concentration (MAC) for an inhalational anesthetic is the concentration of inspired anesthetic producing inhibition of responses to noxious stimuli in 50 percent of the subjects tested. The MAC
   (1) is therefore the ED_{50} for a given anesthetic for inhibition of responses to noxious stimuli.
   (2) is independent of the specific anesthetic agent being used.
   (3) is greater than 100 percent for nitrous oxide at atmospheric pressure.
   (4) is the amount of anesthetic that should be used in all patients.

3. Halothane, an inhalational anesthetic, affects tissues other than nervous tissue. These effects include

(1) dose-dependent depression of the heart.
(2) sensitization of the myocardium to circulating catecholamines.
(3) hepatotoxicity.
(4) relaxation of uterine muscle.

4. Problems involved with certain inhalational anesthetics include
   (1) increases in air-containing spaces within the body (e.g., with pneumothoraxes and pneumoencephalography).
   (2) diffusion hypoxia.
   (3) increased intracranial pressure.
   (4) inability to quickly alter anesthetic concentrations.

5. Short-acting intravenously administered anesthetics include the following:
   (1) ketamine
   (2) ethylhexitol
   (3) thiopental
   (4) methomidate

SECTION III
Pharmacology Related to Other Major Organ Systems

Chapter 9

1. The pharmacological treatment of hypertension has several strategies. Drugs used for control of hypertension include
   (1) direct-acting vasodilators.
   (2) inhibitors of sympathetic nervous system outflow.
   (3) inhibitors of the renin/angiotensin system.
   (4) diuretics.

2. Sympathetic outflow can be modulated by
   (1) agents acting within the central nervous system that modulate the generation of tonic vascular tone.
   (2) ganglionic blockers (nicotinic cholinergic antagonists).
   (3) agents acting to deplete nerve terminals of norepinephrine.
   (4) agents such as antidepressants.

3. Antianginal agents are thought to act in part by decreasing the work of the heart, thereby reducing the myocardial oxygen requirement. Drugs that do this include
   (1) β-adrenergic antagonists.
   (2) calcium antagonists (channel blockers).
   (3) vasodilators such as the organonitrates (e.g., nitroglycerin).
   (4) cardiac glycosides.

4. Arrhythmias occur with the destabilization of certain excitable membranes within the heart. Hence, the following drugs that act to stabilize membranes can be effective in the treatment of arrhythmias:
   (1) phenytoin
   (2) lidocaine
   (3) bretylium
   (4) organonitrates

5. The cardiac glycosides
   (1) have low therapeutic indices and hence may only be beneficial to a small group of patients suffering from congestive heart failure.
   (2) experimentally cause increased contractility of the heart and increased parasympathetic tone.
   (3) have as their presumed mechanism of beneficial action inhibition of the Na^+ -K^+ ATPase ionic pump, resulting eventually in increased intracellular cardiac Ca^{2+} levels, which leads to increased strength of contraction.
   (4) have as their presumed mechanism of toxic action inhibition of the Na^+ -K^+ ATPase, leading to depression of the excitability of cardiac and neuronal membranes.

Chapter 10

1. Thiazide diuretics decrease the plasma concentration of potassium ions;
   (1) hence, patients subject to arrhythmias may require a different diuretic.
   (2) hence, the increase in potassium excretion is what causes a lowering of blood pressure.
   (3) therefore, ingestion of foods rich in potassium (oranges, bananas, prunes) or potassium supplements is suggested.
   (4) and so, if one were to give a potassium-sparing diuretic agent, it would block the diuretic effects of the thiazides.

2. A patient has gout. Reasonable therapeutic measures would be to
   (1) discontinue probenecid treatment.
   (2) take the patient off thiazide diuretics.
   (3) acidify the urine.
   (4) treat the patient with allopurinol.

3. Loop diuretics are thought to act by inhibiting the co-transport of Na^+ and Cl^- in the loop of Henle and by increasing renal blood flow *via* a prostanoid mechanism. Hence,
   (1) the use of nonsteroidal anti-inflammatory agents might be contraindicated when a patient is taking furosemide.
   (2) a contraction acidosis occurs as Na^+ and Cl^- and water are excreted, but bicarbonate is left behind.

(3) what likely occurs is a washout of the osmotic gradient of the kidney, which allows urine to become concentrated.

(4) infarcts of the kidney are more likely to occur with the use of loop diuretics.

4. A patient's hearing is affected following institution of a new drug therapy. Drugs that may have affected the patient's hearing include
   (1) loop diuretics.
   (2) aminoglycoside antibiotics.
   (3) aspirin.
   (4) β-adrenergic blockers.

5. As compared to thiazides, loop diuretics are
   (1) not as effective in treating pulmonary edema.
   (2) useful in the treatment of hypercalcemia.
   (3) more effective as an antihypertensive.
   (4) more efficacious as a natriuretic.

6. Long-term use of the potassium-sparing diuretic, spironolactone, is contraindicated because
   (1) muscle hypertrophy occurs with increased potassium levels.
   (2) it is potentially carcinogenic.
   (3) owing to its lipophilicity, it must be given parentally.
   (4) it has weak androgenic activity leading to masculinization of children and females and feminization of adult males.

7. Primary uses of diuretics include
   (1) the treatment of hypertension.
   (2) reduction of edema/ascites.
   (3) assisting the removal of toxic/irritant substances from the bloodstream and urinary tract.
   (4) increasing renal function in a compromised kidney.

Chapter 11

1. Endocrine disorders are usually due to too much or too little hormone circulating within the body, and so therapy consists of the administration of replacement, facilitation, or antagonism of hormone actions. Drugs correctly matched with hormonal system include
   (1) clomiphene citrate; gonadotrophins.
   (2) thiocarbamides; parathyroid hormone.
   (3) sulfonylureas; insulin.
   (4) bromocryptine; thyroid function.

2. Estrogens, in addition to their use in oral contraceptives, have other effects, which include

(1) increasing motility of the bowel following surgical intervention.

(2) inhibiting endometriosis.

(3) causing a decrease in the rate of blood coagulation by increasing the number of α-lipoproteins.

(4) antagonizing the effects of parathyroid hormone effectively causing a decrease in bone resorption.

3. Gonadotropin-releasing hormone (GnRH) is a hypothalamic peptide that causes the release of gonadotropins from the pituitary. GnRH and agonistic/antagonistic analogs thereof may therefore find clinical uses in the control of

(1) infertility.

(2) precocious puberty.

(3) cryptorchidism.

(4) fertility.

4. Calcium metabolism is directly affected by which of the following substances?

(1) parathyroid hormone

(2) vitamin D

(3) calcitonin

(4) estrogen

Chapter 12

1. Situations in which specific NSAIDs and related compounds should not be used include

(1) NSAIDs in people with bleeding tendencies.

(2) phenylbutazone in the elderly.

(3) when tinnitus occurs.

(4) when a patient is also taking furosemide.

2. Anti-inflammatories with analgesic and antipyretic efficacy include

(1) aurothioglucose, gold thiomalate.

(2) corticosteroids.

(3) acetaminophen, phenacetin.

(4) aspirin, NSAIDs.

3. Toxicity to aspirin occurs

(1) with prolonged use (GI ulcers, renal disease, hepatic dysfunction).

(2) short-term as intolerance to the drug (GI ulcers, vertigo, tinnitis).

(3) with overdose (hepatic damage, decreased lipid synthesis).

(4) with codosage of NSAIDs.

4. Inflammation and all of its acute as well as chronic effects (e.g., redness, swelling, heat, pain) can be reduced by

(1) treatment with glucocorticoids.

(2) aspirin.

(3) NSAIDs.

(4) acetaminophen.

Chapter 13

1. Theophylline's therapeutic index is small. Therefore,
   (1) it is advisable to look for signs of toxicity (CNS, cardiovascular).
   (2) the effects of other drugs on the metabolism of theophylline should be considered before discontinuing their use.
   (3) plasma concentration of theophylline should be determined in a clinical setting and monitored continually, at least until a proper dose has been determined.
   (4) therapeutic doses are much smaller than toxic doses of the drug.

2. Therapy for asthma can be
   (1) chronic bronchodilation, as in theophylline treatment.
   (2) prophylactic, as in cromolyn treatment.
   (3) local and anti-inflammatory, as in inhalational glucocorticoid therapy.
   (4) sympathoinhibitory, blocking "choke-up," as in propranolol therapy.

3. Drugs can be administered in a variety of ways in order to target the tissues being treated, thus limiting the systemic side effects of the drugs. Examples of this include
   (1) the use of cromolyn as an inhalational antiasthmatic.
   (2) the administration of morphine intrathecally, in order to limit the gastrointestinal and respiratory depressant effects of the drug.
   (3) the administration of a local anesthetic with a vasoconstrictor.
   (4) administration of a nonabsorbable compound for treatment of GI tract disorders.

4. Oral absorption of a drug is dependent upon
   (1) whether it is broken down by peptidases.
   (2) its lipophilicity.
   (3) pH, as in the case of aspirin, which is best absorbed from an empty, acid stomach.
   (4) the metabolism of the drug by the liver ("first-pass" phenomenon).

Chapter 14

1. Drugs effective in the treatment of peptic ulcer disease include
   (1) H_2-antihistamines (e.g., cimetidine, rantidine).
   (2) anticholinergics.
   (3) mucosal protectants (e.g., sucralfate).
   (4) adrenergic antagonists.

2. The antihistamines cimetidine and rantidine are used in the treatment of peptic ulcer disease because they are thought to
   (1) reduce the spasmotic hyperactivity of the stomach that occurs following damage, effectively reducing pain and allowing the stomach to heal more quickly.
   (2) reduce the inflammatory effects of histamine release that occur at the site of tissue damage.
   (3) block activation of visceral afferents responsible for signaling gastric acid production.
   (4) reduce HCl secretion in the stomach, which normally occurs in response to the release of histamine.

3. Use of laxatives to promote evacuation of the intestines is desirable for
   (1) the hastening of the excretion of intra-alimentary toxins.
   (2) the presurgical preparation of the bowels.
   (3) the reduction of physical strain in patients with cardiac or GI problems.
   (4) the elimination of intestinal worms with anthelminthic therapy.

4. Various compounds are mixed in antacid formulations. This is to achieve multiple effects, some of which may be opposite to each other. Examples of drug mixes and reasons for the mix include
   (1) use of aluminum hydroxide with magnesium hydroxide in order to offset the renal effects of too much divalent non-calcium ions.
   (2) use of simethecone with gas-producing antacids to act as an anti-flatulent.
   (3) use of aluminum hydroxide with calcium carbonate to offset the constipation it produces.
   (4) the use of calcium carbonate with magnesium hydroxide in order to offset the diarrhea it produces.

5. Laxatives and related compounds may need to be taken with which of the following drugs in order to offset the constipation they produce?
   (1) antidepressants (e.g., imipramine)
   (2) antipsychotics (e.g., chlorpromazine)
   (3) opioid analgesics (e.g., morphine)
   (4) H_2 antihistamines (e.g., cimetidine)

Chapter 15

1. Dicumerol overdose may be treated successfully with
   (1) warfarin.
   (2) vitamin E.
   (3) heparin.
   (4) vitamin K.

2. Leucovorin (formyltetrahydrofolate) can be used to treat folic acid deficiency associated with
   (1) methotrexate.
   (2) chronic alcoholism.
   (3) phenytoin.
   (4) avidin deficiency.

3. Which of the following are correctly matched?
   (1) manganese overdose; parkinsonian symptoms
   (2) iodine overdose; endemic goiter
   (3) vitamin D deficiency; barbiturates
   (4) calcium deficiency; pernicious anemia

4. Which of the following are associated with antioxidative effects?
   (1) tretinoin
   (2) selenium
   (3) pyridoxal phosphate
   (4) vitamin E

SECTION IV
Chemotherapy for Infection and Neoplasm

Chapter 16

1. Which of the following are correctly matched?
   (1) rifampin; inhibition of nucleic acid synthesis
   (2) penicillin; inhibition of cell wall synthesis
   (3) amphotericin B; inhibition of membrane function
   (4) chloramphenicol; inhibition of protein synthesis

2. Acquisition of antibiotic resistance
   (1) is a critical consideration in the judicious use of antibiotics.
   (2) to a specific drug can occur only after exposure to that drug.
   (3) can occur through changes in bacterial metabolic pathways, membrane permeability, or drug receptor sites.
   (4) occurs only when multiple antibiotics are given simultaneously.

3. Ampicillin
   (1) does not readily cross the blood-brain barrier under normal circumstances.
   (2) exhibits a broader antibiotic spectrum than does penicillin G.
   (3) is not resistant to penicillinases.
   (4) does not cross-sensitize to other penicillins.

4. Which of the following is/are characteristics of tetracyclines?

(1) They cannot be given orally.

(2) They exhibit broad-spectrum activity.

(3) They act by inhibiting nucleic acid synthesis.

(4) They can interfere with calcium deposition in teeth and bone in children.

5. Which of the following is/are characteristics of gentamicin?

(1) It is associated with nephrotoxicity and ototoxicity.

(2) It can be inactivated by plasmid-transmitted mechanisms.

(3) It can be used against resistant organisms by combining with penicillin.

(4) It is bacteriostatic only.

6. The acidic nature of the sulfonamides

(1) enables these drugs to concentrate in the urine.

(2) is the basis for their selectivity against bacterial folate synthesis.

(3) can be modified to prevent crystalization of the drug in the urine.

(4) is not a factor in their urinary solubility.

7. Which of the following are considerations in the treatment of tuberculosis?

(1) Multiple drugs are frequently used against tuberculosis to avoid the selection of resistant organisms.

(2) Isoniazid may be used prophylactically against tuberculosis.

(3) Ethambutol is associated with neural toxicity.

(4) Resistance to rifampin can develop rapidly.

8. Which of the following antifungal agents is/are used orally against systemic fungal infections?

(1) clotrimazole

(2) miconazole

(3) nystatin

(4) ketoconazole

9. Which of the following are correctly matched?

(1) niclosamide; antimalarial

(2) vidarabine; systemic herpes infections

(3) primaquine; anthelmintic

(4) metronidazole; amebicide

Chapter 17

1. What characteristic(s) of tumor cells form(s) the basis of many chemotherapeutic approaches to tumor treatment?

   (1) the inability of tumor cells (unlike bacteria) to gain resistance to chemotherapeutic agents

   (2) the existence of entirely novel metabolic pathways in tumor cells

   (3) the property of all tumors to exist in discrete encapsulated sites isolated from normal tissues

   (4) the greater proliferative activity of tumor cells relative to normal tissue

2. The *in vivo* formation of DNA-alkylating species is a spontaneous process for which of the following compounds?

   (1) mechlorethamine

   (2) streptozotocin

   (3) busulfan

   (4) cyclophosphamide

3. Which of the following are side effects of many antitumor agents?

   (1) immunosuppression

   (2) nausea

   (3) carcinogenicity

   (4) bone marrow depression

4. Which properties are shared by the pyrimadine antimetabolites 5-fluorouracil, cytosine arabinoside, and 5-azacytidine?

   (1) All must be biosynthetically activated to ultimate antitumor metabolites.

   (2) All act primarily to inhibit thymidylate synthetase.

   (3) All act on the S phase of the cell cycle.

   (4) All are routinely administered orally.

5. Which of the following are correctly matched?

   (1) vincristine; inhibition of mitotic spindle assembly

   (2) *cis*-platin; DNA cross-linking

   (3) methotrexate; irreversible inhibition of dihydrofolate reductase

   (4) procarbazine; S-phase specific cytotoxicity

6. Bleomycin

   (1) acts in part as a DNA intercalating agent.

   (2) is not limited in use by myelosuppressive effects.

   (3) is used primarily in combination therapies.

   (4) is accumulated in lungs and skin.

7. Which of the following are correctly matched?

   (1) tamoxifen; testosterone antagonist

   (2) steroid receptor; marker of tumor sensitivity

   (3) prednisone; inhibition of erythropoiesis

   (4) diethylstilbestrol; physiological androgen antagonist

SECTION V
Toxicology

Chapter 18

1. Metabolism of a xenobiotic compound can produce
   (1) a reactive metabolite.
   (2) an inactivated metabolite.
   (3) a more readily excreted compound.
   (4) a biosynthetically conjugated metabolite.

2. Which of the following environmental toxins act(s) by directly interfering with oxygen metabolism?
   (1) DDT
   (2) cyanide
   (3) sodium hypochlorite
   (4) carbon monoxide

3. Which of the following compounds would be expected to be a more potent CNS depressant than ethanol?
   (1) n-propanol
   (2) water
   (3) n-butanol
   (4) methanol

4. Which of the following are correctly matched?
   (1) hexachlorobenzene; inhibits heme biosynthesis
   (2) lead; CNS toxicity
   (3) polyhalogenated biphenyls; reproductive systems toxicities
   (4) mercury; successful chelation therapy

5. Which of the following apply to methanol poisoning in primates?
   (1) metabolic acidosis occurs
   (2) ocular toxicity can occur
   (3) elevated plasma formate occurs
   (4) elevated plasma formaldehyde occurs

6. Which of the following apply to ethanol ingestion by humans?
   (1) The rate of disappearance of ethanol from the blood is always a linear function of its initial concentration.
   (2) High doses of ethanol are associated with changes in hepatic lipid metabolism.
   (3) Tolerance to ethanol is thought to be largely metabolic rather than behavioral in nature.
   (4) Aversion therapy with disulfiram depends on inhibition of acetaldehyde metabolism.

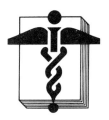

Answers to Review Questions

SECTION I
Fundamental Principles

CHAPTER 1

1. D
2. D
3. B

4. A
5. E

CHAPTER 2

1. E
2. A
3. A

4. E
5. D

CHAPTER 3

1. D
2. C
3. A

4. D
5. B

SECTION II
Pharmacology Related to the Nervous
System

CHAPTER 4

1. C
2. A
3. C
4. D

5. D
6. C
7. A
8. B

9. B
10. A
11. C

12. E
13. C

CHAPTER 5

1. A
2. E
3. B
4. C
5. A
6. D
7. B
8. C
9. D
10. A
11. E

12. B
13. B
14. B
15. A
16. B
17. B
18. C
19. C
20. E
21. D

CHAPTER 6

1. D
2. C

3. D
4. E

CHAPTER 7

1. A
2. B

3. E

CHAPTER 8

1. E
2. A
3. E

4. C
5. A

SECTION III
Pharmacology Related to Other Major Organ Systems

CHAPTER 9

1. E
2. E
3. C

4. C
5. E

CHAPTER 10

1. A
2. B
3. A
4. C

5. B
6. B
7. E

CHAPTER 11

1. A
2. D

3. E
4. E

CHAPTER 12

1. E
2. D

3. E
4. C

CHAPTER 13

1. C
2. C

3. E
4. E

CHAPTER 14

1. C
2. D
3. E

4. B
5. C

CHAPTER 15

1. D
2. C

3. A
4. B

SECTION IV
Chemotherapy for Infection and Neoplasm

CHAPTER 16

1. E
2. A
3. C
4. B
5. C

6. A
7. E
8. D
9. B

CHAPTER 17

1. D
2. C
3. E
4. A

5. C
6. E
7. B

SECTION V
Toxicology

CHAPTER 18

1. E
2. B
3. A

4. C
5. C
6. B

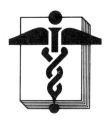

APPENDIX A

Schedules of Controlled Drugs*

Schedule I. Drugs in this class are not available for legitimate use for any purposes other than investigative ones. Clearance from the FDA is required before these drugs (e.g., LSD and marijuana) can be legally obtained.

Schedule II. Drugs in this class have high abuse potentials that may lead to severe psychological or physical dependence or both. No telephoned prescriptions will be filled. Each refill must be reordered with a new prescription.

Examples of Schedule II Drugs

amphetamine	methadone
codeine	methylphenidate
dextroamphetamine	morphine
droperidol with fentanyl	oxycodone
hydromorphone	pentobarbital
meperidine	secobarbital

For hospitalized patients, you must rewrite routine orders for drugs in schedules III, IV, and V every 7 days and prn orders every 72 hours. You must sign phone orders within 48 hours.

Schedule III. Drugs in this class have a lower abuse potential than those in schedule I or II. These prescriptions can be filled by telephone. They must be rewritten every 6 months or after five refills, whichever comes first.

*Adapted from Mathewson, M: Pharmacotherapeutics: A Nursing Process Approach. FA Davis, Philadelphia, 1986.

Example of Schedule III Drugs
codeine (when combined with selected drugs)

Schedule IV. This schedule is similar to schedule III, except for the penalties for illegal possession.

Examples of Schedule IV Drugs

alprazolam	midazolam
chloral hydrate	oxazepam
chlordiazepoxide	pemoline
clonazepam	pentazocine
clorazepate	phenobarbital
diazepam	prazepam
flurazepam	propoxyphene
lorazepam	temazepam
meprobamate	triazolam

Schedule V. According to federal law, this class of drugs has a low abuse potential, does not require a prescription, and is sold over the counter. Most states, however, have a stricter ruling that requires prescriptions and the same refill regulations as in schedules III and IV.

Examples of Schedule V Drugs

buprenorphine	diphenoxylate with atropine
codeine (cough preparations)	paregoric

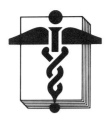

APPENDIX B

Commonly Used Abbreviations

ac	before meals
AD	right ear
AS	left ear
AU	both ears
bid	two times a day
c̄	with
cap	capsule
D5W	5 percent dextrose in water
D10W	10 percent dextrose in water
gm or g	gram(s)
gr	grain(s)
gtt	drop(s)
h or hr	hour(s)
hs	hour of sleep (bedtime)
IM	intramuscular
Inhal or Inhaln	inhalation
I & O	intake and output
IT	intrathecal
IV	intravenous
L	liter

LR	lactated Ringer's solution
M	minim
MAO	monoamine oxidase
mcg	microgram(s)
mg	milligram(s)
ml	milliliter(s)
NS	normal saline (0.9% NaCl)
NSAI	nonsteroidal anti-inflammatory agent(s)
OD	right eye
Oint	ointment
Ophth	ophthalmic
OS	left eye
OU	both eyes
oz	ounce(s)℥
pc	after meals
PO	by mouth, orally
prn	when required
q	every
qd	every day
qh	every hour
qod	every other day
qwk	every week
q2h	every 2 hours
q3h	every 3 hours
q4h	every 4 hours
qid	four times a day
qs	as much as is required
rect	rectally
s̄	without
SC	subcutaneous
SL	sublingual
SR	sustained release
s̄s̄	one half
stat	immediately
supp	suppository
tab	tablet
Tbs	tablespoon(s)
tid	three times a day
Top	topically
tsp	teaspoon(s)

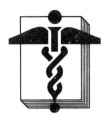

Index

An "F" following a page number indicates a figure; a "T" indicates a table.